Introduction to

Sixth Edition

Radiologic Technology

Introduction to

Radiologic Technology

Sixth Edition

LaVerne Tolley Gurley
PhD, (FASRT)

William J. Callaway
BA, RT(R)

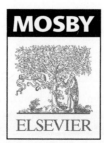

MOSBY

ELSEVIER

MOSBY
ELSEVIER

11830 Westline Industrial Drive,
St. Louis, Missouri 63146

INTRODUCTION TO RADIOLOGIC TECHNOLOGY　　ISBN-13: 978-0-323-03566-8
LaVerne Tolley Gurley, William J. Callaway　　ISBN-10: 0-323-03566-3
Copyright © 2006, 2002, 1996, 1992 by Mosby, Inc.

Notice

Neither the Publisher nor the Authors assume any responsibility for any loss or injury and/or damage to persons or property arising out of or related to any use of the material contained in this book. It is the responsibility of the treating practitioner, relying on independent expertise and knowledge of the patient, to determine the best treatment and method of application for the patient.

The Publisher

Sixth Edition

ISBN-13: 978-0-323-03566-8
ISBN-10: 0-323-03566-3

Acquisitions Editor: Jeanne Wilke
Developmental Editor: Rebecca Swisher
Publishing Services Manager: Karen Edwards
Project Manager: Karen Edwards
Design Direction: Paula Ruckenbrod
Cover Designer: Paula Ruckenbrod

Printed in the United States of America

Last digit is the print number: 9　8　7　6　5　4　3

Authors

LaVerne Tolley Gurley, PhD, (FASRT), is certified in radiologic technology, nuclear medicine technology, and radiation therapy. She is a fellow and life member of ASRT, a life member of AERS, and she is recognized in such international listings as 2000 Women of Achievement, International Scholars Directory, and the World's Who's Who of Women. After nearly 30 years with the University of Tennessee Medical Units, Dr. Gurley transferred to Shelby State Community College to direct the radiologic technology program. She retired from full-time service in 1989 and from part-time service in 1996. She continues her affiliation as Professor Emeritus.

William J. Callaway, BA, RT(R), has been involved in radiography education for nearly 30 years. He has directed both collegiate associate degree and hospital-sponsored programs, as well as teaching the subjects covered in this text. Mr. Callaway is the author of Mosby's Comprehensive Review of Radiography, also published by Mosby-Elsevier, and has had writings published in state and national radiologic technology journals. He has also coauthored a quality customer service guide for radiology and co-founded Radiography Educators of the Midwest (REM).

Educated in Radiologic Technology at Franciscan Medical Center and Black Hawk College in the Illinois Quad-Cities, Mr. Callaway also attended Augustana College there and later received a BA from Western Illinois University.

He is widely known for his highly motivational Key Points Presentations for students, educators, and practicing technologists as conducted at interna-tional, national, state, and local radiologic technology meetings. He has presented more than 500 of his Key Points Presentations that include "Face to Face with Moments of Truth," "You're Not the Boss of Me", "I'd Rather Die...Than Give a Presentation", Practical Physics for the Radiographer (and You Thought Physics Had to Be Boring!)," "Just Be Something . . . The You-Shaped Piece of the Puzzle," and "Motivation's Greatest Hits".

Contributors

Barbara A. Burnham-Rupp, BS, RT(R), FASRT, FAHRA, received her baccalaureate degree in health arts from the University of St. Francis, Joliet, Illinois. Following graduation from the radiologic technology program at Triton College in River Grove, Illinois, Ms. Burnham-Rupp became a clinical instructor at Community Memorial General Hospital. After 10 years as an instructor, Ms. Burnham moved into administration as a chief technologist and served as the administrative director of the Department of Radiology at LaGrange Memorial Hospital in LaGrange, Illinois until 1995. Ms. Burnham-Rupp served as president of Burnham Consultants until 2003 when she assumed the position of Assistant Accreditation Specialist at the Joint Review Committee on Education in Radiologic Technology. Ms, Burnham-Rupp is a fellow in the ASRT and AHRA and has received many awards and much recognition for her work in advancing the profession.

Peggy D. Franklin, BS, RT(R) is the director of Methodist University Hospital School of Radiologic and Imaging Sciences in Memphis, Tennessee. She is a past president of the Tennessee Society of Radiologic Technologists and is currently serving as a member of its board of directors. She has served in the ASRT House of Delegates and is a member of the Association of Educators in Radiologic Sciences, for which she previously served on the board of directors.

Joanne S. Greathouse, Ed.S, RT(R), FASRT, FAERS, received her x-ray education at Methodist Hospital of Central Illinois in Peoria, Illinois, and she holds an EdS degree in higher education administration from the College of William and Mary. Dr. Greathouse currently serves as the Chief Executive Officer of the Joint Review Committee on Education in Radiologic Technology (JRCERT), a position she has held since 1999. She works closely with the JRCERT Board of Directors in carrying out the work of the organization, and she participates in a wide variety of national meetings to educate people about the profession and the role of programmatic accreditation. Before joining the JRCERT, she served as associate professor and chairman of the Department of Radiation Sciences at Virginia Commonwealth University/Medical College of Virginia in Richmond.

Penny S. Mays, RT(ASRT), is an instructor at the School of Radiologic Technology at Southwest Tennessee Community College in Memphis. Ms. Mays was educated in radiologic technology at the University of Tennessee Medical Units in Memphis. She was the founder and educational director of the School of Radiologic Technology and administrative director of radiology services in Huntsville, Alabama. She is the recipient of the Alabama Governor's award, the John B. Cahoon award, and Alabama's Technologist of the Year award, and she is listed in the *Who's Who of American Women*. Ms. Mays is the author of articles in professional publications, and she has participated in numerous radiology research projects.

Neta B. McKnight, BA, RT(FASRT), is a professor and director of the radiologic technology program at Jackson State Community College in Jackson, Tennessee. She was a member of the AART Board of Trustees from 1976 to 1984. Ms. McKnight has a BA in education from Northeastern Illinois University. She is a past board member and fellow of the ASRT and AERS.

James Ohnysty, RT(FASRT), is president of Medical Imaging Operations Consultations Analysis (MIOCA) and chief operations officer of National Vascular Health. He has been actively involved in radiologic technology since 1956. As a member of ASRT since 1959, Mr. Ohnysty's activities have included charter membership of the JRCERT. He has had articles published in *Radiologic Technology,* and he wrote *Aids to Ethics and Professional Conduct for Student Radiologic Technologists.*

Russell A. Tolley, BA, JD, received his BA from the University of Georgia in 1980 and his JD from the University of Georgia School of Law in 1983. He is associated with the law firm of Long, Aldridge, and Norman in Atlanta. In 1999, he took a sabbatical from his legal practice to work as a cowboy at a cattle ranch; he is a frequent lecturer about that experience. He is employed by the New Mexico State Police as a recruit in the New Mexico State Police Academy. His practice is in the area of creditors' rights, lender liability, and bankruptcy.

Wanda E. Wesolowski, RT, MA, Ed, (FASRT) received her training in Radiologic Technology at the Thomas Jefferson University Hospital in Philadelphia, completed her undergraduate degree at LaSalle University in Philadelphia, and her graduate degree from Beaver College/Arcadia University in Glenside, Pennsylvania. From 1974 to 2001 she was chairperson of the Radiologic Technology Program at the Community College of Philadelphia and is currently professor of Diagnostic Medical Imaging at the Community College of Philadelphia. In 1973 she was awarded the ASRT second National Electrical Manufacturer's Association (NEMA) award for her technical paper *Basic Concepts of*

Serial Direct Roentgen Enlargement. In 1981 she was presented with the Alumni Special Achievement Award from the Thomas Jefferson University, College of Allied Health Sciences. In 1977 the Philadelphia Society of Radiologic Technologists presented her with the Berenice Lifetime Achievement Award.

Reviewers

Gregory Lee Bradley, MEd, RT (R)(ARRT)
Program Director and Assistant Professor
Radiologic Technology
McNeese State University
Lake Charles, Louisiana

Karen A. Frazier, MS, RT (R)
Program Director
Columbus Regional Hospital
School of Radiologic Technology
Columbus, Indiana

Gerald L. Graddy, MS, RT(R)
Associate Professor of Radiography
Jackson State Community College
Jackson, Tennessee

Kelli Welch Haynes, MSRS, RT(R)
Assistant Professor/Clinical Coordinator
Northwestern State University
Shreveport, Louisiana

Gail Hoffman, RT (R), MEd
Program Director
Bucks County Community College
Newtown, Pennsylvania

Karen A. Jefferies, BS, RT(R)
Associate Professor
Radiography Program
Wright College
Chicago, Illinois

Terry M. Konn, MPA, RT(R)
Program Director and Associate Professor
Brookdale Community College
Lincroft, New Jersey

Debra L. Letizio, MA, RT (R)(QM)(CV)
Program Director
Swedish American Hospital
Rockford, Illinois

Theresa M. Levitsky, MA, RT (R)(M)(QM)(CV)
Radiography Program Director
St. Francis Medical Center
Trenton, New Jersey

Paula Pate-Schloder, MS, RT (R)(CV)(CT)(VI)
Associate Professor
College Misericordia
Dallas, Pennsylvania

Olive Peart, MS, RT (R)(M)
Clinical Instructor
The Stanford Hospital
Program in Radiography
Stanford, Connecticut

Debra J. Poelhuis, MS, RT (R)(M)
Director-Radiography Program
Montgomery County Community College
Pottstown, Pennsylvania

Mary Jane S. Reynolds, BS, RT (R)(T)
Program Director
Hospital Citizen's Medical Center
Victoria, Texas

Bette Schans, PhD, RT(R)
Professor, Radiologic Technology
Mesa State College
Grand Junction, Colorado

Preface

This sixth edition of *Introduction to Radiologic Technology* has been updated and new material added as suggested by the readers and others who use the text in their programs. The hundreds of programs and thousands of students who have used the previous five editions have confirmed our original belief that a strong introduction and orientation to the profession is vital to a new student embarking on a career in radiologic technology. It is gratifying to attend a conference anywhere in the country and have registered technologists tell us that they began their career with this textbook.

We have, by design, retained the "introductory" nature of this text with the full knowledge that subsequent courses will delve more deeply into the technical aspects of radiography. The chapters have been updated to coincide with trends, technical advances, and changes in the health care system; however, we have taken care, as was suggested by our readers, to maintain the comprehension level and simple style expected of an introductory course.

The purpose of this new edition remains the same as that of previous editions: to introduce the new or prospective student to the profession of radiologic technology and to the body of knowledge required to become a member of the profession. The intent is to inform students early in their study of what they can expect from a career in radiologic technology, options for advancement, and what will be required of them. As the health care environment becomes increasingly more challenging, this goal takes on added significance.

The sequence of chapters has remained essentially the same. Educators who have their course syllabus developed to be consistent with past editions will need to make only minor adjustments.

From the instructor's point of view, perhaps the most helpful features are the multiple-choice review questions (consistent with the Registry-style format), outlines, and key terms developed for each chapter. Another feature is the glossary, which is filled with important terminology that will aid the student in the process of studying. Chapter objectives, which are a popular element among educators, have been included and are fully updated to reflect the new information in each chapter.

The accompanying Instructor's Electronic Resource Manual is designed to help the instructor encourage active student participation in the class. A new feature of this edition is that this Instructor's manual will be available on CD as an added benefit. Included in the manual are problem-solving exercises and critical-thinking activities. In addition to the critical-thinking exercises to involve students, multiple-choice questions have been added to most chapters. This is for the convenience of instructors, who can use them to measure student progress on a daily basis. The instructor materials as well as a course management platform can also be found online at http://evolve.elsevier.com/Gurley/radtech/.

This book is a success because of the thousands who have used it and told us what they found useful and what they would like to see added in future editions. It is our hope that this brand new edition will exceed the expectations of the countless educators who use this book not only for an introductory course but also for many other courses throughout their curriculum.

-LaVerne Tolley Gurley & William J. Callaway

Acknowledgments

Acknowledgment of my indebtedness in preparing this revision is not complete without mentioning the generous help given by the contributors of the previous editions and this current edition. The educators who used the earlier editions and whose suggestions guided me in making the revision were also of great assistance. The readers who reviewed the material deserve a special commendation; their suggestions and comments were often the determining factor in making changes in context and terminology. A special thanks goes to those instructors who gave suggestions and positive—often enthusiastic—comments about the Instructor's Manual; its first edition accompanied the fourth edition of this text and was well received.

I also wish to acknowledge the professional organizations of radiologic technology and the people associated with them for providing an environment for the growth and development of technologists, for maintaining a high level of quality in the accreditation of education, and for certifying individuals for the profession.

My gratitude is extended to Barbara Austin of the University of Mississippi Medical Center. Thanks also to Amy Justice Hill, Tamara Rodriquez, Claudette Moore, Emily Presley, and Ansley Hill. Thanks to the University of Tennessee Health Sciences Center faculty, Diane Wyatt, Medical Technologist, and Beth L. Horn, Dental Hygienist. Nancy Clifton, Program Director in Nuclear Medicine at Methodist University Hospital provided significant technical advice in Nuclear Medicine. I am truly grateful to these institutions, their faculty, and staff.

Thanks to Helen Ronsick, who gave valuable assistance in typing and organizing a portion of the original manuscript. Appreciation is also extended to the faculty and students of radiography at Southwest Tennessee Community College for their continued support.

A special acknowledgment goes to William J. Callaway, my co-editor, valued friend and esteemed professional. I have been privileged and honored to work with this fine professional on each edition, a work that now spans a quarter of a century. This has special meaning for me.

-LaVerne Tolley Gurley

A quarter century of writing and editing this text is a milestone worth celebrating. Many thanks go to the countless educators and students who, since 1982, have placed this text at the forefront of radiography education. I thank my co-author and co-editor Dr. LaVerne Gurley, with whom I've had a unique and productive professional relationship that began with a common vision all those years ago. Special recognition goes to all of the contributors and reviewers that have made these six editions so relevant and student-friendly. In particular, thanks go to my closest friends and colleagues (you know who you are) who have provided encouragement and motivation as this text became a foundation in radiography programs nationwide.

-William J. Callaway

A very special acknowledgment goes to the professionals at the St. Louis office of Elsevier who have carefully guided this project over a quarter century. They once again assembled a great team to bring this project to fruition. Special acknowledgment goes to Jeanne Wilke for her leadership and enthusiastic support of this text. Rebecca Swisher provided expert editing as well as guiding manuscript development throughout this entire project. Christina Pryor kept everything in the right place at the right time. It is always a joy working with Elsevier teams, who are consistently the best at what they do. Given the talents of the entire Elsevier staff, any errors or omissions from this book are solely ours.

-LaVerne Tolley Gurley & William J. Callaway

Contents

PART I   BECOMING A RADIOLOGIC TECHNOLOGIST

Chapter 1   Introduction to Quality Customer Service 3
            William J. Callaway
Chapter 2   Becoming a Better Student 21
            LaVerne Tolley Gurley
Chapter 3   Memorization—A Key to Learning 35
            LaVerne Tolley Gurley
Chapter 4   Critical Thinking Skills 49
            LaVerne Tolley Gurley
Chapter 5   The History of Medicine 57
            William J. Callaway
Chapter 6   Radiology: A Historic Perspective 75
            LaVerne Tolley Gurley

PART II   PRACTICING THE PROFESSION

Chapter 7   Radiography Education: From Classroom to Clinic 91
             LaVerne Tolley Gurley
Chapter 8   The Language of Medicine 109
             William J. Callaway
Chapter 9   Imaging Equipment 119
             William J. Callaway
Chapter 10   Radiographic Examinations: Diagnosing Disease and Injury 127
             William J. Callaway
Chapter 11   Imaging: Life Cycle and Quality 139
             LaVerne Tolley Gurley
Chapter 12   Ethics and Professionalism in Radiologic Technology 167
             James Ohnysty
Chapter 13   Patient Care and Management 181
             Penny S. Mays
Chapter 14   Medicolegal Considerations 191
             Russell A. Tolley
Chapter 15   Organization and Operation of the Radiology Department 205
             Penny S. Mays
Chapter 16   Economics of Radiology 217
             LaVerne Tolley Gurley

Chapter 17 Quality Assurance in Radiology 227
   LaVerne Tolley Gurley
Chapter 18 Radiation Safety and Protective Measures 245
   LaVerne Tolley Gurley
Chapter 19 Allied Health Professions 269
   LaVerne Tolley Gurley

Part III Growing With the Profession

Chapter 20 The American Registry of Radiologic Technologists 285
   Neta B. McKnight
Chapter 21 The Joint Review Committee on Education in Radiologic
   Technology 297
   Joanne S. Greathouse
Chapter 22 Professional Associations 313
   William J. Callaway
Chapter 23 Specialization in Radiologic Technology 325
   Peggy D. Franklin
Chapter 24 Professional Development and Career Advancement 353
   Wanda E. Wesolowski
Chapter 25 Continuing Education for the Radiologic Technologist 371
   Barbara A. Burnham-Rupp
Chapter 26 Status of Health Care Delivery 381
   William J. Callaway

Appendix: Answers to Review Questions 395
Glossary 397
Index 407

Introduction to

Sixth Edition

Radiologic Technology

I

Becoming a Radiologic Technologist

Introduction to Quality Customer Service

William J. Callaway

OBJECTIVES

On completion of this chapter, you should be able to:

- Explain the importance of having a thorough understanding of the technical aspects of radiologic technology.
- Name the sources of information that most patients use when choosing a hospital.
- List the inside and outside customers served by the health care facility.
- Discuss the variety of diversity among patients.
- Describe quality care from the patient's perspective.
- List high-tech and high-touch aspects of health care.
- Explain what is meant by a "moment of truth."
- Outline a customer service cycle for a radiologic examination.
- List ways to enhance telephone conversations.
- Define empathy.
- Be able to use the conflict resolution model in customer service and high-stress situations.

Welcome to the study of radiologic technology! You are about to embark on a series of educational experiences designed to help you work in the

KEY TERMS

conflict resolution
customer service cycle
diversity
effective listening
empathy
events
incidents
inside customers
moments of truth
outside customers

CHAPTER OUTLINE

Overview
The health care service environment
The patient's perspective
   Selected results of the National consumer Trends survey
Inside and outside customers
The benefits of high-quality service
Moments of truth in radiology
Customer service cycles in radiology
Customer service on the telephone
Conflict resolution: opportunities to exceed the customer's expectations
Conclusion

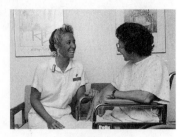

Fig. 1-1

Human concern and empathy, combined with high-quality service, provide total patient care.

intriguing and challenging specialty of medical radiography. The purpose of this book is to introduce you to the many facets of this profession and the educational process you are now beginning.

Radiography is a specialty within the field of radiologic technology. Radiologic technology as a whole includes radiography (all exams using x-rays), radiation therapy, nuclear medicine, sonography, and magnetic resonance imaging. The professionals working in this field are called, collectively, radiologic technologists. Specifically, you are learning to become a radiographer, a medical imaging professional who uses x-rays to produce diagnostic images. It is first and foremost a people-oriented business. It carries with it special opportunities. Patients have entrusted their health to us, and they need to feel that they are in the best of hands. It is up to you, as a new health care professional, to dedicate yourself to providing the highest quality of care and service to your patients (Fig. 1-1).

OVERVIEW

To provide quality service, a thorough understanding of your chosen field is necessary. You must have a command of the technical aspects of radiography so that you are free to concentrate on the health care customer, who is traditionally called "the patient." This book will assist you on your journey. Because education at this level is a complicated task, the majority of the chapters in Part I offer help in understanding the learning process itself. Noted educators share their ideas and suggestions about how to get started with the study habits and personal adjustments required of a new student. Their expertise, based on contact with hundreds of radiography students, provides just the type of information required to establish effective methods of study. Careful attention to this material will help set the stage for all that follows throughout your education in radiography. Keep in mind that lifelong learning is the key to success and that study habits developed now will serve you well in the years to come.

Part I also presents the history and future of health care in general and of radiology in particular. Although volumes have been written on the history of medicine, Chapter 5 provides a concise treatment of this subject. This history of radiology is particularly interesting and exciting, and it is marked by constant change and advances.

The day-to-day practice of radiography is complex. Many new and interesting terms, examinations, and relationships must be learned. Chapters 8 through 11 in Part II introduce you to terminology, equipment, examinations, and radiograph production. These topics are encountered immediately on entering the clinical phase of the educational program, so they are presented here to begin to give you a working knowledge of what is happening in the radiology department. Your early clinical rotations will mean more to you if you already have some grasp of the imaging environment.

Part II also includes discussions about medical ethics and the legal implications of the practice of radiography. These two areas must be taken seriously throughout the duration of the educational process and beyond to ensure that you practice according to established standards and within legal parameters.

The remainder of Part II deals with topics that you must understand as you work within a radiology department or, as it is called in many institutions, an imaging department. The operation of a radiology complex is discussed in terms of its organizational structure. Becoming aware of your surroundings enables you to begin to understand your role. Radiology is a very expensive department; hence, you are also introduced to the complex economic issues involved in its operation. Assuring the quality of services is a serious matter that is presented in its own chapter.

The code of ethics followed by radiologic technologists includes attention to radiation safety and public education. Entering the field of radiography implies that you will accept some exposure to radiation and learn to protect yourself and the public from unnecessary exposure. A complete chapter is devoted to this topic. This knowledge will enable you to feel confident and comfortable as you enter the clinical site, and you will be self-assured as friends, relatives, and patients ask questions about radiation safety. By understanding this material, you will be in a position to properly educate both patients and acquaintances.

The entire field of health care has been advancing at a rapid pace. With this rapid advancement have come the increased specialization on the part of physicians and the emergence of many new health care fields (known collectively as the allied health professions). Part II ends with a description of the roles of the other members of the health care team that you will encounter during your clinical experiences. Why learn about other health care professionals? Total care of the patient depends on the cooperation and mutual respect of all departments. You will provide services to many of these departments, and other departments will provide services to radiology. All of these departments exist to provide high-quality service to patients, families, and physicians. Teamwork requires that everyone understand the role of other members. In this treatment of the subject, you will learn about the educational background and job responsibilities of some of the fellow professionals you will encounter during patient care. You will soon realize that everyone is equally important in providing clinical care and service to the sick or injured.

Part III addresses the professional aspects of radiologic technology. Serious, career-minded professionals need to know as much as possible about the field and the opportunities it provides. Leaders in radiologic technology present the profession as they see it based on many years of experience. The American Registry of Radiologic Technologists is discussed, and its role as the certifying agency for thousands of radiologic technologists is explained. Professional organizations, all dedicated to providing members the finest in continuing education and professional representation, are also described. These organizations play an important role in your education as well as in your career plans.

Part III also deals with career advancement and specialization in radiologic technology. A career in this profession can take you in many directions. Although you are just beginning your career, this discussion will help you to better understand the varied opportunities available in this field; it is never too early to begin setting long-term goals.

A discussion of the current status of health care delivery and the outlook on disease, health, and death in our culture completes the text. This section provides you with a background to help you appreciate some of the major issues in health care and to evaluate your own values regarding such topics. It is also vital that you have a basic understanding of the financing of health care and its impact on you as a professional, a patient, and a taxpayer. You have chosen a fascinating and exciting career—one that is always changing and that never stands still.

Again, congratulations on being accepted to study in the field of health care! In few other careers can you find the potential for doing so much good while achieving satisfaction. Your future studies will be interesting and intriguing as you strive to become a professional in your field. As you study and observe those around you, you will come to know what is meant by the term *professional*. You will see both positive and negative examples of professional performance, and before long, you will be able to decide which of these you want to emulate in your daily work. The title "professional" is earned through dedication and hard work; it is not something you can purchase with your tuition dollars. As you progress in your studies, take pride in what you do, and act appropriately. Your growth as a professional does not end when you become a radiographer; it will continue throughout your career. You must act like a professional and demand to be treated like one, and you must also remember that you, as well as all other health care workers, are important to the patient's well-being.

During the next 2 to 4 years you will have the chance to examine your career goals and personal expectations. Enjoy your studies and your chosen profession. Although much hard work is involved, it can be satisfying. Make the most of this time, and you will construct a secure foundation for a lifetime career in professional health care. Remember that by mastering the technical portions of medical radiography you will be free to concentrate on the reason you came into this field: to help people with the best care that you can provide. The balance of this chapter explains just how to practice value-added, high-touch radiography by understanding all of the variables involved in the delivery of this very important service.

THE HEALTH CARE SERVICE ENVIRONMENT

One of the most important facets of your practice is the realization that you are part of a service industry. Patients and their families are, in fact, customers. Many health care professionals are uncomfortable using the term *customer* for those served in the hospital; therefore the term *patient* is used in this book where appropriate. However, keep in mind that a customer is someone to whom we provide a product or a service and that this definition describes patients perfectly. Although our product is quite different from that of other service businesses, we are nevertheless judged by many of the same criteria. Total patient care must be a balance of human caring and concern, technical expertise, and high-quality customer service. Caring and quality service are not mutually exclusive; in fact, only when these aspects of care are combined in the health care setting are we able to satisfy the needs of our patients and provide the quality they have come to expect. Any one of these traits, on its own, does not provide total patient care.

Keep in mind that patients and the services we offer should never be thought of in exactly the same vein as fast-food restaurants, department stores, hotels, and the like. If quality service is expected and delivered in those service settings, however, we as health care professionals can certainly provide similar levels of service for our patients and practices, which are so much more important.

The Joint Commission on Accreditation of Healthcare Organizations (JCAHO) stipulates that patient and family complaint systems must be in place and made available for use as part of a continuous quality improvement program. Furthermore, the JCAHO specifies that such complaint systems allow complaints relating to the quality of care to be addressed. Hospitals are focusing on delivering the quality of service that an increasingly demanding public expects. Service systems, strategies, and people form the basis for marketing and service delivery in today's successful health care organizations.

A good understanding of the health care delivery system is vital to the student radiographer, because this is the context in which all patient care takes place. You will be a part of this system from the beginning of school and throughout your career. In your role as a student and later as an employee, you must be able to function within the socioeconomic boundaries of health care delivery. These issues are described in Chapter 26. A strong grasp of these concepts is vital to being a productive member of the health care team. Most important, however, are the interactions that you will have with your patients.

The patient's perspective

Just who are our patients? From where do our patients come? What do our patients think, and what do they expect? How do we begin to try to understand them and their specific needs? For the health care professional, this is no easy task. However, a good place to start is with the understanding that, while many differences exist among people of all backgrounds, we are all more alike than different.

Humans respond positively to kindness and respect. People want to feel safe and secure, especially in an unfamiliar environment. They want to be comfortable. Patients want to be free of pain and discomfort. Privacy is important, as is the comfort of family. Humans who become our patients want their individual beliefs, wants, and needs accommodated as much as possible.

Diversity among humans is infinite, for the gene pool of over 6 billion people produces infinite combinations. Each person is unique. Every human is then influenced not only by a specific culture, but by life's experiences. Some studies focus on cultural diversity alone, but such an approach would severely limit your understanding of the patients you will care for. Regardless of a person's cultural background, life will add such things as age, illness, injury, socioeconomics, and so forth. Gender, family tradition, sexual preference, and religious beliefs all are a part of each patient's background.

As you begin working with patients in clinical education, you will come to see that every patient brings to you unique experiences, and a view of life that you have not yet experienced. Patients will also teach you the folly of stereotypes, for no matter the background of the patient, broad judgments must never be made to fit preconceived notions.

Cultural diversity itself is **difficult to define**. In America, the predominant cultures may be a mix of influences from Europe, Hispanic nations, the continent of Africa, the lands of Asia and the Middle East, and American Indian tribes. Some patients may be first-generation immigrants, attempting to assimilate into a new culture while still heavily influenced by their culture of origin. Others may be several generations removed from their family's land of origin, but still be influenced by those beliefs or observe certain traditions or rites. Still others, while bearing physical resemblance to their ancestors, may have broken ties with their family's past. As a health care professional, you will never be sure of your patients' backgrounds, regardless of physical appearances. You will need to be comfortable working with a diverse population.

To make a discussion of diversity relevant, consider the ways in which you add to diversity. Think about (better yet, write a page about) your family heritage, your age, attitudes, socioeconomic status, gender, core religious/moral/ethical values, preferences in life, sense of humor, diseases or injuries that influence how you live your daily life, privacy or openness, land of origin, and so on. Consider your hopes and dreams, successes and disappointments, victories and failures. Now, picture yourself as a patient. Finally, consider all the variations on your beliefs that might come from over 6 billion humans.

Your studies in health care will include further discussion of diversity, beyond the scope of this text. However, consider that there are some basic considerations that should be added to your radiography practice to help you shape your approach to those of diverse backgrounds. Interaction and communication with patients can be enhanced by incorporating the key points in Box 1-1 into your practice. As you read them, keep in mind that references to cultures and limited English-speaking persons can also refer to the elderly, the very young, seriously impaired patients, and others. Consider that these suggestions may be used in a multitude of situations, with a wide variety of patients who may not necessarily be from another country or culture.

BOX 1-1 KEY POINTS FOR DIVERSE PATIENT INTERACTIONS

Tips for Successful Caregiver / Patient Interaction Across Cultures

1. Don't treat the patient in the same manner you would want to be treated.
2. Begin by being more formal with patients who were born in another culture.
3. Don't be "put off" if the patient fails to "look you in the eye" or ask questions about the treatment.
4. Don't make *any* assumptions regarding the patient's concepts about the ways to maintain health, the causes of illness, or the means to prevent or cure illness.

Tips for Communicating Directly with Limited English-Speaking Patients

1. Speak slowly, not loudly.
2. Face the patient and make extensive use of gestures, pictures, and facial expressions. Watch the patient's face, eyes, and body language carefully.
3. Avoid difficult and uncommon words and idiomatic expressions.
4. Don't "muddy the waters" with unnecessary words or information.
5. Organize what you say for easy access.
6. Rephrase and summarize often.
7. Don't ask questions that can be answered by "yes" or "no."

(From Salimbene S: *What language does your patient hurt in?* ed 1, St. Paul, 2000, Paradigm.)

You may be surprised by the suggestion to not treat the patient in the same manner as you would want to be treated. Bear in mind the individuality of each person across ages, cultures, and backgrounds. Certainly a calm and gentle demeanor is universally appropriate, but figures of speech, the use of touch, or overall approach that you might find normal or even desirable may be offensive to someone else. Asking an elderly patient if she wishes to 'hang out' in the waiting room may be misinterpreted. Few health care professionals touch the patient as much as a radiographer. You may appreciate a gentle touch of encouragement, but touch must be approached carefully, whether positioning for a procedure or providing encouragement with a hand on the patient's shoulder. Your preferences may not be the same as those of the patients you serve. The ongoing study of diversity of all kinds will greatly assist you with patient interactions. Age and culture greatly influence how a patient interprets your words and actions. Choose them carefully.

Each of your patients is someone's daughter or son, and perhaps someone's mother or father, grandmother or grandfather, brother or sister. Each is unique, with basic wants and needs quite possibly similar to your own, but each patient may wish to be approached in a special way. You must care for each as a valued member of humanity.

Selected Results of the National Consumer Trends Survey

Service as expected by the patient and delivered by the caregiver is the prime factor in patient satisfaction. Only by knowing what the public perceives about health care delivery can we attempt to focus on how to provide our services.

Consumer organizations regularly interview patients about current issues in health care delivery. Their responses are part of a major survey of the changing health care climate. Selected results of one such survey are presented in Box 1-2. Percentages are rounded to the nearest whole number.

The information in these surveys is not just part of a lesson to be learned; it should be totally integrated into your radiography practice as part of the health care team. In a field that is as rich in modern technology as diagnostic imaging and therapy is, it is imperative that a balance exist between this high technology and the high-touch care that only you can provide.

Surveys indicate a strong reliance on word-of-mouth advertising and peer recommendation when choosing a hospital (see Box 1-2). Furthermore, staff courtesy and quality of care are identified as important factors in patients' initial choice of a hospital and their reasons for returning to that hospital. The balance between high-tech and high-touch care can be a primary **reason for** patient satisfaction.

As can be seen, high-tech and high-touch care continue to be focus areas for an American public that is better informed and more assertive than at any other time in the history of health care delivery. Your success as a radiographer will be determined by how far you can exceed your patients' expectations.

INSIDE AND OUTSIDE CUSTOMERS

The marketing of health care targets both **outside customers** and **inside customers**. Outside customers are those people from outside of the hospital such as patients, their families, physicians, and others within the community; inside customers are members of other departments (e.g., nursing units, the emergency department), coworkers, and radiologists.

When we realize that we serve inside customers, the work environment becomes more cooperative. We are as responsible for providing high-quality service to each other as we are for providing it to the patient. All departments are striving to heal those who come to them; we must work together with support and cooperation.

Everyone in the community is an outside customer. We focus on the patients and their families as our primary outside customers; they are the ones who come to us and place their confidence in our care. The physicians who practice at our facility are important outside customers as well. They admit their patients because of our expertise. These physicians also deserve the best of our service.

BOX 1-2 HEALTH CARE CONSUMER TRENDS SURVEY RESULTS

1. All hospitals offer the same quality of care.
   Agree: 25%
   Disagree: 68%
2. All hospitals have about the same level of technology and equipment.
   Agree: 16%
   Disagree: 75%
3. Hospitals should advertise to inform the public of their services.
   Agree: 77%
   Disagree: 16%
4. Where do you get most of your information about local physicians and hospitals? (choose one)
   Friends/relatives: 50%
   Hospital mailings: 4%
   Family physician: 21%
   Newspapers: 4%
   Advertising: 21%
5. Who chooses the hospital for you?
   Self/family: 52%
   Physician alone: 42%
   Self and physician: 6%
6. What factors are important to you when selecting a hospital in a nonemergency situation for the first time? (Percentage indicates the first choice of responders.)
   Latest technology and equipment: 88%
   Courtesy of hospital staff: 83%
   Variety of specialists: 83%
   Physician recommendation: 65%
   Cost of services: 62%
   Close to home: 48%
   Friend/family recommendation: 27%
   Religious affiliation: 14%
7. For consumers with a hospital preference (those who have used the hospital before), what is the main reason for that preference? In other words, why do you go back?
   Physician recommendation: 9%
   Quality of care: 44%
   Tradition: 13%
   Close to home: 24%

Many others from the outside come to our facility on a regular basis. They may be suppliers, delivery personnel, clergy, or sales and service specialists. Although they may not be customers as such, remember that they spread our reputation by word of mouth and should be regarded as important links to the community.

Understanding that we serve both inside and outside customers by providing the care and service they expect and deserve enhances our self-images as radiographers and emphasizes the importance of the role we play within the organization.

THE BENEFITS OF HIGH-QUALITY SERVICE

Delivering high-quality customer service benefits everyone. The radiographer, inside and outside customers, and the employer all gain when patient care takes place within the context of value-added service. The radiographer can add value by making each interaction special for the person served. Smiles, appropriate touch, using the person's name, explaining the examination, and other examples described in this chapter are all ways of adding value. However, radiographers must be aware that they cannot give away what they do not have; their ability to deliver high-quality care is directly related to self-image, self-esteem, self-confidence, and their values relating to life and the workplace.

MOMENTS OF TRUTH IN RADIOLOGY

High-touch radiography may occur during each moment of an interaction between the patient and the radiographer who is delivering the service. These **moments of truth** can be considered points at which patients form perceptions about the quality of service being given and, in this case, the quality of care. Such moments of truth begin with observations that the patient makes and conclude with inferences being made about the care and service being provided.

Moments of truth can occur in every conceivable circumstance. They may relate to the physical appearance of the work area, the appearance of the radiographer, and the professional behavior of everyone involved.

You must first come to realize that quality must be the hallmark of practicing radiography. Understanding that the patient's experiences are a series of moments of truth sets the stage for clinical excellence.

CUSTOMER SERVICE CYCLES IN RADIOLOGY

The achievement of patient satisfaction is not something that can be left to chance. By viewing the patient's experiences as cycles, we can examine the events and incidents that make up those cycles. Each **customer service cycle** is part of the patient's total experience while at the facility or when interacting over the telephone. Divided into its component parts, the radiographer can manage the cycle like acts in a play to ensure that quality service is delivered to each patient. For example, a patient may be scheduled for an outpatient upper gastrointestinal (GI) series (see Box 1-3). Having the examination performed and being released are the primary

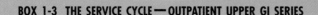

BOX 1-3 THE SERVICE CYCLE — OUTPATIENT UPPER GI SERIES

The Events
Scheduling the appointment
Arriving at the hospital
Being registered
Having the examination performed
Being released

BOX 1-4 EVENT — HAVING THE EXAMINATION PERFORMED

Introducing self to the patient
Instructing the patient how to dress for the examination
Taking the patient to the examining room
Taking a history
Explaining the examination
Introducing the radiologist, if present
Performing the examination
Releasing the patient

events involving the radiographer; they are composed of the following **incidents** (see Box 1-4), each of which is managed by the radiographer.

The key to value-added service is making the patient's experience as pleasant as possible at each step along the way and making it superior to what would be received anywhere else; the challenge is to perform each incident as if you were the best radiographer in the world. As you learn radiographic positioning and procedures, keep in mind that they are but combinations of a series of experiences that can each be enhanced for the patient. Remember that you want to perform each step in the most professional way possible. You want to convey to the patient that you are a competent and reliable professional in whom trust can be placed. Each incident in the list can be enhanced with value-added service as described in the suggestions that follow. Remember that there is no single best way to add value. As a radiographer, you may wish to have many different ways of handling each situation to take into account different patients and examinations and to avoid sounding like a recording.

Each incident may be managed as follows:

1. Use of the patient's name and, if appropriate, his or her title, conveys respect. Adults (those older than about 18 to 21 years of age) should not be greeted by their first names. Greeting people with a smile and a handshake is the accepted business salutation in U.S. culture. It is highly appropriate in health care.

EXAMPLE: "Good morning, Mrs. Davidson, my name is Amy Kim. I am the radiographer who will be performing your x-ray examination today."

2. Instructing the patient about how to dress for the examination makes the patient feel more at ease. Many radiographic examinations require that the patient change into a hospital gown, and this can be very uncomfortable for many people.

EXAMPLE (*On the way to and at the dressing room*): "Mrs. Davidson, an x-ray of your stomach requires that you wear a gown with no buttons or snaps that could show up on the x-ray image. You may change into one here in the women's dressing room. Please remove your clothing from the waist up. A locker is provided for your clothing. Be sure to keep your valuables and the key with you. Please have a seat here when you have changed. I will be back as soon as you are ready."

3. Taking the patient to the radiographic examination room may take seconds if it is nearby or minutes if it is located elsewhere in the imaging department. This time may be filled by asking the patient about the registration process, parking, or ease of finding the department; these questions indicate your desire to see that the moments of truth that the patient has already experienced at your institution have been positive. Even if you are not in a position to change an experience the patient has already had, asking shows that you care about how events have been handled. This gives the patient the opportunity to vent frustration over a mishandled event or to reinforce an already positive experience. In either case, the patient will be more cooperative for you as you perform the examination.

EXAMPLE: "Did you have any problems finding a place to park this morning?" *(The patient's response indicates that there was a problem.)* "I'm sorry to hear that, Mrs. Davidson. I'm sure that was quite annoying. I will let the appropriate department know. They are really trying to improve the situation. When we are finished, I'll give you instructions on getting your parking stub validated."

4. Taking the patient's history greatly assists the radiologist in interpreting the radiographs. It is yet another opportunity to interact professionally with the patient and to provide value-added service.

EXAMPLE: "May I ask why you are having a stomach x-ray, Mrs. Davidson? Have you had any difficulty swallowing, a chronic stomachache, or heartburn? I will share this information with our radiologist so that it may be considered when your images are read."

5. Your careful explanation of the examination gains the patient's cooperation and also builds trust in you as a professional. Speaking to the patient during the examination makes the experience more pleasant and helps the patient remain at ease.

EXAMPLE: *The steps in an upper GI series may be described at this point, and then you can add the following:* "Do you have any questions about the procedure, Mrs. Davidson? I will be here with you throughout the examination."

6. Your enthusiasm about physicians, other departments, or coworkers conveys that the patient is in good hands. The introduction of the radiologist provides such an opportunity.

 EXAMPLE: *(Before the radiologist enters the room)* "Dr. Kailin Rodriguez, an excellent radiologist, will be performing the first part of your examination today." *(When the radiologist enters the room)* "Mrs. Davidson, I would like you to meet Dr. Rodriguez."

7. Performing the examination requires clear communication with the patient. You should include specific instructions about what the patient is to do next, explanations of what the radiographer is doing, and reassurance that the patient is doing well.

 EXAMPLE: "The examination is going fine, Mrs. Davidson. We will be finished in about 3 minutes."

8. A sincere parting comment when the patient is ready to leave the department closes a very positive experience for the patient—an experience that you have successfully managed moment by moment.

 EXAMPLE: "Your examination is finished, Mrs. Davidson. Dr. Rodriguez will interpret your images and send a report to your personal physician, who I see from your chart is Dr. Alex Jacobs. You can call there in a couple of days for the results. May I show you back to the dressing room? Do you know how to find the main lobby and parking area? Cara Adams at the front desk can validate your parking pass. It was nice meeting you today. I hope you are feeling better soon."

The key to the above interactions is that they are delivered in a sincere but timely manner. Taking too much time with one patient delivers poor service to those who are still waiting. One of your most important challenges is to deliver such value-added service in a fairly short period. Once again, having total command of the technical aspects of the procedure will allow you to concentrate on patient interactions.

CUSTOMER SERVICE ON THE TELEPHONE

Enhancing telephone interactions can play a big role in value-added service. Although most imaging departments have clerical personnel who handle many of the daily telephone calls, the radiographer is often called on to deal with inside and outside customers on the telephone. Such calls may be from patients requesting information about an examination or scheduling, physicians needing examination reports or scheduling of tests, or nursing units with questions about patient preparations, scheduling, or examinations. Each such moment of truth can reveal much about the radiographer's level of integrity, knowledge, and professionalism.

A few simple rules to remember about using the telephone go a long way toward improving this often-used method of communication:

1. Keep the number of rings to a minimum. If possible, answer the phone by the third ring.
2. Answer professionally. Identify the department and yourself, and add a phrase such as "May I help you?" or "How may I help you?"

3. Enunciate carefully. Talk directly into the transmitter. Speak clearly. Do not attempt to drink, eat, or chew gum when on the telephone. Make sure your voice is pleasant and unhurried, even if you are in a hurry. Remember, you are there to assist the caller. Keep the tone of your voice alert, pleasant, and expressive. Smiling while you are speaking will automatically make your voice more pleasant. Speak more slowly than normal and with a lower voice.

4. Personalize. Once you know the caller's name, use it. Doing so indicates a desire to assist with the request and brings the interaction to a more personal level.

5. If you have to put the caller on hold, first ask permission to do so and wait for an answer. Indicate to the caller about how long they will be waiting. When you return, thank the caller for holding. If it is necessary to put someone on hold for a long time, come back on the line about every 45 seconds to reassure the caller that the information that is needed will be available shortly.

6. Become comfortable with the telephone system quickly so that you can perform a function such as transferring a call without losing the call. If you must transfer a call, indicate the extension to which you are sending the call, and thank the caller for holding.

7. When terminating a call, thank the caller, and allow the caller to hang up first; that way you will know that the conversation has ended.

CONFLICT RESOLUTION: OPPORTUNITIES TO EXCEED THE CUSTOMER'S EXPECTATIONS

Leaving quality service to chance can be a serious mistake. In this age of consumer awareness and increasing competition, a mishandled patient interaction can result in the loss of patient confidence, and this will reflect negatively on the department and the institution. Because of an increasingly litigious public, unprofessional interactions or mishandled complaints can increase the chances of lawsuits. Most important, exceeding patient expectations improves patient care, and this is a goal to which we all aspire: it makes radiography stimulating and satisfying for the radiographer.

Radiography is a customer-oriented business. Within that business, which is many times typified by high-stress situations and brief encounters, are numerous opportunities for miscommunications and conflict. Other aspects of conflict are addressed in the next chapter, but the following material specifically relates to quality customer service in the radiology department. Highly successful service companies and individuals have at their disposal the **conflict resolution** tools of listening and empathizing, and they also make use of skills that build trust and develop solutions to problems; such tools are equally useful in dealing with coworkers and physicians.

In addition, patients often have special questions for the radiographer. Being comfortable with those questions further enhances our professional standing in the eyes of the patient and increases the patient's confidence in us. Again, such interactions are not left to chance or to spur-of-the-moment answers. By anticipating questions in advance, we can have accurate, truthful, and appropriate answers ready to meet most of our patients' needs.

Most student radiographers have little or no experience in dealing with the public in the health care setting. This relationship is special and quite unlike any other in-service businesses, and it provides all the more reason for thoroughly understanding basic conflict resolution early in your education program.

The two most effective tools you can use for conflict resolution are effective listening and empathizing. **Effective listening** tells other people we respect what they have to say and that we are here to help if we can. It is very important to remember that often the other person is not attacking you personally but rather that he or she is attacking a particular unsatisfactory situation. Effective listening traits are included in Box 1-5.

The second very important step in conflict resolution is empathizing. **Empathy** is understanding and accepting the other person's position without necessarily agreeing or disagreeing. This can be difficult in a high-stress situation, but it is vital that you realize that the person with whom you are in conflict has a right to the feelings involved. Box 1-6 lists phrases that can be used when empathizing.

BOX 1-5 EFFECTIVE LISTENING TRAITS

Establish good eye contact with the customer.
Face the person.
Stay physically relaxed with the arms uncrossed.
Use facial expressions to show concern.
Use vocalizations such as "I see" and "Uh-huh."
Give complete and undivided attention.
Avoid interrupting.

BOX 1-6 EMPATHETIC PHRASES

"I would be upset, too, if I thought . . ."
"It must have been frustrating when you . . ."
"I'm sorry that you are upset."
"I think I understand how you feel."
"I'm sure that was very annoying, wasn't it?"

By empathizing with patients' feelings, you indicate a desire to respect their position and to help deal with the many emotions being expressed. Until you address the feelings, constructive problem solving cannot take place. If you diffuse the tension through listening and empathizing, you will often find that a mutually agreeable solution is at hand.

On occasion, patients may not respond to effective listening and empathy. They may be loud and abusive or simply not interested in an agreeable solution. In such cases, you are wise to seek assistance from another radiographer, a supervisor, or a physician.

Listening and empathizing are also key tools to use when you are faced with the many questions patients may ask. As a new student radiographer, you will soon appreciate how patients feel when confronted with strange technology and uncomfortable situations. The following frequently asked patient questions and radiographer answers come from the actual experiences of student radiographers involved in patient care:

1. How much radiation am I getting?

"With the attention radiation often gets in the media, I can understand your concern, Mr. Brown. Let me assure you that our equipment and procedures give us the information we need with a very small amount of radiation."

2. Will this hurt?

"I can see that you are uneasy about this test, Mrs. Gonzales. There will be a little discomfort, but I will do my best to make you as comfortable as possible."

3. How much will this cost?

"I'm sorry, but I do not know the fee for the examination. If you can wait a few moments, I will obtain the price for you."

4. How many pictures are you going to take?

"I can see you are concerned about the number of images I am taking, Mrs. Olson. It is necessary to see the area of interest from several different angles. After processing the images, I will determine if we need any additional views. We want to give you an accurate diagnosis."

5. When can I leave?

"I'm sure that there are other things you would rather be doing, Mrs. Lightfoot. As soon as I am finished with your examination, I will see that you are released."

6. What do you see on my films?

"I'm sure that you are anxious to find out your test results, Mr. Wong. Interpreting the images is beyond my scope of practice. The radiologist will examine your images and see that your personal physician receives a copy of the results." As you can see from these examples, a direct answer is not always possible. Many times, the patient is expressing fear and anxiety; listening carefully and empathizing are excellent ways to address those feelings. Certainly circumstances such as the concern with which a question is asked, the age of the patient, and the mental condition of the patient may change how the question may be answered; no single answer will work best in every situation. It is wise to have several answers that you can use to handle different circumstances appropriately.

CONCLUSION

Quality customer service is no accident. It is planned for, rehearsed, and used whenever possible. High-quality, value-added service is what the patient/customer expects, and failure to meet those expectations may send the patient elsewhere for future care. Exceeding those expectations satisfies the patient, makes your work more enjoyable, reduces stress, and benefits everyone involved. As a health care professional, you will want to deliver the best care and service possible.

Review Questions

1. Which of the following is the primary source used by patients to obtain information about physicians and hospitals?
   a. Advertising
   b. Newspapers
   c. Physician reference
   d. Friends and relatives
2. When choosing a hospital for care, who is primarily making the selection?
   a. The patient's physician
   b. The third-party payer
   c. The patient and family
   d. The patient and physician together
3. When they are in need of additional care, what is the main reason that patients return to a certain hospital?
   a. Proximity to home
   b. Quality of care
   c. Tradition
   d. Physician recommendation
4. Selecting a hospital is based primarily on what factors?
   a. Cost and courtesy of staff
   b. Physician recommendation and cost
   c. Courtesy of staff and availability of state-of-the-art technology
   d. Proximity to home and religious affiliation
5. What is the ability to appreciate the patient's feelings called?
   a. Sympathy
   b. Effective listening
   c. A moment of truth
   d. Empathy
6. Every interaction between a radiologic technologist and an inside or outside customer is considered to be which of the following?
   a. A moment of truth
   b. A moment of decision
   c. Just part of the job
   d. Conflict

7. When addressing the adult patient for the first time, which of the following should happen?
   a. The first name should be used.
   b. The first name should be used and a formal greeting extended.
   c. The last name with appropriate title should be used, along with a pleasant greeting.
   d. The radiographer should begin the examination quickly, because the patient is probably in a hurry.
8. Examples of inside customers include which of the following?
   a. Patients and their family
   b. Coworkers and other departments
   c. Physicians and vendors
   d. Clergy and counselors
9. Which of the following is the primary outside customer served by the radiographer?
   a. Radiologist
   b. Patient
   c. Coworker
   d. Department supervisor
10. Which of the following is true about conflict?
    a. It must be effectively managed by the radiographer.
    b. It should be avoided at all times.
    c. It always results in a win-lose scenario.
    d. It has little value.

BIBLIOGRAPHY

Callaway W: *Face to face with moments of truth*, Springfield, IL, 2006, lecture.

Callaway W: *Just do something—the you-shaped piece of the puzzle*, Springfield, IL, 2006, lecture.

Organization Dimensions, Inc: *Building organizational excellence*, Wheeling, IL, 1986.

Organization Dimensions, Inc: *That extra touch*, Wheeling, IL, 1986.

Organization Dimensions, Inc: *The healthcare quality service standards system*, Wheeling, IL, 1988.

Organization Dimensions, Inc: *The quality edge*, Wheeling, IL, 1990.

Salimbene S: *What language does your patient hurt in?* ed 1, St. Paul, 2000, Paradigm.

Becoming a Better Student

LaVerne Tolley Gurley

OBJECTIVES

On completion of this chapter, you should be able to:

- Identify needs common to all human beings.

- Describe physiologic needs and their effect on learning.

- Describe psychologic needs and how you maintain a healthy social interaction with others.

- Describe the way you perceive the world and your unique pattern of behavior for satisfying your needs.

- Examine your lifestyle to identify causes of stress and conflict.

- Examine your values and determine what is and what is not important to you.

- Describe ways in which conflict may be resolved.

- Set goals and plan for a lifestyle that has meaning, serenity, and a sense of wholeness.

Making a vocational choice is an explicit statement about the kind of person you are or hope to be. Professional satisfaction will depend on the extent to which you can use your abilities in a productive manner; your work should be consistent with your values and interests and the roles you fulfill in society. Choosing radiologic technology is an exploration. Education in radiologic technology is vastly different from high school or a college liberal arts education; the main difference is that your curriculum requires you to spend much of your time in the clinical setting, where you will learn how to handle sick and injured

KEY TERMS

conflict
controlled environment
emotionality
hierarchy of human
 needs
objectivity
personality
primal stresses
psychologic care
reinforcement behavior
self-discipline

CHAPTER OUTLINE

Knowing your human
 needs
 First level
 Second level
 Third level
 Fourth level
 Fifth level
Physiologic needs
 Nutrition
 Sleep
 Recreation and
 exercise
Psychologic needs
 Emotionality
 Objectivity
Emotional and primal
 stress
Stress and conflict
 Stress
 Conflict
 Managing and
 resolving conflict
Planning
Conclusion

patients. Because patient care is the focus of your curriculum, generally the code of conduct is more rigidly defined and is based on the moral and ethical standards associated with the medical profession. You should expect and understand these differences to avoid frustration or disappointment.

All students experience some frustration, anxiety, and perhaps a degree of disillusionment in preparing for their careers. Fortunately, most students adjust to these irritants with only minor strain. This chapter is provided to help you learn to cope with the rigors of your educational program in your chosen career.

KNOWING YOUR HUMAN NEEDS

Knowledge about yourself is the most important information you can possess at the beginning of your education. You have your own unique pattern of solving problems and your own values, ambitions, aspirations, and experiences in addition to the basic needs common to everyone; these are the qualities that make up your unique **personality**. Indeed, personality is a combination of habitual patterns and qualities of behavior and attitudes. You think, feel, and act according to your perceptions of the world. You are a seeker, and your thoughts, feelings, and actions are purposefully directed toward satisfying your needs.

Human needs are complex. Some are unique to the individual, and others are common to everyone. Abraham H. Maslow, a noted psychologist, described a **hierarchy of human needs** that ranges from basic needs that are essential to life (food, clothing, and shelter) to the highly complex, psychologic, self-actualization needs (Fig. 2-1). He listed the needs in the following order:

First Level

The needs that are essential to life are first in the order of importance. These needs are food, clothing, shelter, and the will to reproduce.

Second Level

A feeling of safety is essential to growing and developing. You can never be completely safe from physical injury or disease. It is important, however, that you feel a degree of safety in your social and physical environment.

Third Level

The need to be loved is inherent. You need the emotional support of others and the warmth and closeness of those important to you. This need also includes the desire to love others, to return affection, and to support and care for those who love you.

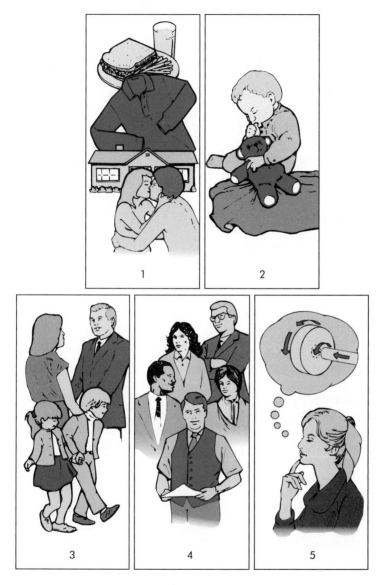

Fig. 2-1

Maslow's hierarchy of needs: (1) food, clothing, shelter, and the will to reproduce; (2) a feeling of safety; (3) love; (4) satisfying relationships; and (5) creativity, self-expression, and achievement.

Fourth Level

You also need satisfying relationships with others in the larger social community. You need to be valued, accepted, and appreciated to maintain self-esteem, self-respect, and a unique identity.

Fifth Level

Creativity, self-expression, and achievement are also needs characteristic of all human beings. Work needs to be useful, productive, and valuable to others.

The higher-level needs are not felt until the first-level needs are satisfied. For example, a drowning man gasping for air does not feel the need to be creative at that moment. A person with extreme hunger and thirst feels the need for love and affection less than the more immediate and urgent need for sustenance. Physical needs must be met before creativity and other higher-level needs are felt.

PHYSIOLOGIC NEEDS

Optimal health and well-being require your attention to nutrition, sleep, relaxation, and exercise. To expect optimal learning performance, you must take optimal care of your body.

Nutrition

Diet, nutrition, and learning are tightly interwoven. Learning is easier with a sound body, and this can help produce a sound mind. Nutritional biochemicals keep body cells healthy and functioning, and these biochemicals come from only one source: what you eat. Proper nutrients are found in foods that contain proteins, vitamins, minerals, carbohydrates, and essential fats. Foods that contain empty calories, preservatives, and artificial additives contribute very little to a healthy diet. In fact, some preservatives and additives can be stored in the body and eventually reach toxic levels. It is best to eat fresh, whole foods and to avoid refined and processed foods.

Breakfast is often considered by nutritionists to be the most important meal of the day. It relieves the long overnight fast and replenishes the body and mind for the planned activities of the day. Usually you should consume one fourth to one third of your daily calorie and protein needs at breakfast. Energy derived from protein is metabolized more consistently and over a longer period of time than energy derived from carbohydrates. A well-balanced breakfast can keep you going through the morning and help you to avoid the "midmorning letdown" that results from a nutritional deficit. Improper diet can also result in unexplained emotional upsets such as crying, depression, and even violent impulses.

Sleep

Your body also requires adequate sleep, which offers rest to the brain and nervous system. In preparing for your career, you want to be relaxed and well rested when you enter classes and laboratories so that you and your body can easily meet the demands placed on you. Without sufficient sleep, you are working against yourself. Lack of sleep can result in inattentiveness, drowsiness, and the inability to retain what you have read and studied in class. Students with inadequate sleep and poor diet may not perform acceptably and are often easily irritated and frustrated. Both sleep and adequate diet are crucial to the learning process.

Recreation and Exercise

Recreation and exercise are important for both the mind and the body. Use of the mind can fatigue an individual. The mind functions better when mental concentration alternates with periods of diversion and exercise. Exercise can reduce frustrations, distract the mind from the concerns of the moment, and enable the mind to recover before study is resumed. Care for the body directly affects the expressions of the mind and the total person.

Proper diet, rest, and recreation are valuable ways to practice personal preventive health care and are essential tools for creating optimal learning conditions.

PSYCHOLOGIC NEEDS

Psychologic care involves developing and maintaining a healthy balance between rational thoughts and emotions. Although your studies will require a great deal of **self-discipline**, it is also important to maintain healthy social interactions with family and friends and to accept your emotions as a natural part of your personality.

Emotionality

Emotionality is the quality or state of a sound emotional balance. Living by values based on a healthy balance between mind and heart and maintaining a sound emotional balance can help you decide what is important and what is not and can help enhance your learning.

You might begin to question the value systems you have learned from parents, religion, and society. As you go through life gaining new experiences and knowledge, you might change some of your beliefs. The important thing is to know what you believe to be right and to live accordingly.

Objectivity

Objectivity is the quality or state of being objective—the ability to interpret a situation from an unbiased point of view rather than from your own subjective view. Learning to use rational thought in making decisions will enhance your objectivity. Being oversensitive can lead to paranoid feelings that others do not like you or are against you, which will lower your performance in the classroom.

If a conflict occurs in the classroom or laboratory, look at it from all points of view and realize that the cause could be something totally unrelated to you or the classroom. It is unfair for you to assume that you are responsible for the unpleasant behavior of others. Learning to be objective about your behavior, as well as that of others, will help you to become a mentally and emotionally healthy person.

EMOTIONAL AND PRIMAL STRESS

You seldom encounter the stress of a life-threatening event as the early cave dwellers did, but your body responds to stress in the same way (Fig. 2-2). Imagine being stalked by a hungry predator. Your heartbeat

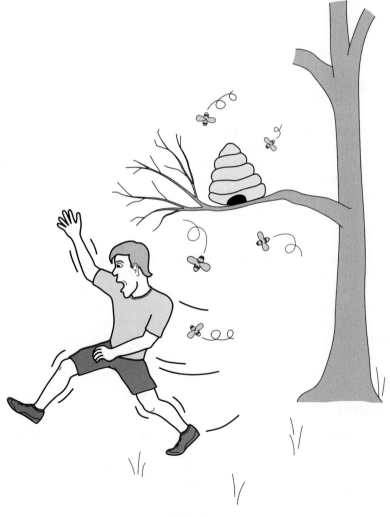

Fig. 2-2
Flight, the body's response to danger.

accelerates, your blood pressure rises, and hormones rush into your bloodstream to send sugar to your muscles and brain. Food digestion temporarily ceases so that more blood is available for energy. In this way, your body prepares to fight the beast or flee to safety. This type of acute stress, which requires a fight-or-flight response, is what McQuade and Aikman call the first **primal stresses**. Because the body does not identify the source of the fear, it reacts in the same way when you get what is commonly known as "stage fright." Stage fright is not life threatening, but for some, the fear they experience when speaking before a group is so intense that the body responds as if it were (Fig. 2-3). McQuade and Aikman also list two other types of acute stress that cause a primal body reaction.

The second primal stress is the basic problem of obtaining food. This type of threat does not elicit a fight-or-flight response but rather persuasion, bartering, searching, and producing. Although the stress resulting from a threat to the food supply is seldom life threatening to us today, it is a psychologic stress that may be as painful as hunger itself. You learned in infancy that while receiving food you also received attention, which you translated as receiving love; you were receiving more than the basic

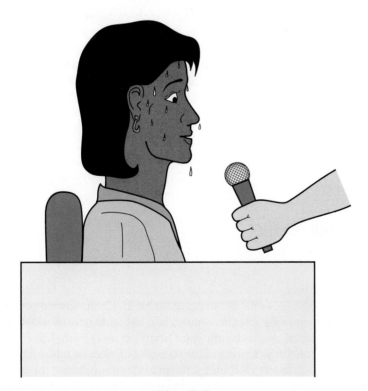

Fig. 2-3

Speaking in a key situation such as before a jury can also be a frightening experience causing the body to respond as if physical danger was present.

nutrients for life. When food is withheld, you may feel that recognition, attention, and love are also being withheld.

Death, the third primal stress, is inevitable. The unalterable truth is that someday you will die. In the meantime, you should make your life worth living; become the person you want to be. For many people, a religious belief provides a strong anchor in times of turmoil and change. Religion will not dispose of all stresses, but it can provide a context of belief that allows a person to deal with those stresses.

Coping with life stresses is not new to you. While growing and developing, you made many adjustments and concessions. You learned to distinguish between your father, mother, brother, and sister, and finally you realized that you were not any of them—this was your discovery of yourself. Later in childhood you began exploring and discovered that you could control parts of your world. You learned what was dangerous and what was safe, what belonged to you and what belonged to others, and that certain behavior brought rewards while other behavior was punished. While you were learning these things, you were developing patterns for coping with life situations. Your behavior was based on your most satisfying experiences. It may sound simplistic, but most people behave in a manner that will give them something in return that will satisfy their basic human needs.

You learned to behave in a certain way because you usually found it rewarding. You continue to behave in that manner as long as you are rewarded. B. F. Skinner, a twentieth-century educational psychologist, studied animal and human behavior. He found that, when placed in a **controlled environment** (an artificial environment to verify the results of an experiment), animals could be taught to perform complex acts by rewarding the desired behavior. He called this **reinforcement behavior**. He found that behavior could also be modified through punishment or merely the absence of a reward. Skinner later worked with humans under less controlled conditions. He found that a form of the reinforcement theory could be applied to shape and modify human behavior.

STRESS AND CONFLICT

Stress

Stress is a response that can occur when others' or your behavior fails to produce the desired or expected results. You should expect a moderate amount of stress throughout life, but there may be a disproportionate amount of stress during your first year away from home. A primary source of stress during adolescence and early adulthood occurs when the need to assert your independence does not produce the expected results in a world that requires a balance between independence and dependence. You must face the problem of needing to be both dependent and independent at the same time. The life situations that require a balance between dependence and independence are many. A financial base is necessary for independent living, but even with wealth, a totally independent existence is impossible. You will always be dependent on others to a certain degree. Most employment opportunities are authoritarian in nature, which means that workers depend on supervisors and supervisors depend on managers. Regardless of how independent you wish to be, you still have dependent needs; therefore, you must accept those aspects of life that involve interdependence. You learn to submit to rational authority and at the same time retain a degree of independence.

Working through the dilemma of dependent-independent relationships is complicated. You have been taught to be submissive and obedient and, at the same time, to despise yourself for being dependent. You must reach a tolerable balance. When this balance is achieved, your energies can be used for creative and productive work.

Conflict

Conflict is tension that results from disagreements between incompatible needs or drives, either within yourself or with others. Conflict does not have to be open warfare or an outbreak of hostilities. It can be as mild and benign as a difference of opinion or diversity in taste. It is an inescapable part of living, and generally speaking, the closer and more intimate a relationship is, the greater the opportunities are for conflict. Conflict can be either healthy and constructive or hostile and destructive. Conflicts occur in families, among close friends, in work relationships, in student groups, and even among strangers.

A type of conflict that is increasingly important concerns identity and role assignment. In the past, roles were often assigned by society; male and female roles were clearly defined. Today, people are questioning their assigned roles and are independently seeking their own identities. This is a source of conflict for both sexes for which there is no magic formula. It calls for understanding, tolerance, and patience.

Another category of conflict concerns your perceptions of encroachment on your territory. For example, nonsmokers may be offended by cigarette smoke, or a roommate may disturb you by playing the radio too loudly. Persuasion, tact, diplomacy, and compromise may be required in these situations.

Managing and Resolving Conflict

Some types of conflict are more easily resolved than others. Factual issues are simpler to resolve than value or identification issues. Once the source of conflict is identified, you can begin to tackle the problem effectively. The most important factor in resolving conflict is to attack the issue rather than the individual. Focus on the issue and resist any temptation to criticize or demean the other person; remember that a true victory is one in which the relationship remains intact and both people are satisfied with the results. Learning to compromise and establish trust can help you to develop the interpersonal skills that are necessary to resolve conflict. Conflict must be resolved in a manner that accommodates your values.

Resolving conflict with casual acquaintances is different from resolving conflict with family and friends. With casual acquaintances, you are less concerned about maintaining good will. The fear of damaging the relationship is slight or perhaps nonexistent. With family and close friends, your desire to maintain the relationship is more intense. Consequently, emotions and feelings influence your behavior. Your behavior can sometimes add more stress to a tense situation. Understanding human behavior will help resolve conflicts in interpersonal relations. Usually you act in what you perceive to be your best self-interest, but your self-interest may conflict with the self-interests of others. Compromise, participation, and allowance for imperfections are elements that you will have to employ in resolving conflicts with others and within yourself.

Internal conflict may be as damaging and destructive as the tense encounters you have with others. With others you can use the inherent fight-or-flight response. Whether you choose fight or flight, your action is clearly defined and directed. It is more difficult to deal with conflict within yourself. You cannot run away from yourself, and to fight yourself is unproductive. To maintain a low-stress lifestyle, you must learn to control the factors that are at the root of tension and anxiety.

Arranging your lifestyle to avoid needless stress and tension helps reduce conflict, but no amount of planning prevents conflict altogether. Conflict can be healthy, constructive, and interesting. You should try to avoid, however, the ill will, hurt feelings, and hostility that often result from conflict. You can improve your skills in interpersonal relationships and often resolve conflict with fewer long-term negative effects.

Silber and Glim (1981) list seven ways people behave when confronted with conflict: they attack, internalize, deny, isolate, manipulate, withdraw, or confront. The authors suggest confronting the problem in a mature manner in open dialogue. Feelings of empathy are created between two people when they share risks, dangers, doubts, and insecurities. Emotions must be dealt with to bring about a change in behavior. Negative emotions serve as a barrier and must be confronted to resolve the conflict. Silber and Glim also state that you must trust the other person when trying to resolve conflict, and you must be open and honest about your objectives, expectations, and needs.

The first step in resolving any conflict is identifying the cause of the conflict. In some cases the cause may be a simple difference of opinion. For example, you may differ with a classmate on when an assignment is due; this can be resolved by asking the instructor for the correct due date. Factual issues can usually be resolved by accepting the opinion of an authority on the issue. Issues involving values, such as differences in religion, politics, or ethics, are more difficult, and a clear-cut answer is unlikely. Facts related to values may be questioned or interpreted differently. For example, a religious writing may be considered to be the authority, but the interpretation of that writing may vary considerably.

Examine the way you have organized your life. Stress and tension can result from the failure to organize your life in a way that is comfortable for you. Are you overextended financially? Are you overcommitted with work or study? Systematic and disciplined work and planning can help prevent the frustrations of unfinished tasks and commitments. In his book *How to Get Control of Your Time and Your Life*, Alan Lakein suggests that it is difficult, if not impossible, to control your life unless you have control of your time. Pacing your work and study will prevent a sense of urgency and help you to keep up with your obligations in a more relaxed manner.

PLANNING

Planning is important. Decide what you want and set goals. You can set short-term goals (for example, completing this radiologic technology course) or long-term goals that involve your family and your status in the community. Once you have established goals, begin listing the activities necessary to achieve each objective. Procrastination ensures stress; reaching your goals requires action. You need self-discipline (control over your emotions and actions), self-motivation, and self-direction to carry out your plan, but it will bring long-term satisfaction. It is unrealistic to expect perfection of yourself; you will only become dissatisfied. It is important to realize that everyone, including you, has flaws and imperfections. You must pursue your goals even though you will not always do things perfectly.

Excessive commitments, whether financial or social, may destroy your best-laid plans. You cannot allow people to make inappropriate or extreme demands of you, and you should not make them of yourself.

When you review your goals and objectives, they may appear overly ambitious; this is because you are looking at the plan as a whole and not in steps. You should accomplish one goal-oriented step at a time. Any undertaking can be broken down into achievable components that can be tackled one at a time. Start on one activity, if only for a short time at first, and you will be amazed at how much you can accomplish.

The pressures of school and work can be dealt with more effectively if you take time out for recreation and relaxation. Because your school schedule will be tight, you must work efficiently so that you will feel good about taking the time you allow for recreation, which can be a reward for work well done. The reward will serve as reinforcement and may, in fact, help you to work more efficiently.

Planning, setting objectives, listing activities for reaching objectives, and scheduling work and recreation should reduce stress (Fig. 2-4). Making improvements in your performance through discipline and motivation should improve your chances of minimizing anxiety, tension, and conflict.

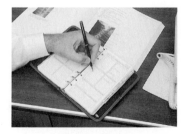

Fig. 2-4

Regular use of a calendar planner is an invaluable tool in the planning and organizing process.

CONCLUSION

Stress is a chemical or emotional factor that causes bodily or mental tension. Stress, as discussed in this chapter, has to do with the mind, because it is with the mind that we confront problems and seek solutions. We try to reach solutions based on logic and wisdom, but emotions creep in and sometimes send the wrong signals to the body, telling it to prepare to flee or fight; these responses are often counterproductive to resolving conflict or reducing stress.

You can, however, learn to handle your own life stresses. You can begin by developing a low-stress lifestyle that employs habits such as exercise and good diet and forces such as religion and philosophy. The aim is to create a healthier, happier self and to find serenity, meaning, and wholeness in your life. The vigorous, expansive personality attempts to handle conflict without confusion and to deal with stress before it becomes intolerable.

Review Questions

1. What are the four human needs essential to survival?
   a. Food, clothing, shelter, and love
   b. Clothing, food, shelter, and the will to reproduce
   c. Shelter, clothing, food, and self-actualization
   d. Self-actualization, food, shelter, and the will to reproduce
2. What are the physiologic needs?
   a. Self-discipline, sociability, and assertiveness
   b. Assertiveness, emotionality, and objectivity
   c. Recreation, sleep, and nutrition
   d. Self-worth, self-discipline, and exercise
3. Psychologic care means maintaining which of the following?
   a. A healthy balance between rational thoughts and emotion
   b. A proper diet, exercise, and sleep
   c. Sufficient recreational activities
   d. Mental concentration training
4. Emotionality:
   a. Is not a normal condition.
   b. Is the state of extreme stress and fear.
   c. Is the state of a sound emotional balance.
   d. Is the source of frustration.
5. What are the three types of primal reaction to stress?
   a. Fight or flight, reinforcement behavior, and religious or philosophic belief
   b. Fight or flight, reinforcement behavior, and persuasion

    c. Persuasion, fight or flight, and bartering and searching

    d. Fight or flight, religious or philosophic belief, and persuasion

6. Which of the following statements is most consistent with the idea of coping with stress?

    a. Coping with life stresses is a new phenomenon brought on by the industrial revolution.

    b. Your pattern for coping with stress is determined almost solely by heredity.

    c. In coping with stress, you behave in a way you found most rewarding in your past experiences.

    d. Coping patterns begin to develop at the time of adulthood.

7. Which statement best characterizes the body's response to stress or threatening situations?

    a. An unnatural calmness and serenity sets in.

    b. The mind responds to stress with logic and wisdom, sparing the physical body of involvement.

    c. Emotions are kept in check because of the mind's clear and realistic reasoning.

    d. Emotions are primitive, and in stress situations they signal the body to prepare for fight or flight.

8. What is the first step in resolving conflict?

    a. Identifying the cause

    b. Negotiating with the other party

    c. Reaching a consensus with all involved

    d. Compromising and establishing trust

9. How is achieving wholeness best described?

    a. A combination of knowledge and skill

    b. An integration of body and mind

    c. Sustaining life with food, clothing, and shelter

    d. Having developed problem-solving skills

10. Which of the following statements about conflict is true?

    a. Proper planning can prevent conflict altogether.

    b. Conflict can be healthy, constructive, and interesting.

    c. Ill will, hurt feelings, and hostility always result in the resolution of conflict.

    d. No amount of planning can eliminate hostility in the resolution of conflict.

11. What is the easiest type of conflict to resolve?

    a. Identity and role assignment

    b. Issues involving values, religion, and politics

    c. Factual issues

    d. Territorial encroachment

12. Why is resolving conflict with casual acquaintances different from resolving conflict with friends and family?

    a. Casual acquaintances are more likely to become hostile.

b. You feel more comfortable with friends and family than with casual acquaintances.

c. You are less concerned with maintaining good will with casual acquaintances than you are with maintaining good will with friends and family.

d. Emotions will not influence the resolution of the conflict with friends and family.

13. A low-stress lifestyle may be characterized as one with which of the following?

   a. Vigorous drive and competitiveness

   b. Impulsive, risk-taking, and erratic behavior

   c. A low level of physical activity and little social interaction

   d. A balance of exercise, good diet, and such forces as religion and philosophy

BIBLIOGRAPHY

Alessandra A, Hunsaker P: *Communicating at work*, New York, 1993, Simon & Schuster.

Charles CM: *Educational psychology: the instructional endeavor*, ed 2, St. Louis, 1976, Mosby.

Fulghum R: *From beginning to end, the rituals of our lives*, New York, 1996, Villard Books.

Gordon S: *Psychology for you*, New York, 1974, Oxford.

Maslow AH: A theory of human motivation, *Psycholog Rev* 50:370, 1943.

McQuade W, Aikman A: *Stress—what it is—what it can do to your health—how to fight back*, New York, 1975, Bantam Books.

Morse R, Furst ML: *Stress for success: a holistic approach to stress and its management*, New York, 1979, Van Nostrand Reinhold.

Memorization— A Key to Learning

LaVerne Tolley Gurley

OBJECTIVES

On completion of this chapter, you should be able to:

- Increase your skills in memory and recall.
- Explain how perception is influenced by your memory of sights, sounds, and events.
- Describe methods to improve your concentration for more effective learning.
- Improve your listening skills and reading effectiveness.
- Practice techniques for memory recall skills.
- Describe the positive and negative aspects of forgetting.
- Examine inaccurate memory and distortions in remembering and explain theories for why they occur.
- List ways to reduce inaccurate recall and fallacies in thinking.
- Use rhymes, mnemonics, associations, and other techniques for memorizing.

This chapter deals with a practical approach to developing memory storage and retrieval skills. It is assumed that you have the ability to remember and that you wish to use that ability more effectively.

REDISCOVERING MEMORY SKILLS

There was a time when **rote memorization**, which means learning word-by-word with little internalization, was a common practice in schools. Students were taught to learn through memorization drills, and much of the

KEY TERMS

attention
long-term memory
memory retrieval
memory storage
mnemonics
perceptions
rote memorization
short-term memory

CHAPTER OUTLINE

Rediscovering memory
  skills
Intentional memorization
  Perception
  Attention
  Improving listening
  skills
  Improving reading
  skills
Retrieving from memory
Forgetting
  Errors in remembering
Conclusion

information was not completely understood. Educators knew that students could memorize a vast amount of information, even though the information was not immediately useful. It was assumed that as the student encountered more life experiences, the stored information would be retrieved and applied. This practice was due, in part, to the economic conditions of the time; only the youth had access to schools, and education ceased abruptly as the youth entered the labor market. Teachers believed they were educating for a lifetime; although the material might not be immediately understood because of the students' limited life experiences, they could rely on the memory-stored information to serve as the need arose.

Some educators thought that memorizing exercised the mind and thus increased learning ability. The analogy was drawn from the effects of exercise on muscular tissue—an analogy that recent research suggests is valid.

Without first understanding it, students could not apply the memorized material to life problems as the educators had hoped; thus, rote memorization has suffered a bad reputation for the past decade.

Recently teachers began trying to instill the understanding of all educational material. Memorization drills were abandoned on the basis that once the students understood what they were learning, they would automatically remember it. However, understanding does not occur without memory. The ability to think depends on information being stored in memory and on the ability to recover it and logically manipulate it. Curriculum design is based on the assumptions that students remember what has been learned and that advanced courses can build on knowledge stored in memory. So memorizing, even rote drilling, has again become respectable when practiced in a meaningful and relevant manner.

INTENTIONAL MEMORIZATION

Many things are stored in memory, some with conscious effort. However, most of the sights and sounds of daily living are stored with no particular effort. Intentional memorization occurs in your deliberate pursuit of knowledge in a systematic or planned study situation. It can be divided into two parts: perception and attention.

Perception

If a scene is presented to a group of observers, each observer will probably perceive it in a different way. To make sense of it, each observer will try to match the scene with a similar scene or scenes stored in his or her memory. The observers are unaware that they are supplying data to make the scene fit into a similar scene or experience in their past. Thus, how you perceive something is heavily influenced by what you have stored in memory. Memory also influences the accuracy of your **perceptions**, which are your observations and resultant mental images. In his experiments in the psychology of perception, Sir Frederick Bartlett found that line drawings that were even vaguely familiar to observers could be perceived and reproduced with greater accuracy than unfamiliar patterns. Thus, the greater the amount of similar information stored in your memory, the more accurate your perceptions and recall of something new.

Suppose you have before you a familiar object, for example, a fish, and are asked to make a line drawing of it. You can probably produce a line drawing that is fairly recognizable to anyone (Fig. 3-1). You perceive the fish with its fins, scales, and gills. Now, suppose marine biology students with a vast amount of knowledge about the particular species of fish undertake the same assignment. Their perceptions of the object will no doubt be different. They will note the lateral fin spread, the positions of the upper and lower fins, the graduated arrangement of the scales, the medially deeply notched tail, and many other details that escape the eye of the untrained observer; their reproductions of their perceptions of the object will be more detailed and accurate (Fig. 3-2). This is an example of how things previously learned and stored in memory affect the perception of objects. It appears that perception depends on organization in human memory. Perception is sharpened when large quantities of related data are organized and stored in memory.

Attention

Attention means concentrating on one activity to the exclusion of others. It is possible to improve your ability to pay attention. In your own experience you have probably found methods that help you. One of the obvious ways is to eliminate interfering thoughts that come from distractions in the environment or from pressing problems. These interfering thoughts produce a state of anxiety that is difficult to ignore. Many of the distractions in the environment can be controlled (for example, loud noises, conversation or chatter, and uncomfortable room temperature). Inner anxiety, fears, and persistent worry about personal and financial

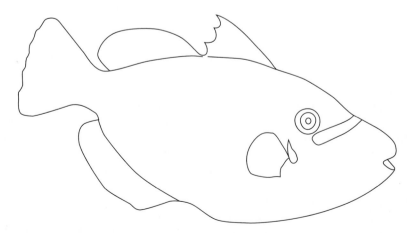

Fig. 3-1
A simple perceptual line drawing.

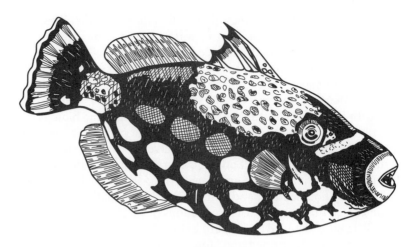

Fig. 3-2

A complex perceptual line drawing.

problems are distractions that are more difficult to handle. It is important to realize, however, that these distractions are probably the ones that are most seriously interfering with your ability to concentrate. Special effort should be made to discipline your mind. You may need to temporarily abandon your problem during learning sessions that require intense concentration. It has been suggested that the best way to overcome mind wandering is to discover the cause. When you are trying to concentrate and distracting thoughts creep in, ask yourself what these thoughts are about. Jot them down, and as you continue to keep a log of the interfering thoughts, you may find that certain thoughts recur with greater frequency. This should help you discover the problem and approach a solution. If the problem itself cannot be solved immediately, practice shelving it by refusing to give it conscious attention during periods that require intense concentration.

You can also improve your ability to concentrate by preparing to pay attention. Preparing involves creating a state of readiness; this means that you must prepare yourself to get the most from a class lecture, a laboratory demonstration, or a reading assignment. You may encounter lectures that seem dull, speakers who are boring, and reading material that is monotonous. You can add interest to a dull lecture by learning something about the subject and the speaker, if possible, before the lecture begins. Becoming reasonably familiar with the subject and the speaker will allow you to add another dimension to the lecture and make the experience more enriching. You can think ahead about what the speaker will say, draw conclusions of your own, and compare your conclusions with the speaker's to create interest.

Working rapidly is another way to improve concentration. By this time, you probably have an idea of what your attention span is, so the objective is to maximize the effectiveness of your span. There is no basis to the adage "what is rapidly learned is quickly forgotten; what is slowly learned is long remembered." In fact, experiments have shown the reverse to be true; rapid learning results in slow forgetting, and slow learning results in rapid forgetting. Working rapidly may require that you increase your listening and reading skills as well as other mental activities.

Improving Listening Skills

Educators have given a great deal of attention to improving reading skills. Only recently, however, has adequate attention been paid to the skill of listening. The research of Ralph Nichols and Ned Flanders of the University of Minnesota exemplifies this interest in listening skills; they report that people rarely listen with near-maximum efficiency. Nichols estimates that listeners operate at about a 25% level of efficiency when listening to a 10-minute talk. He found that Americans average 100 words per minute when speaking informally to an audience. The listener, however, listens at an easy cruising speed of 400 to 500 words per minute. Nichols concludes that the difference between speech speed and thought speed operates as a tremendous pitfall; it allows for increments of time in which the mind can wander.

Educators and psychologists have suggested some ways for improving listening skills:

1. Create an interest in what is being said. You must make an effort to find a motive or reason for listening so that you get in the right frame of mind.
2. Listen without prejudice and with an open mind (Fig. 3-3). You must guard against tuning out individuals whose ideas and beliefs are not congruent with your own. There is no doubt you have had to listen to someone you thought could not possibly teach you anything worthwhile; in that situation, you probably did not listen very well. Psychologists contend that students tend to be selective about what they listen to and to whom they listen. Your perceptions of the significance of the educator have an effect on how well you listen. Master teachers such as John Dewey and Maria Montessori are not encountered every day, but many educators are worth your listening efforts. Listening with an open mind is equally important with regard to subject matter. In this area, too, students tend to be selective. Without being consciously aware of it, they pick and choose those things in a lecture or conversation that are in harmony with their beliefs; furthermore, they remember these pieces of information longer. Details that do not fit comfortably with their notions and values are screened out.
3. Make written notes. Because you cannot remember every part of a lecture and you may unwittingly tune out certain uncomfortable parts, taking notes is important. Although you can assimilate information four times faster than the average speaker can talk, note-taking is much slower; thus you should write down only the most important facts and points to serve as reminders. Review the notes later, and force your concentration to fill in the missing parts.

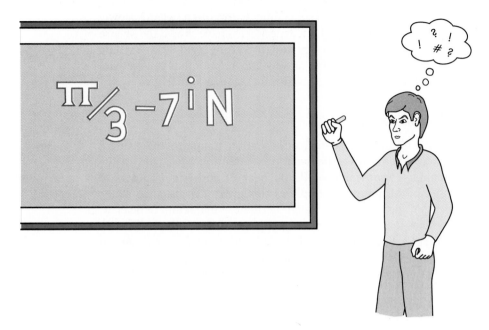

Fig. 3-3

Technical material that is new or appears too complicated requires forced concentration.

Improving Reading Skills

Improving reading skills requires far more than mere speed-reading techniques. **The efficient reader thinks, anticipates, and evaluates while reading.** Reading is a complex intellectual process with no magic formula. There are some basic principles, however, that can be used to increase your reading speed without sacrificing comprehension:

1. Quickly scan through the reading material to familiarize yourself with the organization and structure of the body of thought. By thumbing through the material, you can get a skeletal view of what the information is about and how the thoughts are developed.

2. Develop a clear idea of what you expect to learn. Ask yourself what information you expect to learn and what questions are likely to be answered. This raises your level of anticipation and increases your interest.

3. Search for the main ideas. Generally the first sentence of a paragraph gives the main thought; the sentences that follow are a further development of the idea. This is not always the case, however, so you must be aware of discontinuity in the flow of ideas.

Practice exercises may increase your concentration while reading. Many books on the market describe the mechanics of developing reading skills. Some are quite detailed and include controlling eye motion, using peripheral vision, and avoiding word-by-word reading. These techniques may be helpful, particularly for the reading of nontechnical material. When reading technical and scientific materials, the exercise that will probably be the most helpful is the practice of recall. Recall is a simple exercise performed by reading a page and then, with the page covered, trying to recall as much of the material as possible. Recall what you have read by reciting it aloud. Reciting gives you the benefit of both hearing and voicing the material, and involving the senses enhances the memory. Practice recalling the material in an organized form and searching for the meaning of the material. While reading, ask yourself these questions: What is significant about what I am reading? What have I previously learned that relates to this? In what way does it coincide with what I already know? Could it be explained in a clearer way? How would I explain it to someone else?

Keeping these questions in mind while you read technical or scientific material helps in the search for meaning. Reciting aloud is probably the best test of how well you understand the material. Continue to practice the technique until you feel confident in your progress. You are then ready to increase your reading rate to a level that is right and comfortable for you; this level is reached just before your recall begins to diminish. This exercise not only improves your reading skills, but it is also one of the best ways of increasing your memory power.

In summary, intentional memorization is a function of perception and attention. Perception is influenced by what you have stored in memory. This is your data bank. The richer your data bank, the sharper your perception—but there is more to it than that. The brain has the innate ability to organize and synthesize the stored data into a functional intellect; the intellect determines the responses you make to the situations that you encounter each day. The data that you have stored, organized, and synthesized become an intellect that is unique to you; there is none other like it, because no one else has the combination of your heredity, experiences, and knowledge. Your intellect allows you to act intuitively in problem-solving and decision-making situations.

Attention implies concentration and focusing on specifics. Improving this activity requires effort. It involves a reordering of your external environment to eliminate distractions and ridding your mind of nagging and persistent worry, and it requires a constant vigilance to keep interfering thoughts in check. Finally, it requires that you make a conscious effort to work rapidly to maximize the effectiveness of your attention span.

RETRIEVING FROM MEMORY

Psychologists make a distinction between short-term memory and long-term memory. Remembering a telephone number just long enough to dial it is an example of **short-term memory**. It is transient and fleeting, and it fades rapidly. **Long-term memory** is more permanent **memory storage** (the recording of memory facts, images, sounds, pleasure, pain, and other life experiences), and it is the subject of this discussion about **memory retrieval** (the recalling, recovering, or obtaining of events and experiences stored in memory).

Long-term memory seems to require more activity in the storing process that relates to the organization and association of information. The organizing process is not fully understood, but an analogy may help. Think of your mind as a file into which you place all previously acquired data under the appropriate subject headings. The filing of information continues with each new item placed with the associated data previously stored. In time, some of the files contain large quantities of information, and they expand and bulge with the sheer volume of items; other files may receive only a few items of information, and others may receive none. The files that increase only slightly or that do not increase at all may be displaced to make room for the more voluminous ones. Indeed, an inactive file may become lost or may at least require considerable effort to locate. Storage and retrieval in memory may be similar. This is a simplistic analogy to apply to something as complex as the human memory, but it should serve to make a point: the more facts you associate with an item of information, the more permanent the storage of the item in memory and the more accessible that item becomes. William James observed many years ago that the secret to a good memory lies in forming diverse associations with every fact to be retained. While forming an association with a fact, you are learning more and thinking more about that fact. Memory is improved by learning new facts and organizing and relating them in a systematic way.

Donald and Eleanor Laird, in their *Techniques for Efficient Remembering*, give some helpful suggestions for retrieving from memory. Their first suggestion is to *have a mental set for remembering*. This means that you intend to remember and resolve to remember information that you know will be useful.

The second suggestion is to *react actively*; that is, talk about and think about the information; make an application, if possible; and rehearse, recite, and interpret what you have learned. This activity will help fix the meaning and thus help you with remembering. The authors also state that remembering is enhanced when you react several times, for a long time, with personal interest.

The third suggestion is to *refresh* your memory. Forgetting occurs rather rapidly in spite of your best efforts to remember. Refreshing or touching up fading memory reinforces the learning process; this is particularly important with unfamiliar technical material. Returning to the material at intervals makes the strange become familiar. When studying new and difficult material, it is helpful to give the mind time to organize and assimilate the material. Later, when you return to review it, some of the strangeness will have disappeared, and you will begin to feel more comfortable with it.

The fourth—and probably most important—suggestion is to *search* for meaning. This will increase your concentration and thus aid in memorization.

FORGETTING

Understanding why you forget will help you to understand how you remember. Forgetting is frustrating when you are trying to pass a test, recall the name of an acquaintance, or solve a pressing problem. You must realize, however, that forgetting is essential to survival. Suppose you could not forget. Imagine what life would be like if all the pains of a lifetime remained fresh in your memory. Think of the mental and emotional anguish you have experienced, and add to this the physical pain of illness and trauma. Suppose none of this faded and the sharp reality of every painful experience was as vivid in your memory now as when it occurred. Nature has marvelous ways of protecting you, and forgetting is one method. This survival mechanism allows you to partially—but not entirely—forget pain. When an experience is so painful that you cannot deal with it, you bury it in memory and try to keep it from surfacing. Occasionally it will surface, but often it will be so distorted that you do not recognize it (for example, in dreams). At other times, in your waking hours, it may become more vivid and clear. The sting or cutting edge may be dulled, but the memory of the painful experience may be such that a deep and nagging depression is experienced. However, except in extreme cases, you should be able to hold the painful memories in check and function in a normal and productive way.

The inability to forget painful experiences entirely also has its positive aspects. This, too, is essential to survival. Remembering the painful consequence of touching a hot stove, jumping from an extreme height, or being hit by a moving or flying object gives direction to your action and allows you to order the safety of your environment.

The scale from pain to pleasure is a broad one. In the middle of the extremes lies a neutral ground that cannot be identified as painful or pleasant. Some experiences that are neither painful nor particularly pleasant may be interpreted as merely insignificant; this may account for the common failure to remember names, dates, places, and material you do not understand. You seldom forget the name of a significant person or the date and place of a happily anticipated event. When the pleasure-anticipation level is high, you are able to remember with no difficulty. You can even recall pleasurable experiences that happened years ago. Conversely, you tend to forget events associated with embarrassment, disappointment, or other unpleasant feelings. In effect, you will yourself to forget unpleasant experiences and to remember pleasant ones.

If it is true that you forget, by design, unpleasant things and remember pleasant things, then why do you sometimes forget what you want to remember? What you want to remember is perceived as pleasant in that it will help you pass an examination, solve a problem, or make a decision. So why does it take so much effort? Forgetting and remembering are activities far too complex to fit neatly into a pain-pleasure concept. However, taking a commonsense approach should help you identify and analyze your own pattern of remembering. This does not mean that you have to enjoy all the material you must commit to memory in order to remember it.

Experiments have shown that nonsensical material can be remembered when it is organized into a scheme or pattern. This organization is done by associating the nonsensical with something that makes sense—mentally linking an unknown to a known. This technique, which is called **mnemonics**, is an artificial memory device, but for some material it is quite helpful. If you wish to remember a series of disconnected numbers, letters, or words, you can substitute objects that you can readily visualize for the numbers and memorize rather quickly. For example, if you wish to remember 3637351, you can devise a system for assigning each number a visual object. The visual objects can be held in memory more easily than a string of numbers; thus, you are able to recall meaningless groups of numbers.

Another method for remembering a long series of numbers is to group or arrange them in segments; this is what you do when you recall telephone numbers and Social Security numbers. You can remember a long series of numbers if they are arranged in segments, and you can remember even longer ones when each segment has a meaning. For example, 17016013637351 would be quite difficult to remember as it appears; however, the number is quite easy to remember when grouped and when each group or segment has a meaning. The 14-digit number, when divided into 170-1-601-363-7351, could be a telephone number; the first four digits are the WATS line code for direct dialing, 601 is the area code, and the remainder is the individual number. When grouped this way, each segment has a specific meaning. You can invent your own associations or meanings for groups of numbers.

Rhyming also makes remembering easier, and words that are set to music are also more easily remembered. Making up sentences or phrases that give cues to items to be remembered is helpful. There is no question that artificial methods such as mnemonics help with memorization. These methods have been used for years and are widely accepted for learning certain types of material. However, it is obvious that the range of information that can be committed to memory in this manner is quite limited. For the majority of learning situations, it is best to depend on the methods of purposefully intending to remember, reacting actively with as many senses as possible, refreshing your memory often, and searching for meaning.

Errors in Remembering

Human beings have a way of altering and distorting the details of a remembered event. You seldom remember factual details of an event, a speech, or reading material. Some things are incorrectly remembered: for example, where the car is parked. You correctly remember that the car is parked in the parking garage, but you incorrectly think that it is parked on the third level, when in fact it is on the fourth level. You have noticed how the size of the fish caught by the hopeful fisherman increases with each telling or how the brawl in the beer parlor increases in drama at each recounting. Perhaps the most common example of distortion of memory is in reminiscing about the "good old days." It is not generally remembered that the "good old days" did not include refrigeration, washing machines, television, reliable automobiles, penicillin, polio vaccine, and other things that today's technology makes possible. Memory does not fade uniformly. Some parts of memory remain to hold together the general structure, but the details are often missing or altered.

There must be some motive for twisting and distorting the reality of events and experiences. Indeed, there are two well-confirmed explanations for errors in memory. One is that you distort and retouch memories to make the details more in keeping with what you wish were so; this helps you to support your beliefs, values, notions, and hopes and to defend your prejudices. The second explanation is that you add detail to your recollection of an event in a way that seems reasonable to you to complete and make sense of a sketchy or incomplete recollection; it is simply more satisfying to fill in and round out the missing details to achieve wholeness.

Inaccurate remembering cannot be eliminated altogether, but it is possible to cut down on it to some extent. The most obvious safeguard against inaccurate recall is to memorize well. Taking notes is essential for safeguarding important facts and information that must be recalled precisely. Understand your prejudices and biases as well as your hopes, dreams, and aspirations; you can then guard against wishful remembering. The most important safeguard is to understand clearly from the start so that fallacies in thinking will not occur.

The following is a list of recommended practices that will help you to optimize your memory's performance:

1. Give the cerebral cells an opportunity to rest and rejuvenate. This can be done by getting a sufficient amount of sleep and relaxation.
2. Provide the brain with sufficient nutrients to meet the requirements of the cells. Proper nutrition cannot be overemphasized. Research indicates that the brain fatigues less easily when it receives glucose derived from protein rather than from carbohydrates. Some nutritionists believe that breakfast is the most important nutritional intake of the day for mental alertness and physical stamina.
3. Schedule your study periods at a time when you are most alert and attentive.
4. Organize your environment so that distractions are reduced and attention can be focused on the material to be learned.
5. Read for meaning, and intend to memorize.

CONCLUSION

Increasing memory skills requires memorizing—even rote drilling—for many kinds of material. Most important, it requires that you purposefully will to remember. Intentional memorization involves perception (the way you see an object or interpret an event), and it involves attention that concentrates on one activity to the exclusion of others. It also involves associating one thing with another and realizing that the stronger and more vivid the association, the better the ability to remember.

Forgetting is frustrating in many instances, but the ability to partially forget is essential to your well-being, just like the ability to remember. The key is to remember what will be useful to you. This can be accomplished through a disciplined and serious effort on your part.

Review Questions

1. Rote memory is characterized by the mind's ability to do which of the following?
   a. Organize and process information
   b. Recall information as learned, word for word
   c. Recall the main concept or idea
   d. Repeat the salient parts of the information

2. Which of the following statements about perception is true?
   a. Perception is clouded when large amounts of related data are stored in memory.
   b. The perception of an event is the same for all observers.
   c. How an event is perceived is influenced by what is stored in memory.
   d. Perception of a new event is more accurate if little similar information is stored in memory.

3. Learning may be improved by which of the following?
   a. Eliminating rote memory drills
   b. Slow-paced learning
   c. Concentrating on one activity to the exclusion of others
   d. Avoiding dull reading, lectures, and laboratory activities

4. Which of the following statements about listening skills is true?
   a. We operate at about a 50% level of efficiency when listening.
   b. We speak at a rate of approximately 500 words per minute when lecturing.
   c. We listen at a rate of approximately 500 words per minute.
   d. Speech speed and thought speed are nearly equal.

5. Which of the following should you do when reading?
   a. Quickly scan the material to be read.
   b. Understand each paragraph thoroughly before going to the next.
   c. Avoid making expectations of what is to be learned.
   d. Commit the material to memory word-for-word.

6. Which of the following is not a short-term memory activity?
   a. Remembering a telephone number for dialing
   b. Remembering the gate number for boarding a plane
   c. Remembering a parking space number
   d. Organizing and associating material with other data

7. Retrieving from memory:
   a. Is a fully understood activity.
   b. Is accurate in every detail.
   c. Involves the organization and association of data.
   d. Is mainly a function of short-term memory.

8. Which of the following statements about forgetting is not correct?
   a. Forgetting occurs uniformly.
   b. Partial forgetting is essential to survival.
   c. Painful experiences are forgotten more readily than pleasurable ones.
   d. By design, we tend to forget painful events.
9. Errors in remembering are influenced by which of the following?
   a. What you wish were so
   b. Your prejudices
   c. Your values, beliefs, and hopes
   d. All the above
10. Increasing memory skills requires which of the following?
    a. Memorizing, even rote drill
    b. A purposeful will to remember
    c. Willful attention to events or activities
    d. All of the above

BIBLIOGRAPHY

Charles CM: *Educational psychology: the instructional endeavor*, ed 2, St. Louis, 1976, Mosby.

Cohen G, Kiss G, Voi LM: *Memory current issues*, ed 2, Philadelphia, 1993, Open University Press.

Coles GS: *The learning mystique, a critical look at learning disabilities*, New York, 1987, Pantheon Books.

Coury V: *Personal communication* (compiled for course supplement), Memphis, TN, 1982, University of Tennessee Center for the Health Sciences.

James W: The principles of psychology. In *The works of William James*, Cambridge, 1981, Harvard University Press.

Laird DA, Laird EC: *Techniques for efficient remembering*, New York, 1960, McGraw-Hill.

Nichols RG: Listening is good business, Bureau of Industrial Relations, School of Business Administration, The University of Michigan, Ann Arbor, Mich, Winter 1962, vol 1, no 2.

Small, G *The memory prescription: Dr. Gary Small's 14-day plan to keep your brain and body young*, 2004, Hyperion.

Tye M: *The imagery debate*, Boston, 1991, Massachusetts Institute of Technology.

Critical Thinking Skills

LaVerne Tolley Gurley

OBJECTIVES

On completion of this chapter, you should be able to:

- **Identify the qualities of a critical thinker.**
- **Identify assumptions, ethics, and values in written works.**
- **Discern fallacies in arguments.**
- **Control psychologic impediments to sound reasoning.**
- **Recognize the effects of authors' background beliefs on reasoning.**
- **Present valid facts, evidence, and statistics.**
- **Evaluate advertising claims, statistics, and rhetoric.**

It goes without saying that all health care providers must be able to make logical decisions and wise choices. The care of the patient demands that good judgment is exercised in the selection of technical factors for quality imaging and in other patient care tasks. You will be responsible for giving the physician a radiograph that is diagnostically sound and for providing safe care to the patient while performing the examination.

NEED FOR CRITICAL THINKING

As a professional, you will be making vital decisions regarding your own career. There will be choices to make regarding the route you follow in the profession to meet your own personal needs and goals.

KEY TERMS

critical thinking
emancipation
emancipatory learning
herd instinct

CHAPTER OUTLINE

Need for critical thinking
    What is critical
        thinking?
    The qualities of a
        critical thinker
Factors that hinder critical
    thinking
    Background beliefs
    Faulty reasoning
    Group loyalty
    Frozen mind-set
    Emotional baggage
Becoming a critical
    thinker
    Humility
    Respect for others
    Self-awareness
    Honing your skills
Conclusion

What is Critical Thinking?

Many definitions have been given for **critical thinking**. One definition calls it emancipatory learning. **Emancipation** means freedom from restraint or influence. Things that restrain or influence people can be personal, institutional, or environmental. Personal beliefs, the rules and regulations of institutions, and physical environments can all work to prevent people from seeing new directions and gaining understanding and control of their own lives and of the world around them. **Emancipatory learning** means that learners become aware of the forces that have created the circumstances of their lives and take action to change them.

Another definition focuses on the use of morality and virtues, making wise judgments about aspects of one's life, and recognizing the impact these judgments will have on others. Some stress the importance of recognizing reality in the context of cultural elements and the process of trying to create order in a changing world.

Creating order in a changing world will be a challenge for us all. Never in the history of humankind have changes occurred with such rapidity. There is global information and communication exchange, worldwide exchange of goods and services, and most importantly, an exchange of ideas. Geographic boundaries are becoming blurred, as are the cultures and traditions of separate groups. Learning how to live and work in this changing world makes critical thinking more important than ever.

Although the wording of the definitions of critical thinking may differ, they are all made on the assumption that a set of values exists. They assume that these values are universal; for example, life is better than death, wellness is better than illness, happiness is better than sadness, pleasure is better than pain, and hope is better than despair. Therefore, when we speak of making wise judgments we have to agree on a set of values. These values are not unique to a specific culture or religion, nor are they characteristic of a specific nation or state. These are universal except in rare aberrations of individuals, cult groups, and other deviants.

It is fair to assume you have accepted these values because you have chosen to be a health care provider. We may disagree on the specifics of behaviors that will best accomplish the preservation of these values, but if we disagree on the values, there is no need for further discussion. When we speak of making wise decisions, we are judging decisions made within the framework of a value system that is universally understood. It is equated with logical reasoning abilities and reflective judgment.

The Qualities of a Critical Thinker

Critical thinkers are valued for their ability to look at a situation from a variety of perspectives. They are able to discern the best possible way to react to a situation, making them ideally suited for work in the health care profession. Box 4-1 summarizes the characteristics that a critical thinker needs to possess.

BOX 4-1 DESCRIPTION OF A CRITICAL THINKER

Humane
Analytical
Rational
Open-minded
Systematic
Inquisitive

One of the first traits that one observes in critical thinkers is the presence of heart as well as mind. The definitions regarding critical thinking are reflective of humane values and thus can be expected of critical thinkers. Such a thinker will be able to balance compassion with realism.

The critical thinker must also be analytical. This means finding evidence in unclear and confusing situations. Being alert to the consequences of accepting a course of action and being able to defend that position is very important. Rushing into a plan without examining the ramifications of that action can be very dangerous.

Rational thinkers recognize reality; they can discern what is factual and true from what is opinion or misinformation. Seeking truth and making every effort to be honest with yourself is an important characteristic. To do this, we must recognize the difference between what is true and what we wish were true. This is more difficult than it appears on the surface. It is simple enough to recognize the laws of physics or mathematics as factual. It's when the discussions involve government, religion, evolution, or other similar topics that facts become blurred and clouded with emotion. The truth is often elusive, and the evidence is less convincing. Nonetheless, critical thinkers will seek to make rational judgments and act responsibly.

Open-mindedness is an important quality and necessary in the field of patient care. Disagreements are not uncommon, but a heated confrontation can be diffused by the willingness of the critical thinker to listen and understand. This is especially important in dealing with patients. Making an attempt to understand a patient's point of view will leave him feeling more secure that his health care provider actually cares about him. Dealing with diversity while remaining true to one's values is often complicated, but patience and compromise can lead to a solution.

Patience and organization allow a person time to gather evidence, test ideas, and systematically work through tough problems and complex questions. Rash judgments are less likely to be made when there is time to internalize or ponder the question. During this time, ideas can be tested so that a logical and just decision can be made or appropriate action taken. The critical thinker will resist the desire to reach a solution before all the facts are in.

An inquisitive nature will lead a person to seek knowledge from many sources. This is a quality found in all effective learners. The need to learn, to gather information, and to use that information wisely is a sign of growth and maturity.

In light of the qualities of a critical thinker mentioned above, it becomes obvious that becoming a critical thinker is a process. Unlike a characteristic you are born with, critical thinking is developed throughout life by the experiences you encounter.

FACTORS THAT HINDER CRITICAL THINKING

Background Beliefs

Religious training, attitudes of society, cultural traditions, and the teachings of our parents and schoolteachers form our background beliefs. These beliefs are the stabilizing forces that guide us and the glue that holds our society together. Often, they are the most deeply ingrained beliefs and thus the most intensely defended. There are times, however, when they may be challenged by a conflicting value. If a doctor must choose between performing an abortion to save a mother's life and defending his religious convictions that forbid it, to which does his obligation belong? Although there is usually no clear-cut answer to this question or others like it, examining one's views and beliefs while keeping in mind the reality of the situation enables the critical thinker to choose the right solution.

Faulty Reasoning

Faulty reasoning occurs when biased or false information is stated as fact. This is the aim of advertising. Often, celebrities and famous athletes are used as spokespeople for a certain product or service. The logic here is that endorsement by a public figure will lend credibility to the advertiser's claims that the product is the best. In this case, the ultimate goal is persuading you to buy the product.

If your only evidence of the worth of the information is because of an "authority" endorsement, it is time to examine the information more critically. Even statistics can be used to persuade. We reason that statistics are accurate and unquestionable. But the interpretation of the statistics may be faulty. Statistics must be examined from several aspects, like sample size, evidence of bias, nature of the information, and even how recently the information was gathered. Some statistics, such as those regarding spousal abuse or rape, are by their very nature hard to obtain, since most go unreported. Statistics are also used to predict the future, with the assumption that what happened in the past will be repeated in the future. This assumption may or may not be true. Although some statistics may be suspect, we should not dismiss using them altogether, but it does mean we must critically examine them and understand their limitations.

Group Loyalty

There is a natural cohesiveness in a social group called the **herd instinct**. In such groups, there is a desire to gain status within the group. Generally, all members follow a predetermined set of acceptable behaviors. Success in everyday life depends to a great extent on being accepted by your social group, a concept that is learned early in life. It is this instinct that keeps us loyal to the group, and so we tend to behave in ways that will enhance our status and make us feel comfortable with the group. At a more primitive level, instinct makes us aware that our survival depends on the survival of the group. It is natural to believe what others in the group believe and defend these beliefs without examining or testing them.

For the most part, loyalty is beneficial to the preservation of the group, but when horrifying acts are committed by mobs or street gangs, loyalty becomes disastrous. In recognizing the natural tendency to group loyalty, we must also realize that this tends to make us see everything in terms of our own social group. This may hinder our ability to make just and logical decisions. Unfortunately, creative ideas can be stifled in this environment.

Frozen Mind-Set

Individuals with frozen minds reach frozen solutions. This argument is centered in maintaining the status quo. This they find comfortable because they think, oftentimes rightly so, that they have the consensus and support of the group. Early in childhood, we learn to go along with the group and base our actions on group approval. This is so deeply ingrained in some people that no amount of evidence will change their minds. It takes courage to recognize this within yourself, and it takes discipline to weigh the evidence and create a better solution.

Emotional Baggage

Almost everyone has issues they feel strongly about and will defend vigorously. Emotions run high in the discussions of these issues, and sometimes logic is abandoned. The key to keeping your emotions in check is to identify the issues that cause you discomfort or ire when discussions run counter to your opinion. Some issues that many have emotional ties to are abortion, gun control, the death penalty, censorship—the list goes on and on.

When you have identified the issue that causes you anger or discomfort, it helps to seek out information on both sides of the argument. Learn why those whose position runs counter to yours feel the way they do and on what basis their opinions rest. Make an effort to talk to people whose opinions differ from yours, and read articles on the subject in newspapers and magazines. Understanding both sides of an issue will help sharpen your skills in critical thinking. This in no way means that you should change your opinions to conform to the views of others, but it does mean that you can more calmly weigh the evidence so that logic, rather than emotion, determines your actions.

BECOMING A CRITICAL THINKER

Humility

The first step in becoming a critical thinker is to take a humble approach and be open to learning. It is acceptable, even admirable, to admit that you are not sure or that you need more information. You are living at a time when people are pressured to give quick answers; to examine or consider other points of view is often criticized. Short, quick answers are easy to come by when speaking of things that are certain, such as a mathematical answer. For example, you do not need to seek other points of view to determine that the square root of 144 is 12. Such a factual answer leaves no element of doubt. Answers to other questions are more difficult because of uncertainty or the presence of doubt. In cases in which there is a widely held consensus in your group, it is difficult to give up your belief and accept another view. One example of this is the common belief that more money spent on education will result in higher test scores and, therefore, a better education. Reflecting on this reveals two beliefs that need to be further examined. First, we should question whether money alone is the answer, or if how it is used makes a difference. Second, we should examine the belief that higher scores mean better education. Could higher scores merely be the result of lowering the level of difficulty of the examinations? These two examples, one of certainty, and the other of widely held beliefs, make it necessary to distinguish truths and certainties from beliefs and opinions.

Respect for Others

Another stage in becoming a critical thinker is learning to respect the opinions of others. To live peacefully in a diverse society, we must be tolerant of many different cultures and traditions. Just as there has been a blurring of geographic lines, there is also a blurring of cultural and traditional lines. At times this creates a dilemma because tradition is mingled with religion and is a part of every civilized society. It is at this point that logic and wisdom will be needed.

Self-Awareness

Recognize the things that make you glad, the things that make you sad, and the things that make you mad. Although this is a simplistic way of examining your personality, it is a start. As you grow and develop in your critical thinking ability, the issues that bring forth an emotional response will become more evident, and you will be able to deal with them more effectively. When you are aware of your own standards and ethical values, you can make objective decisions and act responsibly.

Honing Your Skills

It takes practice to become proficient in activities such as sports, music, and dance. Practice also helps to develop your skills in critical thinking. As issues arise, consciously and deliberately look at them from several points of view, and weigh the evidence on the most reliable and convincing basis. This will enable you to resist making instant judgments and taking rash action.

CONCLUSION

Critical thinking is a term used to describe thinking based on a universal value system. Characteristics of critical thinkers are compassion, patience, respect for others' opinions, open-mindedness, and the ability to be analytical. As a health care provider, you will be confronted with many issues requiring logical judgment and rational action. Critical thinkers will be aware of their values and know the reason and consequences of the action taken.

Review Questions

1. The need for critical thinking exists for:
   a. Only supervisors and managers in radiology
   b. All who work in radiology
   c. Only the radiologic technician
   d. None of the above
2. Critical thinking means:
   a. Holding firm to one's traditions
   b. Loyalty to your social group
   c. Loyalty to your country
   d. Thinking logically and wisely
3. Critical thinking requires that you:
   a. Accept the opinions of others in your group
   b. Convince others of your beliefs
   c. Weigh the evidence without bias
   d. Cite statistics to support your beliefs
4. Effective thinking and acting is:
   a. A quality one is born with
   b. A characteristic of specific cultures
   c. Learned from one's parents
   d. A learned process developed over time
5. Statistics are useful in decision making when:
   a. The conclusion agrees with your beliefs
   b. They have been examined and found valid

   c. The research is adequately funded

   d. The funding agency is respectable

6. A desirable trait in critical thinking is:

   a. Inquisitiveness

   b. Loyalty

   c. Self-admiration

   d. Narrow-mindedness

7. Group loyalty is:

   a. Always destructive

   b. Always beneficial

   c. A natural tendency

   d. Easy to deviate from

8. Background beliefs:

   a. Must be defended at all costs

   b. Are usually the most intensely defended

   c. Can easily be cast aside

   d. Never conflict with other values

9. When having a disagreement with another person, a critical thinker will:

   a. Never abandon her position

   b. Try to convince the other person to see her point

   c. Listen to the other person to understand the basis of his argument

   d. Let her emotions cloud her reasoning ability

10. Critical thinkers:

   a. Are persuaded by advertising claims

   b. Recognize that an endorsement by a famous figure is a measure of credibility

   c. Evaluate advertising claims in order to reach the truth

   d. Are persuaded by statistics that are biased

BIBLIOGRAPHY

Coles R: *The moral intelligence of children*, New York, 1997, Random House.

Diestler S: *Becoming a critical thinker: a user friendly manual*, ed 3, New York, 2001, Prentice Hall.

Ellis D: *Becoming a master student*, ed 9, Boston, 2000, Houghton Mifflin.

Kahne H, Cavender N: *Logic and contemporary rhetoric*, ed 8, Belmont, CA, 1998, Wadsworth.

Ormrod JE: *Human learning*, ed 3, New York, Prentice Hall, 1999.

The History of Medicine

William J. Callaway

OBJECTIVES

On completion of this chapter, you should be able to:

- List the main contributions to medicine from ancient Egypt, India, China, and Greece.
- Describe the medical practice of the ancient Hebrews.
- Outline the teachings of Hippocrates.
- Describe the impact of Christianity on medicine.
- List events during the Renaissance that were significant in the progress of medicine.
- Describe important advances in medicine from the eighteenth and nineteenth centuries.
- List the significant developments in medicine during the twentieth century.
- Indicate trends in medicine for the twenty-first century.
- Describe the major issues in medicine at the present time.
- Define disease.
- List the top 15 causes of death in the United States.
- Compare mortality rates among various groups.
- List the primary disabling conditions present in U.S. society.
- List diseases that have been eradicated or targeted for elimination.
- Explain the significance of emerging infectious diseases.

KEY TERMS

disease
emerging infectious
   diseases
epidemic
health
morbidity
mortality
pandemic

CHAPTER OUTLINE

Prehistoric and ancient
   medicine
Ancient Egypt
Ancient India
Ancient China
Ancient Greece
   Pre-hippocratic
      medicine
   Hippocrates
Christianity
The Renaissance
The eighteenth century
The nineteenth century
The twentieth century
The twenty-first century
Health and disease
   Mortality
   Morbidity
   Life expectancy
   Emerging infectious
      diseases
Conclusion

PREHISTORIC AND ANCIENT MEDICINE

The history of medicine abounds with tales of cooperation and confrontation with nature. Disease was present on earth long before human life, and we can only speculate about the human practice of prehistoric medicine. Fractures were probably common injuries. Egyptian mummies and radiographic images of the "ice man" show characteristics of arteriosclerosis, pneumonia, urinary infections, stones, parasites, cavities, teeth erosion, abscesses, pyorrhea, arthritis, and tubercular disease of the spine. Prehistoric people probably treated their wounds similarly to the way animals treat themselves: by immersing themselves in cool water and applying mud to irritated areas, sucking stings, licking wounds, and exerting pressure on wounds to stop the bleeding.

Until well into the nineteenth century, medical treatment was intertwined with religion and magic (Fig. 5-1). Some cultures treated their sick, elderly, and disabled with kindness. Other cultures, during times of famine, sent the elders out into the unsheltered environment; some even killed and ate disabled tribe members. Disease was thought to be caused by gods and spirits, and magic was used to drive away evil forces. Tribal healers held high political and social positions and were responsible for performing religious ceremonies and protecting the tribe from bad weather, poor harvest, and catastrophe. Along with sucking, cupping, bleeding, fumigating, and steam baths, medicinal herbs were used to treat wounds. Surgery was used to treat bone fractures and to sew up wounds. The Mesopotamians studied hepatoscopy, which is the detailed examination of the liver. They believed the liver was the seat of life and the collecting point of blood. Even though gods and magic still played an

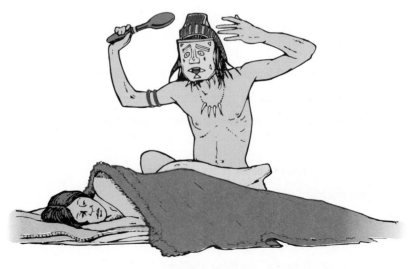

Fig. 5-1

Magic and religion played an important role in medicine well into the nineteenth century.

important role in medicine, rational thought about nature's relationship to health began to increase.

The ancient Hebrews still considered disease to be divine punishment and a mark of sin. Plagues and epidemics such as leprosy were often mentioned in the Bible, and so were medications such as balsams, gums, spices, oils, and narcotics. Surgery was performed only under ritual circumstances.

Hebrew medicine was influenced by the Greeks around the fourth century BC with an emphasis placed on anatomy and physiology, diet, massage, and drugs. Disease was considered an imbalance of the four humors of the body: phlegm, blood, yellow bile, and black bile.

ANCIENT EGYPT

The deities of ancient Egypt were associated with health, illness, and death. Isis was the healing goddess; Hathor was the mistress of heaven and the protector of women during childbirth; Keket ensured fertility.

The embalming practices of the Egyptians have provided much of our knowledge of ancient medicine. The most elaborate embalmings required that the liver, lungs, stomach, and intestines be preserved in stone jars so that they could function for eternity. Cranial contents were removed with hooks through the nostrils. The skull and abdominal cavities were washed with spices; soaked for 70 days in a solution of clay and salts of carbonate, sulfate, and chloride; and then washed. The corpse was then coated with gums and wrapped in fine linen.

The ancient Egyptians linked anatomy and physiology with theology—each body part had a special deity as its protector. They believed that the body was composed of a system of channels, with the heart at the center. They thought air came in through the ears and nose, entered the channels, went to the heart, and was then delivered to the rest of the body. They believed the channels also carried blood, urine, feces, tears, and sperm.

Even though the main water source, the Nile River, was probably clean in ancient Egypt, public health was also a concern. Egyptian homes were immaculate, and personal hygiene was practiced regularly. The prevalent diseases included intestinal ailments, malaria, trachoma, night blindness, cataracts, arteriosclerosis, and epidemic diseases. Diagnoses were made by probing wounds with fingers, taking the pulse, and studying sputum, urine, and feces. Religious rituals were still part of the healing process, and so were drugs administered in the forms of pills, cake suppositories, enemas, ointments, drops, gargles, fumigations, and baths. Drugs were made from vegetable, mineral, and animal substances and imported materials such as saffron, cinnamon, perfumes, spices, sandalwood, gums, and antimony.

ANCIENT INDIA

The ancient Indians believed (as do many contemporary Indians) that life was an eternal cycle of creation, preservation, and destruction. Their

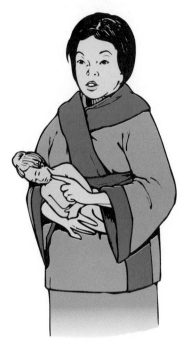

Fig. 5-2

For reasons of modesty, women in ancient China used figurines to indicate the location of their symptoms.

religion allowed secular medicine and sound, rational health care practices, which is remarkable in light of their emphasis on the spiritual over the material. They detected diabetes by the sweetness of the patient's urine and treated snakebites by applying tourniquets. Surgery was a common procedure on the nose, the earlobes, harelips, and hernias; it was also used to remove bladder stones and perform amputations. The Indians also performed cesarean sections.

ANCIENT CHINA

In ancient China, harmony was considered to be a delicate balance between yin and yang, and Tao was considered "the way." Illness was seen as a result of disregard for Tao or acting contrary to natural laws. Chinese medicine focused on the prevention of disease (Fig. 5-2). Because Confucius forbade any violation of the body, dissections were not performed in China until the eighteenth century. According to Nei Ching, there were five methods of treatment: cure the spirit; nourish the body; give medications; treat the whole body; and use acupuncture and moxibustion, which is a treatment similar to acupuncture in which a powdered plant is burned on the skin. Treatment came in the forms of exercise, physical therapy, massage, and administering medicinal herbs, trees, insects, stones, and grains. By the eleventh century, the Chinese had developed an inoculation against smallpox.

ANCIENT GREECE

In the sixth century BC, the Greeks built the healing temples of Asclepios in Thessaly. The temples contained a statue of a god to whom gifts were often given as a sign of worship. There was usually a round building, the tholos, which encircled a pool or sacred spring of water for purification. The abaton was a building considered to be an incubation site, where the cure took place. The patient went to sleep there until visited and cured by the god. The temples usually consisted of a theater, a stadium, a gymnasium, inns, and temporary housing. Healing rituals began after sundown and often involved fasting or abstinence from certain foods or wine.

Pre-Hippocratic Medicine

The ancient Greeks began applying scientific thought to medical theory very early. Thales (625 to 547 BC) professed that the basic element in all animal and plant life was water, from which came the earth and air. Anaximander (610 to 547 BC) believed that all living creatures originated in water. Anaximenes, born in 546 BC, believed that air was the element necessary for life. Heraclitus (540 to 480 BC) believed that fire was the principal element of life. By the sixth century BC, earth, air, fire, and water were accepted as the basic components of life on earth.

Hippocrates

During the sixth, fifth, and fourth centuries BC, the Greeks advanced medicine with their understanding of the place of humanity within the cosmos. Pythagoras, Empedocles, and Democritus approached harmony with the universe in an objective, scientific manner. Mathematics, atomic theory, and the basic elements of nature were used to describe health and disease.

During this period, Hippocrates established himself as the "father of medicine." His approach revolutionized medicine from the ancient past and began turning it into an objective science. Born around 460 BC, Hippocrates believed that people practicing medicine should be pure and holy. He taught that one should (1) observe all, (2) study the patient rather than the disease, (3) evaluate honestly, and (4) assist nature.

"He employed few drugs and relied largely upon the healing powers of nature. . . . The treatment of disease for him was to assist and, above all, not to hinder nature. If succeeding generations had followed his precepts, patients would have been spared countless unnecessary operations and an enormous number of nauseous, disgusting, ineffectual and frequently harmful medicines" (Major, 1954).

Hippocrates' writings addressed mental illness, anxiety, and depression. His teachings reached a peak in Alexandria and then eventually penetrated the Roman Empire.

CHRISTIANITY

The dawn of Christianity changed many attitudes about medicine. Christians sought to bring the "healing message of Christ" to those in need. The Church dominated medicine during the Dark Ages, and practices involved prayer, exorcism, holy oil, relics of saints, supernaturalism, and superstition. At the same time, medical schools separate from the Church were established and soon became part of major universities.

During Jesus' personal ministry and that of his immediate followers, "healing" was not differentiated into physical, mental, or spiritual categories. The author of one of the Gospels was known as Luke the Physician. The content of the Christian faith, with its emphasis on compassion, forgiveness, and concern for the unfortunate and the dispossessed, led the followers of Christianity to provide facilities for the care of the orphaned, the elderly, the outcast, and the poor.

The Roman Emperor Constantine founded a hospital in the fourth century. Others were established by Christian communities in Caesarea, Edessa, and Bethlehem within the same century.

With the Crusades came the distribution of disease. In the twelfth century AD, Europe was inundated with leprosy, typhus, and smallpox. In 1347, bubonic plague spread through Europe and claimed nearly one fourth of its population.

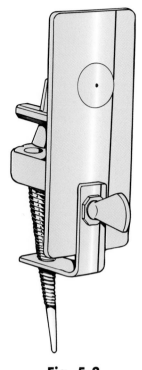

Fig. 5-3

An illustration of Leeuwenhoek's first microscope.

THE RENAISSANCE

The Renaissance brought new beginnings in medicine. Paracelsus, the "father of pharmacology," combined alchemy with the treatment of disease to produce a new science. Jean Fernel professed that physiology, pathology, and therapeutics were the standard disciplines of medicine; he was also the first to suggest that gonorrhea and syphilis were two separate diseases. Ambroise Pare was a forerunner in clinical surgery. An explosion of knowledge of human anatomy was led by Andreas Versallus; his dissections and drawings prompted his designation as the "father of anatomy."

The seventeenth century was an age of scientific revolution. Latrochemistry, a combination of alchemy, medicine, and chemistry, was practiced by followers of Paracelsus. Jan Baptisa van Helmont made the first measurement of the relative weight of urine by comparing its weight with that of water. Galileo presented the laws of motion in a mathematical manner that could be applied to life on earth; Isaac Newton discovered gravity. William Harvey found that there is a continuous circulation of blood in a contained body system. Christian Huygens developed the centigrade system of measuring temperature; Gabriel Daniel Fahrenheit developed the system named after him for measuring temperature. Marcello Malpighi and Anton van Leeuwenhoek were forerunners in the invention of the microscope (Fig. 5-3). Quinine was discovered as a treatment for malaria. Leonardo da Vinci explored human anatomy through dissection; his anatomic sketches disseminated his findings.

THE EIGHTEENTH CENTURY

Significant discoveries continued into the eighteenth century. Albrecht von Haller did in-depth studies of the nervous system, discovered the relationship of the brain cortex to peripheral nerves, and became the founder of modern physiologic theory. Lazzaro Spallanzani discarded the theory of spontaneous generation and became a pioneer in experimental fertilization. Stephen Hales demonstrated the dynamics of blood circulation, stressed the importance of the capillary system, and became the first person to record blood pressure with a manometer.

The "father of pathology," Giovanni Battista Morgagni, correlated anatomy with pathology. His research and writings laid the foundation for much of modern pathology.

Edward Jenner formulated the smallpox vaccination, which was considered one of the greatest discoveries in medical history. William Hunter, a specialist in obstetrics, founded the Great Windmill Street School of Anatomy, the first medical school in London. His brother, John Hunter, was a giant of the eighteenth century. An experimental surgeon, John Hunter developed a method of closing off aneurysms, thus eliminating many unnecessary amputations. Hunter turned surgery into a respected science and became a pioneer in comparative anatomy.

The eighteenth century also saw dramatic changes in the care and treatment of mentally ill patients, with Phillipe Pinel demanding that a more humane regimen be instilled at Bicetre Asylum near Paris.

THE NINETEENTH CENTURY

Autopsies were the major focus of medicine during the nineteenth century. Carl Rokitansky was the most outstanding morphologic pathologist of his time. Rudolf Virchow professed that "all cells come from other cells" and revolutionized the understanding of cells. Claude Bernard was the founder of experimental physiology and discovered the principle of homeostasis, clarified the multiple functions of the liver, studied the digestive activities of the pancreas, and was the first to link the pancreas with diabetes; he pioneered and established the specialty of internal medicine.

Rene-Theophile Hyacinthe Lainnec contributed to the pathologic and clinical understanding of chest diseases including emphysema, bronchiectasis, and tuberculosis; he was also a pioneer in the invention and use of the stethoscope.

Surgery advanced in Paris during the French Revolution and Napoleonic wars. Ephraim McDowell performed the first successful abdominal operation to remove a huge cyst from an ovary. J. Marion Sims laid the foundation for gynecology and founded the Women's Hospital of the State of New York, the first institution of its kind; he also invented the Sims' position and later the speculum and the catheter.

By 1831, ether, nitrous oxide gas, and chloroform had been discovered but not yet applied to medical practice. After Joseph Priestley had discovered nitrous oxide gas, Humphry Davy suggested that it be used in surgery, but he was ignored. Although Crawford W. Long used sulfuric ether during surgery in 1842, he did not publicize its use. When anesthesia finally entered the world of surgery, surgical procedures multiplied in number and complexity. Joseph Lister discovered that bacteria were often the origin of disease and infection; thus safe surgical procedures were introduced to minimize the risks of surgery. Louis Pasteur discovered that the decay of food could be forestalled by heating the food and destroying harmful bacteria; he formulated the germ theory of disease and explained the effectiveness of asepsis and antisepsis.

Robert Koch performed extensive research into microorganisms and founded bacteriology. Psychiatry gained considerable respect from the work of Benjamin Rush, the first American psychiatrist. Based on his involved clinical studies of the human gastrointestinal tract, William Beaumont became the first prominent American physiologist. The foundation of modern genetics was laid by Gregor Mendel in 1886 with his experiments involving the heredity of plants.

November 8, 1895, forever changed the course of diagnosis of disease and injury. As will be explained more fully in Chapter 6, Wilhelm Roentgen discovered and described x-rays. Within months, the significance of these "new kind of rays" in medicine was realized. Pierre and Marie

Curie discovered radium 3 years later and provided the foundation for the use of radioactivity in the treatment of diseases.

Incredible as the discoveries of the previous centuries were, the twentieth century took medicine far beyond the dreams of the heartiest optimists of the past.

The twentieth century

Remarkable developments continued as the century turned, and they built upon previous achievements. Major Walter Reed led a U.S. Army board in discovering the cause of yellow fever, and this led to its eradication. Paul Ehrlich became the father of chemotherapy, which would have ramifications throughout the century. Pavlov conducted extensive research not only about the conditioned response but also about the process of digestion.

In 1913, Abel, Rowntree, and Turner invented the first artificial kidney, and this led to kidney dialysis. World War I provided the opportunity to explore wound infection in detail and advanced the prevention of surgical infections. Willem Einthoven made the first electrocardiogram, and Hans Burger used similar technology to invent the electroencephalogram. Lind, Eijkman, Hopkins, Zent-Gyorgyi, and Funk defined and isolated vitamins and described their role in the life process; this would have a profound effect on diet and, late in the century, on the possible prevention and treatment of chronic diseases.

Surgical techniques were refined, and diagnostic procedures became more accurate. The invention of the electron microscope in 1930 (Fig. 5-4) made possible the study of viruses and advances in the fields of biochemistry, biophysics, physical chemistry, and immunology.

The Salk vaccine virtually eliminated the scourge of polio. Watson and Crick won a Nobel Prize in 1962 for accurately describing the DNA molecule as a double helix and identifying its components. In 1967, Christiaan Barnard performed the first successful human heart transplant. In the ensuing years, other organs were successfully transplanted, adding another valuable tool to improving and saving lives.

Microminiaturization invented for space travel soon found its way into medicine. Coupled with evolving computer technology, the final four decades of the century vastly extended our abilities to diagnose and treat an entire array of medical conditions. Such electronics are used to monitor heart and brain activity with extreme accuracy. The marriage of computers and imaging equipment has provided digital radiography, computed tomography, and magnetic resonance imaging, and it has enhanced nuclear medicine and medical sonography. Treatment planning for radiation therapy is incredibly precise because of the use of computers.

Major organ transplants involving the heart, liver, lungs, and kidneys are performed today. Coronary bypass surgery is commonplace. Arthroscopic surgery works in the joint spaces of the body without major incisions. Laparoscopic surgery became commonplace for incisions into the abdomen for conditions affecting the gallbladder, kidneys, adrenal glands, and female reproductive system. Lithotripsy allows the

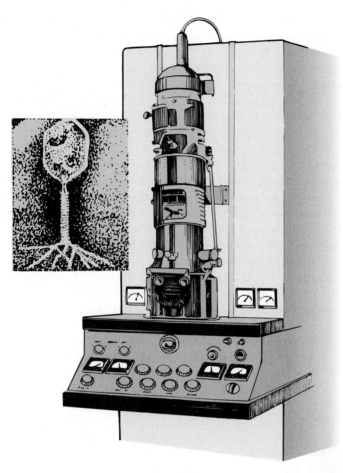

Fig. 5-4

The electron microscope has made possible the study of viruses, which cannot be seen with other microscopes.

painless passing of stones from the urinary system by first blasting them with sonic waves. Lasers are used routinely in countless procedures as a clean, painless way of removing growths; their accuracy allows their use in areas of the body where precision is indispensable.

Artificial hips and knees are inserted to replace those that are degenerating as a result of age or arthritis or that have been destroyed by injury. Plastic surgery allows the reconstruction of most areas of the body that have been disfigured as a result of disease or injury; it is also used extensively for elective cosmetic procedures.

THE TWENTY-FIRST CENTURY

The second millennium AD continues with a rapid expansion of technology and information. The accumulation of knowledge accelerates at an unprecedented pace, doubling every 15 to 18 months. Balancing this technologic explosion in medicine, a trend has emerged toward a more personal aspect of health care. The need for the human touch, caring, and concern has never been more important. More personal aspects of care such as the hospice movement for the terminally ill and the reemergence of family practice as a specialty are but a couple of examples (Fig. 5-5). As you begin your studies in this intriguing profession, keep in mind that the human aspect of patient care and quality service must be ever present in your practice.

Research into genetics has greatly expanded our knowledge about heredity. The entire DNA code has now been deciphered, and this has opened a new era in the treatment and prevention of disease. The unfortunate affliction of Alzheimer's disease has prompted extensive research; its cause remains elusive, and treatment is still in its infancy. Prevention and treatment of HIV infection and AIDS have increased in importance as the condition has become global.

Biotechnology has opened frontiers in treatment that were unimagined when this text was first published. Increasing numbers of surgeries and other interventional procedures are being made obsolete by the introduction of biotechnology into mainstream health care. Robotic surgery permits more precise incisions and excisions than ever before possible. Carefully guided by three-dimensional video, the surgeon probes

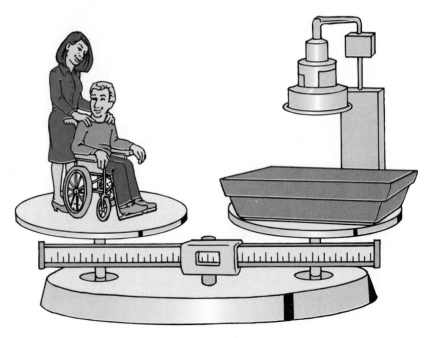

Fig. 5-5

Although technologic advances in radiography have been monumental, human-driven care is equally important in delivering the highest quality of care possible.

deep into the body with a small computer-assisted "hand." Robotic surgery is leading the way to improved patient outcomes when compared with open and even laparoscopic surgery. Advantages of robotic surgery include less blood loss, faster recovery for the patient, and fewer overall complications. It may be used for heart surgery, urinary system procedures, and prostate surgery.

The electrical conduction system of the heart has now been mapped. Patients suffering from tachycardia or atrial fibrillation benefit from ablation procedures that use radiofrequency catheters to burn away errant pathways and permanently restore normal heart rate and rhythm.

The International Space Station is staffed full time and, as a result, new and ongoing research is taking place in the fields of human physiology and pharmacology that will have extensive applications back on Earth.

HEALTH AND DISEASE

Before moving on to discussing morbidity and mortality, it would be wise to consider the definitions of health and disease. The World Health Organization defines **health** as "a state of complete physical, mental, and social well-being, and not merely the absence of disease or infirmity." Sheldon defines **disease** as "the pattern of response of a living organism to some form of injury"; he goes on to explain that disease "should be viewed as disordered function rather than only as altered structure."

Because measuring health status is a time-consuming, complicated, and often subjective process, we have continued to rely on data that indicate rates of **mortality** (death rate) and **morbidity** (occurrence of disease or conditions). It is apparent that Americans live longer and have fewer acute episodes of illness than ever before, but we also have more chronic conditions than ever. Our population is afflicted with arthritis, chronic respiratory diseases, heart and circulatory problems, cancer, allergies, chronic digestive disorders, and alcohol and drug abuse.

Before moving on in this chapter, it must be noted that, at best, statistics are but a snapshot of a moment in time. While all data in this chapter are accurate as of the date of publication, it is up to you, the radiography student, to remain current in your knowledge of health statistics by frequently visiting the websites listed on the following page.

Mortality

Early in the twenty-first century, mortality statistics reveal much about life and death in the United States. The Centers for Disease Control and Prevention (CDC), through its National Center for Health Statistics (NCHS), gathers and publishes such data. The mission of the CDC is to promote health and quality of life by preventing and controlling disease, injury, and disability. The primary sources of health statistics are the following websites:

Centers for Disease Control and Prevention: www.cdc.gov

Centers for Disease Control and Prevention National Center for Health Statistics: www.cdc.gov\nchs

The 15 leading causes of death in the United States, including all races, both genders, and all ages are as follows:

1. Cancer
2. Heart disease
3. Cerebrovascular diseases (stroke)
4. Chronic lower respiratory diseases
5. Accidents (unintentional injuries, including motor vehicle fatalities)
6. Diabetes mellitus
7. Influenza and pneumonia
8. Alzheimer's disease
9. Nephritis (kidney diseases)
10. Septicemia (blood infection)
11. Suicide
12. Chronic liver disease and cirrhosis
13. Hypertension (high blood pressure)
14. Parkinson's disease
15. Pneumonitis (inflammation of the lungs)

Causes of death vary by age group, race, gender, and socioeconomic status.* Key points from National Center for Health Statistics data include:

General Population:

ages 1 to 44 – the leading cause of death is accidents

ages 45 to 64 – the leading cause of death is cancer

ages over 65 years – the leading cause of death is heart disease

cancer and heart disease account for more than half of all deaths in the United States

declines in death from:
    cancer
    heart disease
    stroke
    suicide
    influenza/pneumonia
    chronic liver disease and cirrhosis
    accidents
    firearms
    HIV
    alcohol
    drugs

increases in death from:
    Alzheimer's disease
    kidney disease

---

*The Centers for Disease Control and Prevention use the following terms to describe the three major population groups in the United States: white, black, Hispanic-origin. The terms Caucasian and African American are not used.

hypertension

Parkinson's disease

HIV mortality has declined by more than 70% since 1995

HIV no longer ranks among the top 15 causes of death in the United States

homicide no longer ranks among the top 15 causes of death in the United States

among all women, the number of annual deaths from breast cancer is over 40,000

maternal mortality (death from complications of pregnancy, childbirth, and the postpartum period) is nearly 8 deaths per 100,000 live births

maternal mortality among black women is four times higher than among white women

among all men, the number of annual deaths from prostate cancer is over 30,000

mortality rates are higher for men for each of the fifteen leading causes of death

autopsies are performed after approximately 10% of deaths

most autopsies are performed for traumatic causes: homicide, suicide, accidents

the highest percentages of autopsies performed for nontraumatic causes of death are for infant mortality and chronic liver disease and cirrhosis

Blacks:

have higher death rates from hypertension and homicide

have lower death rates from lung disease, suicide, and Alzheimer's disease

Hispanics:

leading causes of death are homicide, chronic liver disease, and perinatal conditions

have lower death rates from heart disease and cancer

have higher death rates from homicide in age groups 15 to 24 years and 45 to 64 years

rate of death from HIV infection is higher between the ages of 1 and 64 years

rate of death from diabetes mellitus, chronic liver disease, and cirrhosis ranked higher for the population that is 45 years old and older.

Specific causes of death:

Firearms:

59% are white males

25% are black males

10% are white females

3.5% are black females

ages 15 to 34 years —the largest number of deaths from firearms

Drugs:

death rate is approximately 4.3 per 100,000 persons

death rate among males is more than twice the rate of females

death rate for the black population is nearly twice that of the white population

Alcohol:
death rate is approximately 6.8 per 100,000 persons
death rate among males is 3.5 times higher than the death rate for females
death rate for blacks is nearly 2.5 times higher than the death rate for whites

Infant mortality:
just below 7 deaths per 1,000 live births, the lowest rate ever in the United States
increasing order of mortality: Hispanics, whites, blacks (more than twice the rate for whites)
top five causes of infant deaths are:
  congenital malformations, deformations, chromosomal abnormalities
  short gestation/low birth weight
  SIDS (sudden infant death syndrome)
  newborn affected by maternal complications
  newborn affected by complications of placenta, cord, and membranes

Morbidity

In addition to death, morbidity takes its toll. Previously defined as the rate of occurrence of diseases or conditions, the following are the primary causes of disablement, medical intervention, health care expenditures, and overall lack of wellness in the United States:
Obesity
Mental and emotional disorders, including alcohol and drug abuse
Diseases of the cardiovascular system
Arthritis
Epilepsy
Cerebral palsy
Multiple sclerosis
Parkinson's disease
Muscular dystrophy
Hearing and visual impairments
Mental retardation
Diabetes mellitus
Cancer

Life Expectancy

Overall life expectancy in the United States is the highest in its history: 77.6 years. The female-to-male gap has closed to 5.3 years. At birth, the life expectancy by gender and race is as follows for those being born early in the twenty-first century:
  White females: 80.5 years
  Black females: 76.1 years
  White males: 75.4 years
  Black males: 69.2 years
  At age 65, life expectancy is as follows:

All Americans: an additional 18 years
All males: an additional 16 years
All females: an additional 20 years

Emerging Infectious Diseases

Modern medicine has triumphantly eradicated smallpox and is nearing the elimination of polio. Other diseases targeted for worldwide eradication, severe limitation, or elimination by region include guinea worm, onchocerciasis, syphilis, rabies, measles, tuberculosis, and leprosy.

However, the threat from emerging and reemerging infectious diseases has become the leading cause of death and disability worldwide. Dramatic changes in society, technology, and the environment and a diminished effectiveness of some approaches to disease control have allowed this to occur.

It is important for the health care professional to understand two key terms when discussing infectious diseases – epidemic and pandemic. An **epidemic** is a widespread infectious disease within a given geographical area. A **pandemic** is an infectious disease of global proportions. Health care leaders and researchers are trying to contain increasing numbers of emerging infectious diseases in order to prevent a pandemic.

The term **emerging infectious diseases** refers to diseases of infectious origin whose incidence in humans has either increased within the past two decades or threatens to increase in the near future. Such diseases increasingly threaten public health and substantially increase the cost of health care. Infectious diseases account for 25% of all visits to physicians each year, and antimicrobial agents are the second most frequently prescribed class of drugs in the United States. For example, childhood ear infections are the leading cause of visits to pediatricians, and the incidence of visits for such infections has increased by 150%. Direct and indirect costs of infectious diseases exceed $120 billion.

Emerging infections are especially serious in people with lowered immunity, such as those who are HIV-positive, those receiving immunosuppressive chemotherapy, and those receiving transplanted organs; these are all growing populations. Other large groups affected by this threat are the elderly, those cared for in institutions, people with inadequate access to health care, and more than 11 million children in day care centers. Box 5-1 lists examples of emerging infectious diseases.

Disease emergence can be related to many factors. Newly emergent infectious diseases may result from changes in or the evolution of existing organisms; known diseases may spread to new geographic areas or human populations; or previously unrecognized infections may appear in people living or working in areas undergoing ecologic changes (for example, deforestation or reforestation) that increase human exposure to insects, animals, or environmental sources that may harbor new or unusual infectious agents.

Furthermore, infectious diseases may reemerge because of either the development of antimicrobial resistance in existing agents (such as gonorrhea, malaria, and pneumococci) or breakdowns in public health

BOX 5-1   EMERGING INFECTIOUS DISEASES

Diseases in the United States

Anthrax infections (bioterrorism)
Coccidioidomycosis
Cryptosporidiosis
Drug-resistant *Mycobacterium tuberculosis*
Drug-resistant pneumococcal disease
Drug-resistant *Staphylococcus aureus*
Escherichia coli O 157:H7 disease
Hantavirus pulmonary syndrome
HIV/AIDS —global
Influenza A/Beijing/32/92
Vancomycin-resistant enterococcal infections
West Nile fever

Diseases Outside the United States

Avian influenza viruses (bird flu)—Asia
Cholera—Latin America
Dengue—Costa Rica
Diphtheria—Russia
E. coli O 157:H7—South Africa and Swaziland
HIV/AIDS—global
Multidrug-resistant *Shigella dysenteriae*—Burundi
Rift Valley fever—Egypt
SARS – severe acute respiratory syndrome—Asia
Vibrio cholerae O139—Asia
Yellow fever—Kenya

measures for previously controlled infections (such as cholera, tuberculosis, and pertussis). Such infections can affect people in geographically widespread areas regardless of lifestyle, cultural or ethnic background, or socioeconomic status.

Surveillance of infectious diseases in the United States depends on voluntary collaboration among the CDC and state and local health departments, which in turn depend on reporting by health care professionals. Such reporting is frequently incomplete.

The CDC has established the following goals for dealing with the threat of emerging infectious diseases:

Goal 1: Detect, promptly investigate, and monitor emerging pathogens, the diseases they cause, and the factors that influence their emergence.

Goal 2: Integrate laboratory science and epidemiology to optimize public health practice.

Goal 3: Enhance communication of public health information about emerging diseases, and ensure prompt implementation of prevention strategies.

Goal 4: Strengthen local, state, and federal public health infrastructures to support surveillance and implement prevention and control programs.

Implementation of these goals and their accompanying objectives are relevant to health care delivery and its reform. Relevant issues include prolonged hospitalization due to nosocomial (hospital-acquired) infections, increased morbidity and treatment costs resulting from antimicrobial drug resistance, and excessive burdens placed on public and private health care delivery facilities because of community-wide outbreaks of food-borne and waterborne infections.

CONCLUSION

The history of medicine is being recorded even as you begin your studies in radiologic technology. Medicine is advancing at a rapid pace. National goals for the overall improvement of health have been set in the report Healthy People 2010, which will be discussed in Chapter 26. The possibilities for improvements in the quality and longevity of life are only as limited as the dreams and hard work of all involved in health care, including you in your studies and lifestyle choices.

Review Questions

1. Disease may be defined as which of the following?
   a. The pattern of response of a living organism to injury
   b. Disordered function
   c. The absence of health
   d. Any condition more serious than the common cold or influenza
2. Morbidity is defined as which of the following?
   a. Death rate
   b. Diseases that cause death
   c. Rate of occurrence of disease or conditions
   d. Death rate in Third World countries
3. In the United States, statistics on health and disease are tracked by which of the following organizations?
   a. The Department of Health and Human Services
   b. Medicare
   c. Medicaid
   d. Centers for Disease Control and Prevention
4. What is the leading cause of death in the United States?
   a. Cancer
   b. Cerebrovascular disease
   c. Heart disease
   d. AIDS

5. What is the leading cause of death in the United States in the 1- to 44-year-old age group?
   a. AIDS
   b. Accidents
   c. Leukemia
   d. Heart disease
6. What is the occurrence of firearm injury deaths?
   a. Black males, white males, white females, black females
   b. Black males, white males, all females
   c. White males, black males, black females, white females
   d. The same across all groups
7. The rate of HIV infection in males is:
   a. higher than that of females.
   b. lower than that of females.
   c. equal to females.
   d. Fixed at current level.
8. Morbidity is caused most often by which of the following?
   a. Heart disease
   b. Cancer
   c. Mental and emotional disorders, including alcohol and drug abuse
   d. Arthritis
9. A pandemic is:
   a. an infectious disease spread out over a continent.
   b. a worldwide infectious disease.
   c. not infectious.
   d. not as serious as an epidemic.
10. Total knowledge and information on this planet doubles approximately every:
    a. Month.
    b. 15 to 18 months.
    c. 3 years.
    d. 5 years.

BIBLIOGRAPHY

Bettman O: *A pictorial history of medicine*, Springfield, IL, 1979, Charles C Thomas.

Centers for Disease Control and Prevention, www.cdc.gov

Fauci AS, Touchette NA, Folkers GK: Emerging infectious diseases: a 10-year perspective from the National Institute of Allergy and Infectious Diseases. *Emerg Infect Dis.* April, 2005.

Green J: *Medical history for students*, Springfield, IL, 1968, Charles C Thomas.

Lyons AS, Petrucelli RJ: *Medicine: an illustrated history*, New York, 1978, Harry Abrams.

Major R: *A history of medicine*, vol. 1, Springfield, IL, 1954, Charles C Thomas.

Radiology: A Historic Perspective

LaVerne Tolley Gurley

OBJECTIVES

On completion of this chapter, you should be able to:

- List the pioneers in radiology and describe their contributions to the field.
- Describe the events leading to the discovery of x-rays.
- Give a short history of Wilhelm Conrad Roentgen.
- Describe the works of Marie and Pierre Curie in radioactivity.
- List the events leading to the development of nuclear medicine.
- Describe the modern radiology department, including equipment, specialized tasks, and staff development through continuing education.

Few discoveries have so profoundly affected the world as the discovery of the x-ray. This development has changed almost every aspect of medical practice. However, the diagnosis and treatment of disease is not the only area influenced by the discovery. Other uses have also had a dramatic effect on the way we live and work, for example, providing security at airports, developing improved strains of grain, controlling some kinds of insects, detecting flaws in industrial materials and equipment, identifying counterfeit art, and, recently, irradiating food to extend its shelf-life.

KEY TERMS

cyclotron
fiber optics
fluoroscopy
nuclear radiology
radioactivity

CHAPTER OUTLINE

Pioneers of radiology
   Wilhelm Roentgen
Early days in the
   discovery
Advanced
   experimentation of the
   roentgen rays
Nuclear radiology
Modern radiology
Conclusion

PIONEERS OF RADIOLOGY

The development of radiology is, in large measure, a story of the development of technical hardware. The work of early scientists and craftspeople made possible the production of x-rays. There is even evidence of experimentation with the chemical as well as the physical properties of matter as early as the first century AD. Archimedes, for example, explained the reaction of solids when they are placed in liquids. Democritus described materials as being composed of ultimate particles, and Thales discovered some of the effects of electricity.

More recently, three specific aspects of physical science helped pave the way to the discovery of x-rays—electricity, vacuums, and image-recording materials. Evangelista Torricelli produced the first recognized vacuum when he invented a barometer in 1643. In 1646, through many hours of scientific experiments, Otto van Guericke invented an air pump that was capable of removing air from a vessel or tube. This experiment was repeated in 1659 by Robert Boyle and in 1865 by Herman Sprengel. Their techniques considerably improved the amount of evacuation, thus making better vacuum tubes available for further experimentation by other scientists.

From the seventeenth century on, the main interest of scientists seemed to be experimentation with electricity. William Gilbert of England was one of the first to extensively study electricity and magnetism. He was also noted for inventing a primitive electroscope. Robert Boyle's experiments with electricity earned him a place among the serious investigators. Most such scientists had to build their own equipment. Isaac Newton built and improved the static generator. Charles DuFay, working with glass, silk, and paper, distinguished two different kinds of electricity.

Abbé Jean Antoine Nollet made a significant improvement in the electroscope, a vessel for discharging electricity under vacuum conditions. The electroscope was a forerunner of the x-ray tube. Of course, Benjamin Franklin conducted many electrical experiments and should be mentioned in any discussion of pioneers in electricity. William Watson demonstrated a current of electricity by transmitting electricity from a Leyden jar through wires and a vacuum tube.

While conducting experiments with electrical discharges, William Morgan noticed the difference in color of partially evacuated tubes. He noted that when a tube cracked and some air leaked in, the amount of air in the tube determined the coloration.

In 1831 Michael Faraday induced an electric current by moving a magnet in and out of a coil. From this experiment evolved the concept of electromagnetic induction, which led to the production of better generators and transformers and higher voltages for use in evacuated tubes. The most significant improvement on induction coils was made by H.D. Ruhmkorff of Paris.

Johann Wilhelm Hittorf conducted several experiments with cathode rays, streams of electrons emitted from the surface of a cathode. William

Crookes furthered the study of cathode rays and demonstrated that matter was emitted from the cathode with enough energy to rotate a wheel placed within a tube. Hittorf's works were repeated and further developed by Crookes. Philipp Lenard furthered the investigation of the cathode rays. He found that cathode rays could penetrate thin metal and would project a few centimeters into the air. Lenard did a tremendous amount of research with cathode rays and determined their energies by measuring the amount of penetration. He also studied the deflection of rays due to magnetic fields.

William Goodspeed produced a radiograph in 1890. His achievement was recognized only in retrospect, after the discovery of x-rays by Wilhelm Conrad Roentgen, and Goodspeed was not credited with the discovery of x-rays.

The image-recording materials, that is, the photographic recording techniques, were very important to the investigators of the cathode rays. The first photographic copy of written material was produced by J.H. Scholtz in 1727. This technique was tested further and greatly improved in later years. In 1871, R.L. Maddox produced a film with a gelatin silver bromide emulsion that has remained the basic component for film. In 1884, George Eastman produced and patented roll-paper film. With this significant improvement of image-recording material and the improvement in the cathode ray tube, the basis for modern-day radiography was established.

Wilhelm Roentgen

Wilhelm Conrad Roentgen was born on March 27, 1845, in Lennep, a small town near the Rhine River in Germany (Fig. 6-1, *A*). He was the only child of Friedrich Conrad Roentgen, a textile merchant whose ancestors had lived in or near Lennep for several generations. Wilhelm Roentgen married Bertha Ludwig in 1872 (Fig. 6-1, *B*), and in 1888 he was offered employment at the University of Wurzburg. He readily accepted the offer, knowing of the university's new physics institute and its impressive facilities. Roentgen was elected rector at the university, although he continued to work in the physics department and on his personal research projects. He became interested in cathode ray experiments with the Crookes tube, which he worked with until his discovery of x-rays.

Discovery of X-rays

On November 8, 1895, Wilhelm Roentgen discovered x-rays while working in his modest laboratory at the university. While operating a Crookes tube at high voltage in a darkened room, he noticed a piece of barium platinocyanide paper on a bench several feet from the Crookes tube. He noticed a glowing or fluorescence of the barium platinocyanide after he passed a current through the tube for only a short period. Knowing the parameters of this particular experiment, Roentgen realized that the fluorescence was some kind of ray, rather than light or electricity, escaping the Crookes tube.

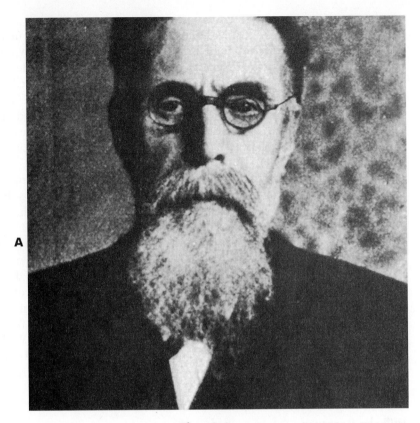

Fig. 6-1

A, Wilhelm C. Roentgen a few weeks before he died.

Roentgen proved that by continuously producing the fluorescent effect of the barium platinocyanide, he had produced some type of x-ray (x being a mathematical symbol for an unknown quantity). By performing several more tests with the mysterious rays, he determined that the x-rays had a degree of penetrative power dependent on the density of the material. On December 28, 1895, Roentgen submitted a report entitled "On a new kind of rays" to the Wurzburg Physico-Medical Society. He realized there could be potential medical use for this new type of ray. Putting this thought to action, Roentgen discovered that by placing his hand between the tube and a piece of cardboard coated with barium platinocyanide, he could actually visualize the bones of his hand, thus demonstrating the primitive fluoroscopic screen. He knew he had discovered something that could revolutionize the world of science, but he still did not know whether his observations were correct. This prompted him to further test the cathode rays so that he could prove the validity of his previous experiments. After several weeks of working in virtual seclusion, Roentgen did prove that his previous work was, in fact, valid. He tried another experiment in which he convinced his wife to place her

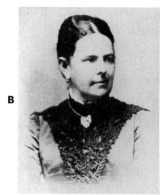
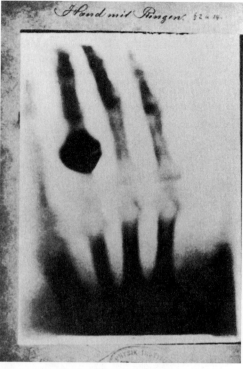

B

C

Fig. 6-1, cont'd

B, Roentgen's wife, Anna Bertha Roentgen (1839-1919). **C**, Roentgen's first radiograph, showing his wife's hand and two rings on her finger. (From Glasser O: Wilhelm Conrad Röentgen and the early history of the roentgen rays, Springfield, 1933, Charles C Thomas.)

hand on a cassette loaded with a photographic plate upon which he directed the x-rays from the tube for approximately 15 minutes. Development of the plate proved again that Roentgen's experiments were successful. The bones in his wife's hand, as well as the two rings on her finger, were clearly visible (Fig. 6-1, *C*).

Roentgen continued to study the effects of x-rays, and he presented his notes to different societies. In addition to many other awards and honors, Roentgen received the first Nobel Prize in Physics in 1901 in Stockholm and became a member of the Physical Society of Stockholm. In 1902, he received an invitation from the Carnegie Institute in Washington, D.C., to use its laboratory for special experiments, but he did not accept the invitation. On February 10, 1923, Wilhelm Conrad Roentgen died in Munich.

EARLY DAYS IN THE DISCOVERY

The discovery of x-rays offered much hope in the discipline of science, but few discoveries have been so little understood by the general public. The nature of the rays is partly responsible for this. They cannot be sensed by sight, touch, taste, smell, or hearing. Thus, explaining them is difficult. In 1895, when Wilhelm Roentgen discovered the as yet unknown rays and published his findings, the western world immediately reacted and clamored for more information. Through newspapers, Thomas Alva Edison attempted to explain the nature of the rays to the citizens in the United States. However, no one fully understood the effects of radiation. This did not prevent entrepreneurs from taking risks and developing schemes for profit in the market place. Scientists and others produced a flurry of publications, and while some seriously attempted to explain the nature of the rays, some were vague, some comic, and some clearly dishonest. There were also jokes and cartoons, as well as ludicrous advertisements appearing in newspapers (Fig. 6-2).

Circuses used x-rays for entertainment in guessing the contents of women's purses. Department stores and fairs offered "bone portraits," like the one shown in Fig. 6-3. A manufacturing company produced lead underwear for modest women and men. England passed a law against opera glasses with x-ray vision. Some wealthy persons purchased x-ray

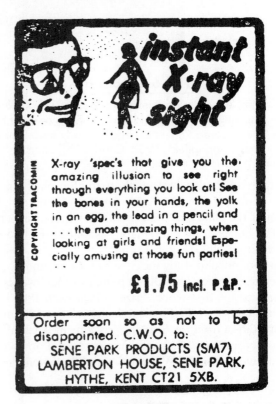

Fig. 6-2

An advertisement that capitalizes on use of x-rays for profit. (From Eisenberg RL: Radiology: an illustrated history, St. Louis, 1992, Mosby.)

units for their homes to entertain guests by imaging their skeletons with the fluoroscope (Fig. 6-4).

Abuses of these rays were rampant, and in time the latent effects on tissues began to show degenerating results. Thomas Edison, one of the most knowledgeable persons on the subject, took notice and questioned the effects of x-rays. He complained that his eyes were sore and red after working with a fluorescent tube. Although it was not clearly established that this was caused by x-rays, later reports coming from other workers in his laboratory confirmed a direct relationship between their injuries and x-ray exposure.

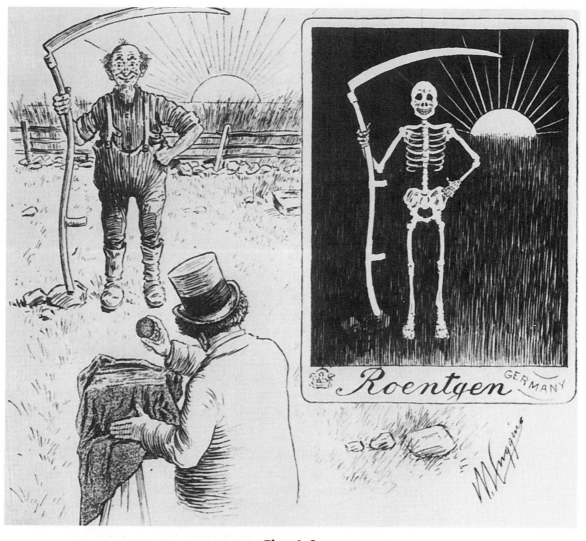

Fig. 6-3

An x-ray photograph like the ones taken at circuses or fairs.

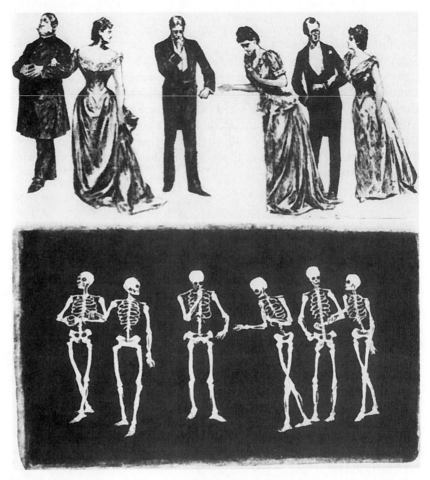

Fig. 6-4

A dangerous party game. (From Glasser O: Wilhelm Conrad Roentgen and the early history of the roentgen rays, Springfield, 1933, Charles C Thomas.)

When these reports began to emerge both in Europe and the United States, serious efforts were made to protect those who worked with the rays and those who would be exposed to them. These efforts have been successful; today, a career in radiology is as safe as any other career.

ADVANCED EXPERIMENTATION OF THE ROENTGEN RAYS

After Roentgen's discovery, most investigators based their experimental priorities on the relationship between x-ray exposure and tissue injury. When the discovery of the roentgen rays was announced throughout the world, several of the investigators who had also been working with the cathode rays began to publish literature on their own experiments. It is thought that the first known radiograph produced in the United States was made on January 2, 1896, by Michael Idvorsky Pupin, a professor at Columbia University. Pupin's production of the radiograph was thought to have occurred approximately 2 weeks after Roentgen discovered x-rays.

Soon after the announcement of Roentgen's discovery, Thomas Edison started his experiments with the Roentgen rays. His primary concern was working with **fluoroscopy**, a procedure using x-rays to image inner parts of the body in movement and motion. Only after Edison and his staff had performed a large number of experiments did they discover the use of calcium tungstate, a great improvement over barium platinocyanide. Edison promoted the use of calcium tungstate coating in fluoroscopy, with the hope that the vast improvement would increase sales of the fluoroscope. He also became interested in trying to develop a tube in which energy could be transformed into light rather than x-rays. However, he immediately stopped all his research in fluoroscopy, which involved extensive use of radiation, when one of his assistants, Clarence Madison Dally, suffered severe radiation damage as a result of the work.

During the time of Roentgen's work, another field of study evolved. It resulted in the discovery of **radioactivity**, the property of certain elements to spontaneously emit rays or subatomic particles from matter. Three of the most prominent persons credited with this work were Pierre and Marie Curie and Henri Becquerel, who were jointly awarded the Nobel Prize for Physics in 1903. While experimenting with radium on animals, Pierre Curie noticed that the radium killed diseased cells, which was the first suggestion of the medical utility of radioactivity. Marie Curie refined the knowledge of radioactivity and purified the radium metal. In 1911, she received a Nobel Prize for her work in chemistry. She continued to study radioactivity until she suffered a severe illness and required a kidney operation. After her health improved, she became acquainted with Albert Einstein and resumed her experiments with radium. However, her efforts were halted because of World War I. Unable to work in her laboratory, she made radiographic equipment for the French military medical service. She developed approximately 20 mobile radiographic units and 200 installations for the army. After training herself as an x-ray technician, she trained French soldiers and gave x-ray classes to American soldiers.

The demand for x-ray equipment and technicians continued to rise through the years. With the onset of World War II, there was a shortage of roentgenologists and equipment in the United States because the army was sending technicians and supplies overseas. The U.S. Army established the Army School of Roentgenology at the University of Tennessee at Memphis in 1942. The army continued to train x-ray personnel at John Gaston Hospital in Memphis and trained more than 900 enlisted technicians. These graduates greatly helped to relieve the need for qualified technicians.

NUCLEAR RADIOLOGY

Continuous improvements in x-ray equipment brought about several other studies in radiology, including **nuclear radiology**, the branch of radiology using radioactive materials for medical diagnosis and treatment. In 1932, Ernest Lawrence invented the **cyclotron**, a chamber that made it possible to accelerate particles to high speeds for use as projectiles. The cyclotron first made radioisotopes available in large quantities. Enrico Fermi made a significant breakthrough when he induced a successful chain reaction in a uranium pile at the University of Chicago in 1942. The results of this breakthrough were first demonstrated when atomic devices were detonated experimentally in 1945 at White Sands, New Mexico. Shortly thereafter, these devices were introduced as weapons when atomic bombs were dropped on Hiroshima and Nagasaki, Japan. Ironically, from the same basic research that ushered in the age of nuclear arms emerged the highly beneficial medical applications of radioisotopes.

MODERN RADIOLOGY

The technical advances in radiology since Roentgen's discovery of x-rays in 1895 have been phenomenal. Today's imaging departments consist of an impressive array of diagnostic and therapeutic devices. Many specialties have emerged, including computed tomography, magnetic resonance imaging, nuclear medicine, radiation therapy, ultrasound, neurovascular radiology, digital imaging, and, of course, routine diagnostic radiography (Fig. 6-5). It would be difficult to diagnose or treat many medical problems without this team of radiology services.

The equipment in contemporary radiology departments is made with extreme precision. The tubes are capable of producing accurate multiple exposures. The development of **fiber optics**, that is, man-made fibers with the unique characteristic of allowing light to turn a curve, has had a significant impact on radiology and indeed all disciplines of medicine. This plastic-like material that will transmit light through curves and bends has been used in radiology imaging equipment and instruments for diagnostic tests and treatment.

Films are capable of resolving structures smaller than the human eye can see. Improvements in cassettes and film holders have made them more durable and have provided a tighter closure that allows better screen-film contact. Intensifying screen speeds are five to six times those of previous screens, making it possible to decrease exposure factors. Lowering exposure factors not only reduces radiation exposure to patients and personnel, it also prolongs the life of x-ray equipment. Film processors routinely produce radiographs in 90 seconds, 60-second and 45-second machines are also available.

Continuing education has played an important role in the development of radiology and is essential to keeping abreast of the rapid changes

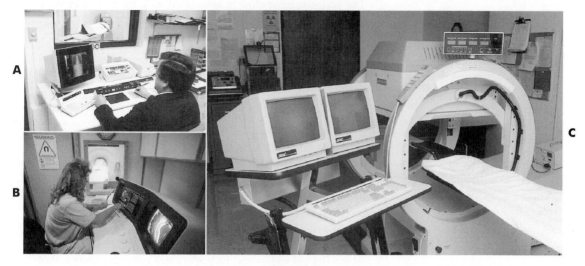

Fig. 6-5

A, Computed tomography is conventional x-ray combined with radiation detectors and a digital computer. **B**, Magnetic resonance imaging (MRI) is one of the newest of the medical imaging modalities. Instead of x-ray, MRI uses non-ionizing radiofrequency waves, a strong magnetic field, and a computer to produce an image. **C**, Nuclear medicine uses ionizing radiation to produce physiologic images or to visualize the functioning of a specific organ.

and innovations in the field. Radiology, in its short history, has proved its capabilities and will continue to serve patients in the years to come.

CONCLUSION

It can be seen that the history of radiology is a story of how creative individuals built on the discoveries and inventions of others, adding their own inventive techniques to create the radiologic practices we have today. From the earliest scientists and craftspeople, such as Archimedes and Democritus, to the more current scientists, such as Faraday, Hittorf, Roentgen, and Edison, we see each one's work building on another's in the development of radiology. In addition, we witness the continuing development of radiologic advances, with improved imaging equipment for more accurate diagnosis and advanced therapeutic units for the treatment of diseases.

Review Questions

1. Marie Curie is best known for her work with:
   a. Radiation-absorbed dose standards
   b. The cyclotron and nuclear particle acceleration
   c. Radium and the refinement of radium
   d. Electric capacitance and induction

2. The scientist most closely associated with the atomic bomb is:
   a. Pierre Curie
   b. Michael Faraday
   c. Thomas Edison
   d. Enrico Fermi
3. Wilhelm Conrad Roentgen:
   a. Discovered the x-ray
   b. Developed silver bromide–coated film
   c. Established the international unit of x-ray quantity
   d. All the above
4. Three scientists credited with early research in the development of the x-ray tube are:
   a. Hittorf, Faraday, and Fermi
   b. Crookes, Hittorf, and Goodspeed
   c. Crookes, Hittorf, and Lenard
   d. Hittorf, Goodspeed, and Fermi
5. In the field of radiology, Edison's chief contribution was the:
   a. Platinocyanide coating for fluoroscopic screens
   b. Promotion of a vacuum tube for generating x-rays
   c. Use of lithium fluoride for fluoroscopic screen coating
   d. Use of calcium tungstate for fluoroscopic screen coating
6. The World War II military experiments resulted in a new radiology discipline called:
   a. Computed tomography scanning
   b. Nuclear medicine imaging
   c. Magnetic resonance imaging
   d. Cardiovascular radiography
7. The first radiograph produced in the United States is thought to have occurred _____ after the discovery of x-ray.
   a. 6 months
   b. 6 weeks
   c. 2 months
   d. 2 weeks
8. The early experiments with fluoroscopy were made by:
   a. Michael Idvorsky Pupin
   b. Thomas Edison
   c. Marie Curie
   d. William Crookes
9. The Army School of Roentgenology was established to aid in the war effort of:
   a. World War I
   b. World War II
   c. The Spanish-American War
   d. The Korean War

10. The development of mobile x-ray units for military medical service in World War I was the work of:
   a. Thomas Edison
   b. Albert Einstein
   c. Marie Curie
   d. Ernest Lawrence

BIBLIOGRAPHY

Coates JB: *Radiology in World War II*, Washington, DC, 1966, Office of the U.S. Surgeon General, Department of the Army.

Dewing S: *Modern radiology in historical perspective*, Springfield, IL, 1962, Charles C Thomas.

Eisenberg RL: *Radiology: an illustrated history*, St. Louis, 1992, Mosby.

Glasser O: *Dr. W.C. Roentgen*, ed 2, Springfield, IL, 1972, Charles C Thomas.

Glasser O: *Wilhelm Conrad Roentgen and the early history of the roentgen rays*, Springfield, IL, 1933, Charles C Thomas.

Grigg ERN: *The trail of the invisible light*, Springfield, IL, 1965, Charles C Thomas.

Harris EL, et al: *The shadowmakers: a history of radiologic technology*, Albuquerque, NM, 1995, American Society of Radiologic Technologists.

II

Practicing
the Profession

Radiography Education: From Classroom to Clinic

LaVerne Tolley Gurley

OBJECTIVES

On completion of this chapter, you should be able to:

- **Describe the essentials for patient/radiologic technologist interaction.**
- **List and describe the basic courses essential to the education of radiologic technologists.**
- **Explain the relationship between clinical education and the theory component of the radiologic technology curriculum.**
- **Explain what is meant by "clinical competency evaluation."**
- **List and describe the competencies evaluated in clinical education.**
- **Describe what is meant by "optimum patient care."**

KEY TERMS

affective learning
clinical competency
   evaluation
cognitive learning
independent clinical
   performance
interaction
maudlin
passive participation
psychomotor learning
solicitous

CHAPTER OUTLINE

The patient as our guest
Your responsibilities in
   health care
   Radiologic technology
      basic curriculum
From the classroom to the
   clinical setting
   Clinical competency
      evaluation
Clinical participation
   Competency
      evaluations
   Criteria for
      performance evaluation
Continuing education
Conclusion

Few professions are as diverse as radiologic technology. Daily tasks range from communications and psychology to artistic expression in the production of the radiographic image to physics, anatomy, physiology, and chemistry.

To the novice, the work performed by a well-educated registered technologist may seem methodic, repetitive, and lacking challenge. However, on closer examination it becomes apparent that the technologist must possess complex knowledge and apply it to the radiologic examination of patients.

If a particular occupation or task looks easy, it is because the person doing the job has learned the many intricacies involved. This is particularly true of radiologic technology. The educated technologist provides every patient with optimum patient care, which includes interaction with the patient, positioning procedures, and the selection of exposure factors that produce the best diagnostic radiologic examination. Therefore, the performance of various tasks might look easy to the patients and others outside the profession.

This chapter introduces the student to the work of the radiologic technologist, provides the minimum core curriculum necessary for entry-level performance, and evaluates the student during the learning process.

THE PATIENT AS OUR GUEST

The key individual in the health care setting is the patient. This means that we must think of the patient as our guest. It is imperative to examine this phrase and understand how the patient is a guest. The patient is the recipient of the many services provided in medical facilities. On admission to the hospital, clinic, or physician's office, the patient is abruptly introduced to an unusual environment filled with wondrous, unnamed machines and a variety of people, all waiting for the guest—the patient.

When a qualified physician requests a radiographic examination, it becomes the radiologic technologist's responsibility to:
1. Interact with the patient.
2. Establish and maintain an atmosphere of caring and empathy for the patient.
3. Treat the patient as a guest in a home.

Essentially, this treatment should be respectful without being familiar, empathetic without being **maudlin** (tearful, emotional), considerate without being **solicitous** (fearful, overly concerned), and professional without being cold and clinical.

This all sounds like a tall order, especially when the workload is heavy, the hour grows late, and there are more things to be done; but you need only to put yourself in the place of the patient to understand the importance of a health care professional's responsibility (Fig. 7-1).

When caring for the very young or the very old, the terminally ill, or the handicapped, this responsibility might be difficult to handle. These cases do not, however, change the importance of these responsibilities. This is the basis of being in a helping profession. Above all, every patient who comes to radiology is *a guest*!

YOUR RESPONSIBILITIES IN HEALTH CARE

There is no substitute for the knowledge necessary to perform the tasks of a radiologic technologist with confidence, effectiveness, and efficiency.

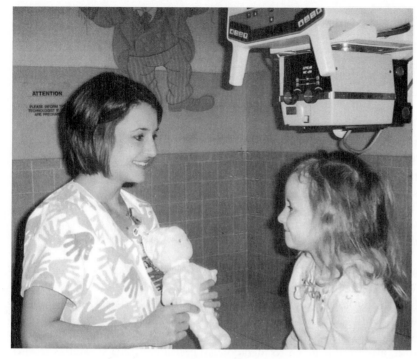

Fig. 7-1

Technologist interacting with young patient. (Courtesy University of Mississippi Medical Center, Amy Justice-Hill and Ansley Hill.)

This confidence is a direct result of being prepared. Students are confronted with quizzes, competency tests, and finally, the certifying examination. Yet the greatest tests will come with every radiologic examination you perform. Educators in radiologic technology are aware of the need for well-prepared radiologic technologists.

The field of radiology is continually changing in the wake of technology, recently accelerated by the space age. However, it is imperative that the student radiologic technologist learn the basic principles of the production of x-radiation and how to make these principles work. What does the radiologic technologist need to know to perform the responsibilities of radiologic technology?

To answer this question, you need to look at the course recommendations for approved programs in radiologic technology, as well as the unique goals and needs of the sponsoring institutions and clinical affiliates.

Essentially, the courses listed here are considered basic. The titles and brief descriptions of topics are based on the curriculum guide published by the American Society of Radiologic Technologists (ASRT). More complete information is available from the ASRT.

Radiologic Technology Basic Curriculum

The radiologic technology curriculum is composed of several courses taught over a period of two consecutive calendar years. The courses listed here are not inclusive, and each is under continual study and review by the professional organizations responsible for recommending the basic curriculum.

Introduction to Radiography

This course is designed to introduce the student to the basic aspects of the department of imaging, radiologic technology, and the health care system in general. The basic principles of radiation protection are introduced. The student should gain a better understanding of the structure and function of agencies through which medical services are delivered.

Medical Ethics and Law

What are the moral, legal, and professional responsibilities of the radiologic technologist? This course helps the student understand how to deal with confidential information and the interpersonal relationships, or **interaction**, with patients and other health care team members. In addition, attention is given to medicolegal considerations, as well as to professional guidelines and codes of ethics.

Principles of Diagnostic Imaging

This course introduces the student to various methods of recording images. These images result from the fluoroscopic and radiographic application of the principles of image production. The student is expected to comprehend and apply the principles to the various imaging systems. Some special techniques, such as magnetic resonance imaging (MRI), digital radiography, and ultrasonography, are discussed.

Imaging Equipment

This course describes the process of radiographic image production and the specific equipment needed to produce the radiographic image.

Radiographic Processing

The design, structure, function, and application of the various rooms and equipment needed to obtain a radiograph are presented. Darkrooms, processing and materials, and radiographic film, including its storage, handling, characteristics, and possible artifacts, are discussed.

Human Structure and Function

This course refers to the anatomy and physiology of the human body. For the radiologic technologist to do radiologic procedures on various anatomic parts, it is necessary to know the location and function of all body parts.

Medical Terminology

The written and spoken language of medicine incorporates many uncommon words, meanings, and symbols. For the radiologic technologist to work effectively in radiology, it is necessary to understand the language of medicine.

Principles of Radiographic Exposure

What are the technical factors required to produce high-quality diagnostic radiographs? What kinds of accessory equipment are used? This course involves the use of the mathematic principles used in producing a radiograph.

Radiographic Procedures

Every radiology department has a routine for performing procedures specific to that department. These procedures range from simple radiographic imaging to more complex tasks requiring contrast media, special radiographic equipment, and accessory materials.

Principles of Radiation Protection

The technologist must know how to use ionizing radiation in a safe and prudent manner. Patients, as well as radiologic technologists and coworkers, must be protected from radiation as much as possible. Therefore, radiologic technologists must know how exposure factors affect radiation dose, what the maximum permissible dose is, and the methods of exposure monitoring. The objective is to practice the "as low as reasonably achievable" (ALARA) concept in diagnostic radiography.

Radiographic Film Evaluation

What is the difference between an optimal-quality radiograph and a nondiagnostic one (Fig. 7-2)? This course integrates all of the material

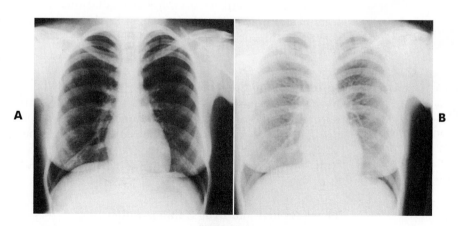

Fig. 7-2

A, An optimal-quality radiograph. **B**, A nondiagnostic radiograph.

previously learned. Although radiologic technologists do not interpret radiographs, they do evaluate them for diagnostic quality; this includes consideration of pathologic conditions.

Pathology

The student needs to be acquainted with the various disease conditions that may affect the resulting radiographic image. In addition, knowledge of disease entities is helpful in working with patients.

Methods of Patient Care

Through information presented in this course, the radiologic technologist prepares to deal with patients, regardless of their health conditions, in a manner that does not cause them additional injury or discomfort or hinder their recovery.

Quality Assurance

Optimal-quality radiographs achieve many important benefits: they minimize the patient's exposure to radiation, provide the physician with the best possible image for diagnosis, and contain health care costs. Students must know the regulations that govern quality assurance as well as the techniques, equipment, and procedures for attaining it.

Radiation Physics

To help the student understand how radiation works as well as the interaction of radiation with matter, this course concentrates on basic information about the physical properties of radiation, how it is produced, how it is measured, and how it is used in the medical environment. Also included is information about electrostatics, electric safety, x-ray tubes and transformers, and x-ray circuits and equipment.

Radiobiology

The hazardous effects of ionizing radiation on living tissue have long been known. The student must be thoroughly familiar with the reactions that occur when a single living cell or an entire organism is irradiated.

Introduction to Computer Science

Many of the technical innovations that are constantly changing the nature of radiology rely on computers. The capacity of computer storage and image manipulation is basic to many of the newer imaging systems, such as computed tomography, digital imaging, and MRI. This course introduces the student to basic computer applications (Fig. 7-3).

Pharmacology and Drug Administration

In this course, the student learns about pharmaceuticals used in radiology, including their nature, effects, routes of administration, and signs of adverse effects.

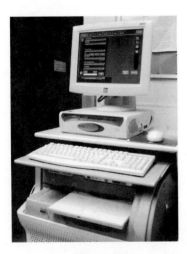

Fig. 7-3

Computers are an integral part of radiography equipment. (Courtesy University of Mississippi Medical Center.)

FROM THE CLASSROOM TO THE CLINICAL SETTING

After classroom preparation, the clinical experience is the opportunity for the student radiologic technologist to find out whether all the things he has learned about the production of x-rays are true.

However, there is more to the clinical experience than proving that widely held theories are indeed true. There are patients with differing health problems to encounter, hundreds of procedures to experience, and rules of behavior and ethics by which to abide. In this situation, students have the opportunity to prove their understanding of the classroom material by competently performing various radiologic procedures (Fig. 7-4).

Throughout the classroom preparation, the student is eased into the clinical setting through a series of lectures and demonstrations. A student has the opportunity to observe the activities of an imaging department, from office procedures and day-to-day operation to watching the performance of various radiologic examinations. Before beginning clinical participation on a full scale, the student has a good understanding of the functions of an imaging department and its importance in the delivery of health care services.

A basic guideline for evaluating the competency skills of a student radiologic technologist in the clinical setting has been developed and approved by the ASRT. This document is entitled *Clinical Competency Evaluation*. Although other methods of clinical competency evaluation may be available and in use, the information in this document is the focus of our discussion because it has been accepted by the ASRT, which is the profession's official organization.

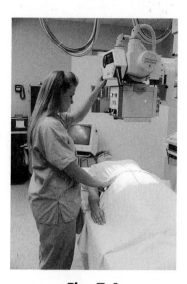

Fig. 7-4

Following classroom instruction, clinical education provides the student with the opportunity to practice what has been learned.

Clinical Competency Evaluation

Simply defined, **clinical competency evaluation** is a method of standardizing the evaluation of a student radiologic technologist's performance in the clinical setting. The student must fully appreciate and understand the importance of a standard evaluation concept and methodology. There are three specific aspects in this evaluation of performance: cognitive, affective, and psychomotor learning.

Cognitive learning refers to classroom lectures and demonstrations of theories, as well as to facts and background information necessary to understand a specific body of knowledge. Once this fundamental information has been learned, the student has the opportunity to participate in the clinical setting. It is in the clinical setting that each student has the opportunity to apply the knowledge gained from the classroom setting.

Affective learning involves attitudes, values, and feelings. The clinical environment provides the opportunity to develop pride in one's work as well as feelings of self-worth, skills in interpersonal relationships, and personal, moral, and ethical beliefs for daily practice.

Psychomotor learning is the actual hands-on phase—the application of previously learned material. Didactic information is put to actual use in the clinical situation.

CLINICAL PARTICIPATION

Clinical participation is the integration of the cognitive, affective, and psychomotor aspects of radiologic technology education. The student participates by:

1. Assisting the practicing radiologic technologist and observing each detail of the radiographic procedure. This is considered **passive participation** because the student is observing.
2. Performing various assigned tasks associated with procedures after becoming familiar with them. The performance of any task depends on the student's ability to understand the responsibilities involved with the assigned tasks and to perform these tasks correctly.
3. Progressing into the **independent clinical performance** phase. This means that the student will perform all aspects of the procedure with remote supervision of a radiologic technologist.

During this time, the student's learning ability and performance are evaluated. The student now has the opportunity to demonstrate knowledge of the subject material and how well each task can be accomplished.

This evaluation is designed to be a positive experience. It is an opportunity for the student to gain confidence by becoming thoroughly familiar with each detail of the assigned tasks.

As the student makes the transition from a classroom environment to one that combines both classroom and clinical experience, the learning process becomes integrated and more complex. The student is expected to be more aware of the responsibilities in learning. This means he must determine:

1. What do I know?
2. What must I learn?
3. How well have I learned the basic material?
4. Can I apply the classroom information in the clinical setting?

During this phase of radiologic technology education, the student also learns the importance of meeting the objectives of the educational process. Because competency levels vary from individual to individual, these objectives are self-paced. However, there is a great deal of coordination between classroom learning and clinical application. This coordination is facilitated by the program director and the clinical supervisors and coordinators. These people plan the course work and clinical participation that provide an optimal learning environment for the student (see Box 7-1).

Competency Evaluations

Examinations vary in emphasis depending on the teaching institution. However, the final objective is always that each student be able to successfully perform all examinations, regardless of specific emphasis, because routines for procedures vary from institution to institution. Student radiologic technologists must have a well-rounded preparatory

BOX 7-1 SAMPLE CLINICAL EDUCATION CHECKLIST

Orientation to Room

1. Become familiar with the full operation of the x-ray table (tilt, floating tabletop, raise and lower, footboard, operation of Bucky tray with insertion of cassettes, etc.).
2. Become familiar with full operation of the x-ray tube (longitudinal, vertical, transverse, collimator, etc.).
3. In fluoroscopic rooms, become familiar with image intensifier and spot film device (loading and unloading cassettes, loading and unloading cut film cartridges, etc.).
4. Become familiar with x-ray control panel (setting kVp, mA, time, mAs, focal spot size, fluoroscopic timer, Bucky selection, phototimer with backup time, chamber selection, operation of on-off switch, and performance of warm-up procedure, etc.).
5. Be aware of all types of procedures that are performed in this room.
6. Locate all appropriate supplies in the room.
7. Become familiar with the full operation of the wall Bucky for chest x-rays.
8. If contrast media are used for any procedures in this room, become familiar with their preparation.
9. Locate storage areas for all cassettes and stationary grids.

Tasks to Be Performed

1. Set up the room for each procedure before the patient is brought into the room.
2. Assist with or perform all imaging procedures in the assigned room.
3. If it is necessary to consult your notes, do so before you bring the patient into the room. At no time let the patient see you consulting your notes.
4. You are an adult pursuing a new career. Take charge to the best of your ability. If in doubt, ask the radiologic technologist, but not in front of the patient.
5. Courtesy is essential when providing service to the patient during the greeting, the procedure, and the dismissal phases of the examination.
6. Position the patient professionally and confidently. Position the part to be radiographed, adjust it, and make the exposure.
7. Initially you may have to ask the radiologic technologist with whom you are working what exposure technique to set.
8. After completion of the procedure and dismissal of the patient, critique the radiographs with the radiologic technologist. You should be able to identify all pertinent anatomy.
9. Immediately prepare the room for the next patient.

Things to Do With Free Time During Clinical Hours

1. Stock additional supplies wherever necessary.
2. Clean x-ray tabletop, footstool, control panel, wall Bucky, and any other equipment used.

Continued

BOX 7-1 SAMPLE CLINICAL EDUCATION CHECKLIST — CONT'D

3. Make sure there is an adequate supply of proper lead markers in the room.
4. Practice positioning using the radiologic technologist as the patient.
5. Go through your notes reviewing positioning and making sure that you have exposure techniques written in for all of the examinations you have performed so far.
6. Check to see what other procedures are scheduled for that room later in the day and familiarize yourself with them so you can take the initiative in performing them.
7. Familiarize yourself further with the darkroom (where film is stored, how to feed films into the processor, operation of the film duplicating machine, etc.). **CAUTION**: *Film bin may only be opened with the door closed, the safe light on, and white light off.*
8. Generally, clinical hours are for clinical education. Textbook studying generally should not occur during this time. However, during slow periods or equipment breakdown in your assigned area, studying is expected.

---

education in the professional program to enable them to practice radiologic technology in any type of medical facility.

The American Registry of Radiologic Technology (ARRT), the organization certifying Radiologic Technologists, produced a document, *Radiography Didactic and Clinical Competency Requirements*, listing the rules and regulations for meeting certification. A significant rule is that your program director or designated faculty member must verify that the didactic and clinical skills have been satisfied. Therefore, you may expect that frequent testing and evaluation will occur throughout your course of study.

Criteria for Performance Evaluation

To provide a basis for minimal performance evaluation criteria, the ASRT has developed a general, comprehensive list to help make performance evaluation as objective as possible for a wide variety of programs. The remainder of this chapter is taken directly from the *Clinical Competency Evaluation* document (with permission from the ASRT) so that the integrity of this process, as defined by the ASRT, is maintained.

The entire evaluation process is outlined in a flowchart (Fig. 7-5), and a model competency evaluation grade sheet is provided (Fig. 7-6). These criteria for performance evaluation might be more demanding at some teaching institutions. The criteria are:

Evaluation of Requisition
Student was able to:
    Identify procedures to be performed
    Recall the patient's age and name
    Identify mode of transportation to the clinical area
    Pronounce the patient's name (within reasonable limits)

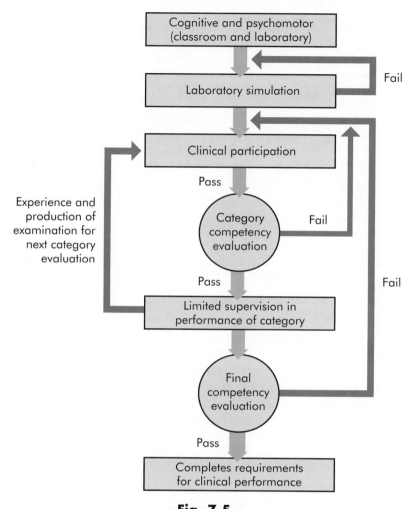

Fig. 7-5

A flowchart of the clinical evaluation process.

Physical Facilities Readiness

Student was able to:

Provide clean table

Exhibit orderly cabinets and storage space

Have appropriate size cassettes available

Have emesis basins and drugs ready

Locate syringes and needles as necessary

Turn machine on and be prepared for exposures

Turn tube in position necessary for the examination

Find and re-supply linens if appropriate

PROGRAM IN RADIOLOGIC TECHNOLOGY   **CLINICAL EDUCATION**

Student: _____   Final Grade: _____
Evaluator: _____   Date: _____
Type of Evaluation: _____ Category   Final(   )
(Identify Specific)

PERFORMANCE EVALUATION: **A.** Sufficient evaluation of requisition   Yes ( )   No ( )
        B. Adequate physical facilities readiness   Yes ( )   No ( )

EXAM/VIEW:	A				B				C			
	0	1	2	3	0	1	2	3	0	1	2	3
1. Patient-technologist relationship												
2. Positioning skills												
3. Equipment manipulation												
4. Evidence of radiation protection												
IMAGE EVALUATION:												
5. Anatomical part(s)												
6. Proper alignment												
7. Technique manipulation												
8. Film identification												
9. Radiation protection												
TOTAL												

Comments; Please list comments by number and view

_____

_____

_____

_____

COMPETENCY EVALUATION GRADE SHEET

The Competency Evaluation Grade Sheet has been designed for evaluating a maximum of three views per radiographic examination. Each exam requested necessitates a separate grade sheet, except for the Final Competency Evaluation which will represent multiple nonrelated views.

0 = unacceptable
1 = requires major improvement
2 = requires minor improvement
3 = acceptable

The evaluator will mark each area with a check (√) or X to indicate that point value.

Fig. 7-6

A competency evaluation grade sheet.

Patient/Technologist Relationship
Student was able to:
    Select the correct patient
    Assist patient to radiographic room
    Assist patient to radiographic table
    Keep patient clothed and/or draped for modesty
    Talk with patient in a concerned, professional manner
    Give proper instructions for moving and breathing
    Have patient gowned properly
    Follow proper isolation procedure when appropriate

Positioning Skills

Student was able to:

Position the patient correctly on table (head at the appropriate end, prone or supine)

Align center of part to be demonstrated to the center of the film

Position the central ray (CR) to the center of the film

Oblique patient correctly if required

Angle the CR to center of film

Restrict the size of the radiation field (collimation, cones, shields) and be certain that non-pertinent anatomic parts are not in the radiographic exposure area

Equipment Manipulation

Student was able to:

Turn tube from horizontal to vertical (and vice versa)

Move the Bucky tray and locks

Identify and use tube locks

Insert and remove cassettes from Bucky tray and spot film device

Operate film advance for automatic changers (e.g., chest)

Select factors at control panel

Use a technique chart

Measure the patient

Identify the film with right (R) and left (L) markers and other appropriate identifications (e.g., time, tube angle, name, date)

Fill syringes using aseptic technique

Direct mobile unit

Operate controls for mobile unit

Select proper cassette size

Adapt for technique changes in source-image distance (SID) or focal-film distance (FFD), grid ratio, collimation, etc.

Evidence of Radiation Protection

Student was able to:

Cone or collimate to the part

Use gonad shields, if appropriate

Demonstrate utilization of lead aprons and gloves, if appropriate

Produce the film badge as required by the institution

Select proper exposure factors

Adjust exposure technique for motion, when appropriate

Radiograph Demonstration—Image Evaluation

Anatomic part(s):

Part is shown in proper perspective

No motion is present

Proper alignment:

Film centered

Part centered

Tube centered
Patient obliqued or rotated correctly

Standard Radiographic Exposure—Image Evaluation
Radiographic techniques:
    Chart was used correctly (proper contrast and density)
    Compensation made for factors for pathology
    Correct exposure used to produce image
Film identification and/or other identifications:
    R and L in correct position on film
    Minute or hour markers visible
    Patient information and date can be identified
Radiation protection:
    Cone or collimation limits visible
    No repeats
    Gonad shields in place (if used)

CONTINUING EDUCATION

In 1997, the American Registry of Radiologic Technologists (ARRT) began requiring continuing education for all ARRT registrants. Each ARRT registrant must either obtain 24 continuing education credits acceptable to ARRT or pass an examination in an additional discipline.

It is imperative that each student considers education in radiologic technology a continuing process. These courses are an indication of the basic responsibilities of every radiologic technologist. This material must be learned and understood before you can correctly and safely operate the complicated equipment. You need to know not only how the equipment works but also why it works as it does. You must also be able to provide the physician with the best diagnostic radiographic study possible, regardless of the patient condition presented.

Look closely at each task as it is encountered, and study not just the work involved, but the concepts behind the tasks. You should not be surprised to learn that radiologic technology education must be an ongoing process.

CONCLUSION

Educators in radiologic technology are aware that, for the student radiologic technologist, the transition from classroom to clinic can be not only demanding but also, at times, confusing. In approved programs, every effort is made to ensure that students are better prepared to accept and deal with this transition. In addition, educators work to ensure that each student is evaluated on a fair and objective basis according to acceptable standards and institutional requirements for completion of the program.

From time to time, changes are made in the current procedures as new ideas and developments in radiologic technology occur. These changes are incorporated into the curriculum so that students are familiar with new concepts and procedures.

There is no substitute for being well prepared to practice your chosen profession. For the student, this time must be spent preparing for the challenges presented with each radiologic procedure. Each radiologic procedure is, after all, a test of your ability to perform the assigned tasks in an efficient, cheerful, and professional manner.

Review Questions

1. What kind of information is necessary to legally identify a radiographic film? (Check answer that is appropriate for your facility/state/country.)
   a. Right or left marker, complete name, identification number, physician's name, date, name and address of medical facility
   b. Right or left marker, date, identification number
   c. Right or left marker, date, identification number, physician's name, medical facility
   d. Right or left marker, identification number, physician's name, name and address of medical facility, technologist's identification
   e. None of the above
   f. A combination of the above choices; please list
2. What other information may be required or useful for the film? (Check all that apply.)
   a. Angle of tube (i.e., degree of angle, vertical, horizontal, etc.)
   b. Position of the patient (e.g., erect, supine, prone, angle of obliquity, etc.)
   c. Radiographic room number
   d. Equipment used
   e. Techniques used
   f. Collimator number
   g. Amount of contrast media injected
   h. Time of day
   i. Processor number
   j. Stretcher/wheelchair number
   k. Bed and room number
3. Where can you obtain specific and accurate information about the content of the curriculum used in approved programs in radiologic technology?
   a. American Hospital Association
   b. Joint Review Committee on Hospital Accreditation
   c. American Registry of Radiologic Technologists
   d. American Society of Radiologic Technologists

4. Understanding the process of radiographic image production and the specific equipment used in the processes is generally taught in which section of the curriculum?
   a. Principles of radiographic exposure
   b. Imaging equipment
   c. Radiographic processing
   d. Radiographic film evaluation

5. To help student radiologic technologists understand how to work with sick and injured patients of all ages and sizes, regardless of ethnic or cultural background, the student will study information presented in the following course work:
   a. Radiobiology
   b. Quality assurance
   c. Methods of patient care
   d. Human structure and function

6. Pathology is the study of:
   a. The normal structure and function of the various anatomic structures of the body
   b. The abnormal structure and/or function of the various anatomic structures of the body
   c. The study of any abnormal structures found on the resulting radiographic image
   d. The study of any abnormality associated with radiographic procedures

7. The written and spoken language of medicine is taught in the following: (Select all that apply.)
   a. Radiographic procedures
   b. Medical terminology
   c. In the clinical radiology laboratory only
   d. In conduction with methods of patient care only

8. Which of the following areas of study is included in "quality assurance"?
   a. Quality assurance procedures and regulations
   b. Principles of cost accounting procedures for containment of department costs
   c. Radiographic anatomy and positioning
   d. Radiographic evaluation of pathologic diagnostic procedures

9. The three most important specific aspects in evaluating a student's clinical performance are:
   a. Radiographic positioning, anatomy, and psychomotor learning
   b. Affective understanding, clinical participation, and radiation physics
   c. Cognitive, affective, and psychomotor levels
   d. Cognitive and affective performance levels and quality assurance

10. Passive participation occurs when the student is:
    a. Performing and assisting the practicing radiologic technologist during the radiographic procedure

b. Taking notes about the performance and execution of the work as it is done by the practicing radiologic technologist

   c. Assisting the radiologic technologist and the radiologist in doing the radiographic examinations

   d. Performing the various tasks associated with specific radiographic procedures

11. Interaction with the patient and with coworkers includes:

   a. Using intuition to figure out what the other person is saying and wishing to have done

   b. Referring to textbooks to assess the psychologic state of the patient and coworkers

   c. Evaluation of the radiographic procedure based on directions from coworkers and the condition of the patient

   d. Listening, understanding, and responding appropriately to information exchanges with the patient and with coworkers

12. Classroom lectures and demonstrations of theories and facts relating to a specific body of knowledge can usually be considered:

   a. Psychomotor knowledge

   b. Affective learning

   c. Cognitive learning

   d. Memorization only

BIBLIOGRAPHY

American Registry of Radiologic Technologists: *Radiography didactic and clinical competency requirements*, St. Paul, MN, 2005, The Registry.

American Society of Radiologic Technologists: *Essentials and guidelines of an accredited educational program for the radiographer*, Albuquerque, NM, July 1, 1994, The Society.

American Society of Radiologic Technologists: *Radiography clinical competency requirements*, Albuquerque, NM, 1999, The Society.

Ballinger P: *Merrill's atlas of radiographic positions and radiologic procedures*, ed 10, St. Louis, 2003, Mosby.

Bontrager KL: *Textbook of radiographic positioning and related anatomy*, ed 5, St. Louis, 2001, Mosby.

Joint Review Committee on Education in Radiologic Technology: *Standards for an accredited program in radiologic sciences*. Chicago, 1996, The Committee.

The Language of Medicine

William J. Callaway

OBJECTIVES

On completion of this chapter, you should be able to:

- **Define the prefixes, roots, and suffixes that comprise medical terms.**
- **Interpret the abbreviations commonly used in medicine.**
- **Name titles and organizations when given their abbreviations.**
- **Define terms and phrases in general usage in radiography.**

A newcomer to the field of health care is often overwhelmed by medical terminology. As with any specialized field, the medical profession comes with a language of its own. Medical terminology is simultaneously intriguing and frustrating: the intrigue lies in the fact that you will be learning, in effect, a new language that you will use to communicate with your health care colleagues; the frustration is the same as you would experience in learning any foreign language. If you have had previous exposure to a second language, medical terminology may come easily to you. If not, this will be an exciting new endeavor, although it may be somewhat confusing because of the unfamiliar combinations of word parts used to form the medical vocabulary.

Everyone working in health care should know some medical terminology. Each medical specialty, including radiologic technology, has its own unique terms. Both general and specific terminologies are covered in this chapter, but it is not possible to explore the entire collection of terms that you will need to learn. Early exposure to this nomenclature, however, will greatly aid in your understanding of the language you will soon be hearing. As with any other foreign language, the best method for first learning this material is probably memorization.

KEY TERMS

prefixes
roots
suffixes

CHAPTER OUTLINE

Word parts
Medical abbreviations
Titles and organizations
Radiographic
  nomenclature
Conclusion

As you study the words and combining forms in this chapter, keep in mind that most of them are of Latin or Greek origin. To those who have spoken English since childhood, there may seem to be little relation between these words and the concepts they represent. The student who is interested in an in-depth study of medical terminology can refer to any reputable medical dictionary or terminology textbook for further information about the words presented in this chapter.

WORD PARTS

The following section presents the word parts that are used to make new words; these include **prefixes**, **roots**, and **suffixes**. They are presented in alphabetical order in each category (see Box 8-1).

BOX 8-1 WORD PARTS

Prefixes

ab-	*away from*	hyper-	*above or greater*
a-, an-	*without*	hypo-	*below or lesser*
ante-	*front*	infero-	*below*
anti-	*against*	megal-	*large*
bi-	*two*	pan-	*all*
co-	*together*	peri-	*around*
contra-	*against*	poly-	*many*
decub-	*side*	post-	*back, after*
dors-	*back*	pre-	*before*
dys-	*difficult*	pseudo-	*false*
ect-	*outside*	retro-	*backward*
en-	*in*	scler-	*hard*
endo-	*within*	sub-	*below*
epi-	*upon*	super-	*above*
ex-	*out*	trans-	*across*
hemi-	*half*	tri-	*three*
hydro-	*water*	vent-	*front*

Roots

angio	*vessel*	enter	*intestine*
arth	*joint*	gastr	*stomach*
cardi	*heart*	hem	*blood*
cephal	*brain*	hepat	*liver*
cerebro	*head*	hyster	*uterus*
cerv	*neck*	leuk	*white*
chiro	*hand*	lith	*stone*

Continued

BOX 8-1 WORD PARTS — CONT'D

chole	*bile*	nephr	*kidney*
chondr	*cartilage*	osteo	*bone*
cost	*rib*	phren	*diaphragm*
crani	*skull*	pneum	*air*
cysto	*bladder*	pyel	*pelvis (renal)*
derm	*skin*	radi	*ray*
encephal	*brain*	viscer	*organ*

Suffixes

-algia	*pain*	-oid	*like*
-centesis	*puncture*	-oma	*tumor*
-dia	*through*	-osis	*condition*
-ectomy	*excision*	-pathy	*disease*
-emia	*blood*	-plasty	*surgical correction*
-ectasis	*expansion*	-pulm	*lung*
-genic	*origin*	-pyel	*pelvis (renal)*
-iasis	*condition*	-rhaphy	*suture*
-itis	*inflammation*	-scopy	*inspection*
-megaly	*enlargement*	-tomy	*incision*
-myel	*spinal cord*		

MEDICAL ABBREVIATIONS

Abbreviations are as much a part of medical communication as words. Listed here are the most common abbreviations that you may encounter during examination requisitions, on surgery schedules, and in patients' charts:

AIDS	acquired immunodeficiency syndrome
ARC	AIDS-related complex
ASAP	as soon as possible
ASHD	arteriosclerotic heart disease
BE	barium enema
BID	twice daily
BP	blood pressure
bx	biopsy
c–	with
CA	cancer
CAD	coronary artery disease
CBC	complete blood count
cc	cubic centimeter
CCU	coronary care unit
CHF	congestive heart failure
cm	centimeter

CNS	central nervous system
COPD	chronic obstructive pulmonary disease
CPR	cardiopulmonary resuscitation
CS	central supply
C-section	Cesarean section
CSF	cerebrospinal fluid
CT	computed tomography
CVA	cerebrovascular accident (stroke)
CXR	chest x-ray
DOA	dead on arrival
DOB	date of birth
DX	diagnosis
ECG, EKG	electrocardiogram
EEG	electroencephalogram
EMG	electromyogram
ENT	ear, nose, and throat
ER/ED	emergency room / emergency department
FUO	fever of undetermined origin
GI	gastrointestinal
HH	hiatal hernia
HHS	United States Department of Health and Human Services
HIPAA	Health Insurance Portability and Accountability Act of 1996
HIV	human immunodeficiency virus
H/O	history of
HX	history
ICCU	intensive coronary care unit
ICU	intensive care unit
IM	intramuscular
I/O	intake and output
IV	intravenous
IVP	intravenous pyelogram
KUB	kidneys, ureters, and bladder
lat	lateral
LMP	last menstrual period
mets	metastases
MI	myocardial infarction (heart attack)
mm	millimeter
MRI, MR	magnetic resonance imaging
NG	nasogastric
noc	night
npo	nothing by mouth
OB	obstetrics
OP	outpatient
OR	operating room
OTC	over the counter
PAR	postanesthesia recovery

PE	physical examination
peds	pediatrics
PID	pelvic inflammatory disease
p/o	postoperative
post-OP	after surgery
pre-OP	before surgery
prn	as needed
PT	physical therapy; prothrombin time
pt	patient
QID	four times daily
R/O	rule out
req	requisition
ROM	range of motion
RX	treatment or prescription
s–	without
SIDS	sudden infant death syndrome
SOB	short of breath
S/P	status post
STAT	immediately
STD	sexually transmitted disease
Sx	symptoms
TB	tuberculosis
TIA	transient ischemic attack
TID	three times daily
TKO	to keep open (refers to IV line)
TPN	total parenteral nutrition (IV feeding)
TPR	temperature, pulse, and respiration
Tx	treatment
UA	urinalysis
UGI	upper gastrointestinal series
URI	upper respiratory infection
UTI	urinary tract infection
VD	venereal disease
y/o	years old

TITLES AND ORGANIZATIONS

You will be seeing and hearing the abbreviations for various titles and organization names in the literature you read and in use throughout the hospital. Listed here are many that you will encounter:

ACERT	Association of Collegiate Educators in Radiologic Technology
ACR	American College of Radiology
AERS	Association of Educators in Radiological Sciences
AHA	American Hospital Association
AHRA	American Healthcare Radiology Administrators

AMA	American Medical Association
ANA	American Nurses Association
ARDMS	American Registry of Diagnostic Medical Sonographers
ARRT	American Registry of Radiologic Technologists
ASRT	American Society of Radiologic Technologists
CDC	Centers for Disease Control and Prevention
CNA	certified nursing assistant
EAP	employee assistance program
EMT	emergency medical technician
HMO	health maintenance organization
ISRRT	International Society of Radiographers and Radiologic Technologists
JCAHO	Joint Commission on Accreditation of Healthcare Organizations
JRCERT	Joint Review Committee on Education in Radiologic Technology
LPN	licensed practical nurse
MD	medical doctor/physician
MT	medical technologist
NCRP	National Council on Radiation Protection and Measurements
NIH	National Institutes of Health
NMTCB	Nuclear Medicine Technology Certification Board
OSHA	Occupational Safety and Health Administration
PPO	Preferred Provider Organization
RDMS	registered diagnostic medical sonographer
RN	registered nurse
RPH	registered pharmacist
RPT	registered physical therapist
RRT	registered respiratory therapist
RSNA	Radiological Society of North America
RT(N)	registered technologist in nuclear medicine
RT(R)	registered technologist in radiography
RT(T)	registered technologist in radiation therapy
SDMS	Society of Diagnostic Medical Sonographers
SI	international system of units
SMRI	Society of Magnetic Resonance Imaging
SNM	Society of Nuclear Medicine
WHO	World Health Organization

RADIOGRAPHIC NOMENCLATURE

Terms relating to your chosen specialty are of paramount importance if you are to function comfortably in the clinical setting. Here are the most common terms that you will need to know, including those related to digital imaging as well as film-screen imaging:

ADC Analog-to-digital converter; converts image information into numerical data

anode The positive electrode in the x-ray tube

automatic collimation Also known as positive beam limitation (PBL); the ability of the radiographic equipment to automatically collimate the x-ray beam to the same size as the image receptor resting in the Bucky tray; this prevents unnecessary exposure to the parts of the patient outside the area covered by the image receptor

blur The effect of motion on the radiographic image

Bucky Short for Potter-Bucky diaphragm; a moving grid used to remove scatter radiation from the remnant beam, which can cause fog on the image receptor

cassette A light-proof container holding the image receptor, either an imaging plate for CR or x-ray film and intensifying screens

cathode The negative electrode in the x-ray tube

collimator A box-like structure attached to the x-ray tube containing lead shutters that limits the x-ray beam to a specific area of the body

Computed Radiography (CR): Digital radiographic imaging using a cassette containing an imaging plate

contrast The differences in densities on a processed image; contrast allows detail to be seen

CRT Cathode ray tube (video monitor)

density The opaqueness or degree of blackening on an area of the processed image

DICOM Digital imaging and communications in medicine, a standard protocol used for blending PACS and various imaging modalities

Direct Digital Radiography (DR) Uses fixed detectors that communicate directly with a computer

distortion Misrepresentation of the size or shape of the object as recorded in the radiographic image

exposure indicator s-number or exposure index that describes the status of the exposure and diagnostic value of the digital image

film Refers to film before exposure to radiation

focal spot (focal track) The area of the anode in the x-ray tube from which x-rays emanate

grid A device that is placed between the patient and the image receptor that absorbs scatter radiation that is exiting the body

HIS Hospital information system

histogram A graphic display of the distribution of pixel values

image receptor In radiography, a general term applied to any device or medium that captures the remnant beam

Imaging plate (IP) Device that is made of a photostimulable phosphor that absorbs the photon energies exiting the patient; located inside a CR cassette

intensifying screens Mounted in the cassette singly or in pairs, these screens glow with visible light when struck by radiation and expose the film contained in the cassette

kVp The peak kilovoltage that is applied to the x-ray tube; this determines the wavelength of the x-ray beam, its ability to penetrate the body, and the overall contrast of the radiographic image

lead aprons Coverings worn by radiographers who are in a radiographic/fluoroscopic room with the x-ray beam turned on; the lead absorbs most of the scatter radiation that strikes the apron

mAs Milliampere-seconds; the product of milliamperage and time; the mA is the current that is passed through the x-ray tube that is converted to x-rays when it strikes the anode; it determines the number of x-rays produced and consequently the overall darkness of the resulting radiograph; radiation exposure to the patient is directly proportional to the mAs used

matrix Digital image comprised of rows and columns of data

object-to-image receptor distance (OID) The distance from the part being examined to the device that is detecting the radiation; this term is preferred over object-film distance (OFD) because some imaging modalities do not use film as the primary image receptor

PACS Picture archiving and communications system

pixel Picture element; the smallest component of a matrix

postprocessing image enhancement Digital manipulation of a radiographic image after its acquisition by the computer

processor A machine that automatically develops x-ray film

radiograph The x-ray image as viewed after it has been exposed and processed

radiographic position The specific position of the body or body part in relation to the table or image receptor

radiographic projection The path that the x-ray beam takes as it passes through the body; described as if the body is in the anatomical position

radiographic view The term used to explain how the image receptor sees the body image; the opposite of the radiographic projection

recorded detail The sharpness of structural lines as recorded on the radiograph

remnant beam (exit radiation) The x-ray beam that exits the patient; comprised of image-forming rays and scatter radiation

RIS Radiology information system

source-to-image receptor distance (SID) The distance from the source of radiation to the device that is detecting the radiation; this term is preferred over focal film distance (FFD)

source-to-object distance (SOD) The distance from the source of radiation to the part being examined; this term is preferred over focal object distance (FOD)

voxel Volume element; section of tissue represented by a pixel

window level Midpoint of densities in a digital image; used to adjust digital image brightness

window width Adjusts contrast of the digital image

CONCLUSION

Many other terms relating to radiography will be presented in appropriate classes during the course of your education. This listing is by no means complete, but it will give you a good start as you begin your studies. To assist with your comprehension of this material, be sure to complete the exercises at the end of this chapter.

Review Questions

1. Most medical terms have their origin in what languages?
   a. English and French
   b. Greek and Latin
   c. Egyptian and Middle Eastern
   d. English only
2. "CXR R/O COPD, HX MI" is an example of the use of:
   a. suffixes and prefixes.
   b. Greek in medicine.
   c. medical abbreviations that the radiologic technologist must know.
   d. medical abbreviations that are used only by physicians and nurses.
3. RT(R) stands for:
   a. radiologic technologist.
   b. radiologic technologist in radiography.
   c. registered technologist in radiography.
   d. routine radiography.
4. A procedure that has been ordered "STAT" should be performed:
   a. only by a physician.
   b. immediately.
   c. only when the patient has been held NPO.
   d. twice each day.
5. A cassette containing an imaging plate would be used in which of the following?
   a. CR
   b. DR
   c. film-screen
   d. CT
6. An organization to which radiologic technologists may belong is which of the following?
   a. JCAHO
   b. CDC
   c. ACR
   d. ASRT
7. A CXR would likely be performed for which of the following?
   a. URI
   b. UTI
   c. ROM
   d. PID
8. Because some imaging modalities do not use film, what term is preferred when referring to the destination of the image?
   a. Intensifying screen
   b. Processor

    c. Image receptor

    d. Radiograph

9. Electricity moves through the x-ray tube as a function of:

    a. SID and OID.

    b. kVp and mAs.

    c. PBL.

    d. SOD.

10. The visual radiographic image is comprised of which of the following?

    a. SID and OID

    b. Film and intensifying screens

    c. Density and contrast

    d. Recorded detail and processing

BIBLIOGRAPHY

Ballinger P and Frank E: *Merrill's atlas of radiographic positions and radiologic procedures*, ed. 10, St. Louis, 2003, Mosby.

Bushong S: *Radiologic science for technologists*, ed. 8, St. Louis, 2004, Mosby.

Callaway W: *Mosby's comprehensive review of radiography*, ed. 4, St. Louis, 2006, Mosby.

Fauber T: *Radiographic imaging & exposure*, ed. 2, St. Louis, 2004, Mosby.

Imaging Equipment

William J. Callaway

OBJECTIVES

On completion of this chapter, you should be able to:

- Describe the x-ray tube and name its two main components.
- Explain what energy conversion produces x-rays at the anode.
- Describe screen-film systems.
- Describe the function of the fluoroscope.
- Describe the function of computed tomography.
- Explain two advantages of digital imaging.
- Explain how an image is made in nuclear medicine.
- Describe the use of portable radiographic and fluoroscopic units.
- Discuss how an image is formed in sonography.
- Describe tomography, and explain its significance in imaging.
- List the two types of information obtained by using MRI.
- Explain the primary use of PET.

Imaging the human body is the major thrust of radiography. In-depth knowledge of the equipment is essential for making proper exposures. Such studies are covered in detail in physics and equipment courses. This chapter will summarize the types of equipment used in imaging to help you understand what you will be seeing early in your educational program.

KEY TERMS

anode
cathode
digital imaging
image intensifier
intensifying screen
x-ray film
x-ray tube

CHAPTER OUTLINE

X-ray tube
Digital Imaging
Film-screen system
Fluoroscopy
Specialized imaging
    equipment
    Computed tomography
    Magnetic resonance
        imaging
    Positron emission
        tomography
    Nuclear medicine
    Portable radiography
        and fluoroscopy
Tomography
Sonography
Picture archiving and
    communication system
Conclusion

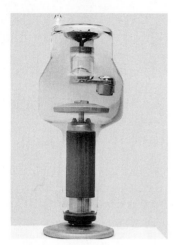

Fig. 9-1

A typical x-ray tube, showing cathode (top) and anode (bottom) within the glass envelope.

X-RAY TUBE

X-rays are not stored, nor do they come from radioactive materials. The radiologic technologist manufactures x-rays for each exposure using technical factors manipulated on the x-ray control panel. X-rays are produced by a series of energy conversions. The primary items needed for the production of x-rays are (1) a source of electrons, (2) a means to accelerate the electrons, and (3) a way to bring the electrons to a sudden stop. This is all accomplished in the x-ray tube. Details about the process of imaging are presented in Chapter 11.

The **x-ray tube** is an evacuated glass bulb with positive (anode) and negative (cathode) electrodes (Fig. 9-1). The **anode** is an electrode toward which negatively charged electrons migrate. The **cathode** is a filament that gives off electrons when heated (the source of electrons). As several thousand volts of electricity are applied to the tube, these electrons are driven across a short distance at very high speed (the means to accelerate the electrons) and strike the anode with high kinetic energy (the way to bring the electrons to a sudden stop). Because energy can neither be created nor destroyed, an energy conversion takes place; this energy conversion is the result of the sudden deceleration of the electrons at the anode. The primary by-product (>99%) of this energy conversion is heat. However, x-rays are also produced (<1%), and they emanate from the tube in all directions. The x-rays exit the tube housing through a device consisting of open lead shutters called a *collimator*.

DIGITAL IMAGING

Digital imaging equipment enhances images of the body, but it does not provide cross-sectional views. The primary advantages of digital equipment include the ability to post-process images in a variety of ways to provide multiple views of the anatomy. In digital radiography, the density and contrast of the image can be altered any time after the completion of the study without re-exposing the patient. In digital fluoroscopy, most of the follow-up "overhead" films are eliminated. The images are stored in a computer and can be transferred to multiple locations on a network. In digital imaging studies of arteries, for example, it is possible to remove the tissue and bones from the image.

FILM-SCREEN SYSTEM

After traversing the patient, the x-rays continue to a cassette that contains the intensifying screens and x-ray film. The primary means of making a radiographic image is through the use of a film-screen system. The **intensifying screen** is a sheet of plastic that is embedded with crystals called *phosphors*. When struck by radiation, phosphors glow with visible light; this light from the phosphors exposes the x-ray film, which is sandwiched between intensifying screens in the lid and the base of the cassette. The phosphors produce thousands of light rays for each x-ray striking them, thereby significantly reducing the amount of radiation necessary to make a good exposure. In the interest of patient safety, it is imperative that dosages be kept as low as possible. Approximately 95% of the image on the film is made by light from the intensifying screens; only 5% of the image is made directly by the x-rays.

The **x-ray film** is a sheet of polyester plastic coated with a thin layer of gelatin and silver compounds (Fig. 9-2). The image contained in the film is made visible by developing the film; the finished radiograph then becomes a permanent record of the examination and is considered a legal document.

Some cassettes contain only one intensifying screen and a sheet of x-ray film that is coated on only one side. This film-screen system provides excellent recorded detail (resolution) and is used primarily in radiography of the extremities.

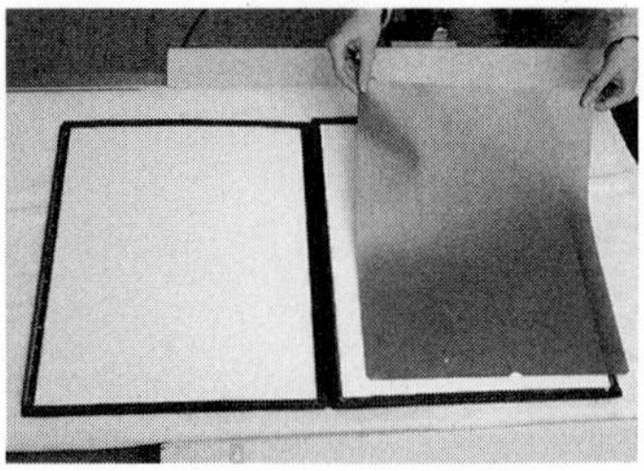

Fig. 9-2

Placement of a sheet of x-ray film into a cassette sandwiched within a pair of intensifying screens.

FLUOROSCOPY

Certain examinations in radiology require the use of fluoroscopy, which provides a "live-action" view of the interior of the body. There is no need to wait for film to be developed, because the image is immediately displayed on a television monitor. In fluoroscopy, the x-ray tube in most installations is located inside the x-ray table. The radiation passes through the tabletop and the patient, and it strikes the fluoroscopic screen to produce an image of the patient's body part. The image is dim at this stage. A device known as an **image intensifier** electronically improves and enhances the image and transmits it to the television monitor. Usually the radiologist operates the fluoroscopy unit while the radiologic technologist assists with the procedure. If the radiologist wants to make a permanent record of the image, digital fluoroscopy allows an image to be captured, saved in a computer, and post-processed in a variety of ways. On older equipment, a spot-film device, which is attached to the fluoroscope, is used. This device allows the image to be transferred to x-ray film, which is later processed and kept for analysis.

SPECIALIZED IMAGING EQUIPMENT

This section presents other imaging equipment used to perform radiographic procedures in special situations.

Computed Tomography

Computed tomography (CT) units provide cross-sectional views of the body. This imaging equipment greatly improves diagnoses and, in many cases, eliminates the need for exploratory surgery. With the patient lying

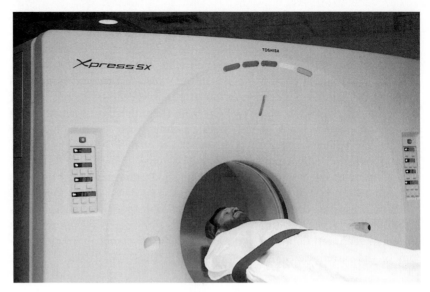

Fig. 9-3

The CT scanner, shown here with a patient in position through the gantry, has become a routine diagnostic tool.

on a movable couch, an x-ray tube and a radiation detector rotate around the table; this rotation provides the computer with a "slab" of information about the patient's body. The computer reconstructs the information into an image that is viewed on a television screen and stored for later retrieval and interpretation. CT scanners are able to obtain several dozen slices" of information with one exposure (Fig. 9-3).

Magnetic Resonance Imaging

Magnetic resonance imaging (MRI) units allow cross-sectional views of the body to be made without the use of ionizing radiation. With the patient lying on the couch in the cylindrical imager, the body part in question is exposed to a magnetic field and radio wave transmission. The images are produced in the computer by reconstructing the information that was received from the interaction of radio waves and magnetism with the body part. The information and images provide the physician with data about both the anatomy and the physiology of the body part being examined (Fig. 9-4).

Positron Emission Tomography

Positron emission tomography (PET) is similar to nuclear medicine in that it uses a radiopharmaceutical injected into the circulatory system to image the area of interest. However, PET is used to evaluate the physiology or function of an organ or system in the body. The radiation

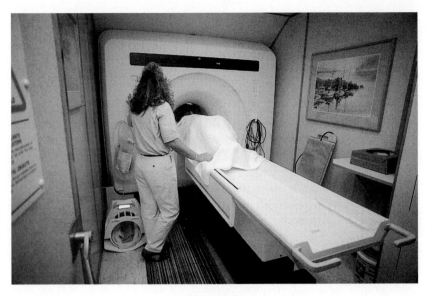

Fig. 9-4

The MRI unit is fast becoming a supplement to—or a replacement for—
other imaging procedures.

emanates from the body and is received by radiation detectors. The resulting images are cross-sectional and indicate how the radiopharmaceutical was taken up and used by the body. Because this chemical is treated by the body much like its own naturally occurring components, the information acquired is a highly accurate representation of the function of the area in question.

Nuclear Medicine

In nuclear medicine, radioactive materials introduced into the body are used to produce images of major organs. The radioactive material concentrates in the area of interest and emits radiation; this radiation is then detected by a sensing device and is computed into an image.

Portable Radiography and Fluoroscopy

Portable radiography and fluoroscopy can be performed if the patient cannot be moved to the radiology department. Mobile radiography units operate from conventional electrical circuits or battery power. The quality of images of some body parts is equivalent to that obtained in the radiology department. However, many radiographic procedures cannot be performed with a portable unit. Portable radiography is used in such areas as the OR, PAR, ICU, CCU, burn unit, orthopedic unit, and morgue.

Mobile fluoroscopy (C-arm) is used primarily in the operating room, where the surgeon must see the images immediately. Portable fluoroscopy must be used with great care to prevent those involved—both workers and patients—from being unnecessarily irradiated.

Tomography

Tomography is a technique used to obtain radiographs of a section or slice of a body part, as in the use of computed tomography. In conventional tomography, however, a computer is not used; the x-ray tube and film are connected by a rod and set in motion in opposite directions during the exposure. All structures above and below a particular level of the body are blurred while the particular level being studied remains in focus. Once used extensively, the current primary use of conventional tomography is during intravenous urograms (x-ray studies of the kidneys).

Sonography

Sonography uses high-frequency sound waves, which is a form of nonionizing radiation, to obtain sectional images of the body. Originally used by the military to detect enemy submarines, sonography is a useful diagnostic tool in certain areas of radiology. The sound waves bounce off interior structures of the body and return as echoes to a probe from which images can be electronically displayed on a television screen; permanent images can then be made from the screen. Cross-sectional images of the body are obtained using this method. Evaluation of moving organs can also be made with sonography. A type of sonography known as the Doppler technique is used to evaluate blood flow through the arteries.

Picture Archiving and Communication System

After reading the descriptions of imaging equipment presented in this chapter, you can see that computers play a vital role in radiologic technology. Computed imaging procedures such as digital radiography, computed tomography, nuclear medicine, digital sonography, and magnetic resonance imaging can be combined into a network. The picture archiving and communication system (PACS) brings digital imaging together with hospital and radiology information systems; it allows for the total management of a patient's case. Conventional radiographs can also be digitized and entered into the system.

Digital images and patient information form a computer network that can be accessed from any workstation that is connected to the system. Data are stored on optical disks. Information can be transmitted from the computer storage device via cable throughout the hospital and vicinity or via satellite across the world. A total PACS eliminates the need for x-ray film. Because the images are ultimately viewed on monitors, resolution is of the utmost importance.

PACS continues to grow in use as the cost of technology decreases. The ability to manage all imaging procedures—as well as examination interpretations, scheduling, patient history, cost analyses, demographics, and billing—makes PACS an invaluable tool in total patient care. Digital imaging and communications in medicine (DICOM) is a standard protocol used for blending PACS and the various imaging modalities discussed here. This is another exciting area in which the technologist must become proficient.

Conclusion

Radiographic imaging can be one of the most exciting activities in any hospital, but keeping abreast of the continual advances in imaging equipment is a challenge for all radiologic technologists. An in-depth knowledge of physics and equipment is a necessary basis for understanding the latest technologic advancements in radiography. All imaging occurs at the atomic level in the body. Physics is not a topic to be feared; it should be seen as the basis for all of diagnostic imaging. It is also apparent that the computer is a vital component of diagnostic imaging; study of the operation and uses of computers in medicine is mandatory for anyone entering the field of radiography, and this is why an introduction to computer science is required in the radiologic technology curriculum. With all of this knowledge and understanding, you will be prepared for the inevitable changes in imaging techniques and equipment.

Review Questions

1. What are the two main parts of the x-ray tube?
   a. Glass bulb and cathode
   b. Cathode and electrode
   c. Anode and cathode
   d. Collimator and glass bulb
2. The conversion of energy that produces x-rays is a result of _____ striking the _____.
   a. protons, cathode
   b. x-rays, anode
   c. electrons, cathode
   d. electrons, anode
3. Most of the image produced on radiographic film comes from:
   a. electrons.
   b. x-rays.
   c. light from intensifying screens.
   d. protons.
4. Live action radiography describes which of the following?
   a. CT scanning
   b. MRI
   c. PET
   d. Fluoroscopy

5. A system using telecommunications, digital imaging, and total management of radiology services describes which of the following?
   a. Total quality management (TQM)
   b. PACS
   c. Continuous quality improvement (CQI)
   d. Quality circles

6. Which of the following is an imaging modality that uses sound to see?
   a. MRI
   b. PACS
   c. Sonography
   d. PET

7. Substances that emit visible light when struck by radiation are called:
   a. image receptors.
   b. phosphors.
   c. contrast agents.
   d. electrodes.

8. The energy conversion that takes place in the x-ray tube primarily produces which of the following?
   a. X-rays
   b. Sound waves
   c. Visible light
   d. Heat

9. Radioactive materials are used in which of the following imaging modalities?
   a. X-ray production
   b. Magnetic resonance imaging
   c. Computed tomography
   d. Nuclear medicine

10. Imaging equipment that allows for manipulation of the image after exposure is called:
    a. image intensifier.
    b. intensifying screen.
    c. x-ray film.
    d. digital imaging.

BIBLIOGRAPHY

Ballinger P, Frank E: *Merrill's atlas of radiographic positions and radiologic procedures*, ed. 10, St. Louis, 2003, Mosby.

Bushong S: *Radiologic science for technologists*, ed. 8, St. Louis, 2004, Mosby.

Callaway W: *Mosby's comprehensive review of radiography*, ed. 4, St. Louis, 2006, Mosby.

Snopek A: *Fundamentals of special radiographic procedures*, ed. 5, St. Louis, 2006, Saunders.

Radiographic Examinations: Diagnosing Disease and Injury

William J. Callaway

OBJECTIVES

On completion of this chapter, you should be able to:

- **Describe internal and external patient preparation.**

- **Describe examinations that use iodine, barium, or air as a contrast agent.**

- **Describe what is included in skull and headwork.**

- **Describe what is included in thoracic radiography.**

- **Describe what is included in extremity radiography.**

- **Describe what is included in spinal radiography.**

- **List conditions for which abdominal radiography may be performed.**

- **Briefly explain esophagograms, upper GI series, small bowel studies, and barium enemas.**

- **List and describe the examinations that are referred to as special procedures.**

Radiography is one of the primary methods of diagnosing disease. Positioning and procedures will be covered in depth during your education, but this chapter provides an excellent overview of what you will observe and experience in the clinical setting. Not all institutions

KEY TERMS

arteriogram
arthrogram
barium
barium enema
contrast media
cystogram
esophagram
excretory urography
external preparation
fluoroscopic studies
hysterosalpingogram
internal preparation
iodine
mammogram
myelogram
sialogram
tomography
upper gastrointestinal (GI)
    series
venogram

CHAPTER OUTLINE

*Patient preparation and
    contrast media*
Radiographic studies
    Skull and headwork
    Thoracic cavity
    Extremities
    Spine
    Abdomen
            Continued

Fluoroscopic
   examinations
   Esophagram
   Upper gastrointestinal
      series
   Barium enema
   Urinary system studies
   Endoscopic retrograde
      cholangiopancreato-
      graphy
Special radiographic
   procedures
   Arteriogram
      (angiogram)
   Arthrogram
   Hysterosalpingogram
   Lithotripsy
   Mammogram
   Myelogram
   Sialogram
   Tomography
   Venogram
Conclusion

perform all of the procedures described here, because hospital services vary. However, you should be familiar with all types of studies, because your actual employment may be elsewhere. In addition, as a student radiographer, you must become competent in the many procedures performed by diagnostic radiographers.

The radiographic examinations discussed in this chapter are divided into radiographic, fluoroscopic, and special procedures. Bear in mind that these procedures may be performed using digital fluoroscopy, digital radiography, or film-screen imaging. There are two important components of most radiographic examinations: patient preparation and contrast media.

PATIENT PREPARATION AND CONTRAST MEDIA

Depending on the examination to be performed, patient preparation is done either internally or externally. **External preparation** requires removing clothing and jewelry that may be covering the area of the body through which the x-rays must pass. Many types of clothing material show up on film as obscure shadows. Buttons and zippers may hide small disease processes or fractures. If a region of the head is being radiographed, false teeth must be removed, because they interfere with the passage of x-rays through the mouth. Rings and watches must be removed when radiographing the hand and wrist. One of the most common mistakes is forgetting to remove a necklace before performing a chest examination (Fig. 10-1, *A*). Always ask each patient to remove jewelry before beginning an examination. If there is any chance that an area of the body to be radiographed is pierced, be certain to ask the patient about that as well, and have piercing jewelry removed from the part. Failure to do so results in a double dose of radiation to the patient, because the radiographs must then be retaken. Note if there is a tattoo in the area being radiographed. If the ink used in the tattoo contains metallic pigmentation, it may show as a faint shadow on the radiographic image. Proper examination of the patient is the responsibility of the radiographer. Checks for unwanted objects should be verbal, visual, and tactile.

Internal preparation for some examinations includes cleansing enemas; these are performed so that structures in the abdomen are not obscured by gas and fecal material. Most of these preparations are performed on the nursing units or by the patient at home; however, awareness of the hospital procedure aids in explaining the importance of this preparation and answering any questions the patient may have. As a competent radiographer, you must be aware of all aspects of patient care that relate to the examination, regardless of whether you perform them.

Contrast media are solutions or gases introduced into the body to provide contrast on a radiograph between an organ and its surrounding tissue. There are three general types of contrast media used in radiography: iodine-based media, barium-based media, and air.

The element **iodine** has a relatively high atomic number. Because x-rays do not readily pass through iodine, solutions that contain this element are placed in organs and blood vessels to provide a contrast between these structures and their surrounding tissues. The radiographer must be alert to possible adverse reactions the patient may experience when using iodinated contrast media. The use of nonionic contrast media greatly reduces the occurrence of such side effects, but it does not eliminate them.

The element **barium** has approximately the same contrast qualities as iodine, but the similarity ends there. Barium sulfate is inert and cannot be absorbed by the body; this makes it the medium of choice for gastrointestinal studies (Fig. 10-1, *B* and *C*). Patient allergic reaction to barium is almost nonexistent because of its inert properties.

However, there are exceptions: for example, if surgery appears imminent or if a perforated stomach or intestine is suspected, barium would not be used, because it cannot be absorbed. In such cases, a water-soluble iodine contrast agent is used, because it is readily absorbed should spillage into the abdominal cavity occur.

Air is used as a contrast agent primarily in chest radiography. Unlike iodine and barium, air is easily penetrated by x-rays, thus providing contrast between lung tissue, vessel markings, and the air sacs themselves. Air may also be used with barium-based or iodine-based contrast media to provide a double contrast; this is done in air-contrast colon studies and arthrography.

A   B   C

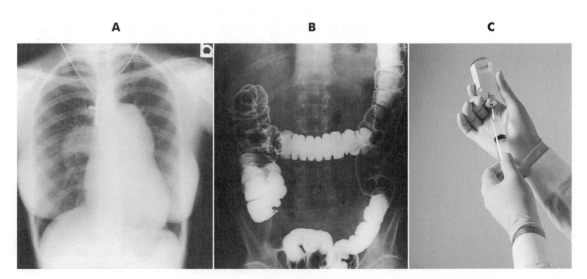

Fig. 10-1

A, Failure to remove a patient's jewelry results in the retaking of a radiograph. **B**, Contrast medium provides contrast between an organ and surrounding tissue. **C**, A radiographer prepares an injection of an iodinated contrast agent.

RADIOGRAPHIC STUDIES

Radiographic studies are examinations performed by the radiographer on particular regions of the body with the use of the x-ray tube. The images are recorded on an imaging plate or radiographic film and subsequently interpreted by the radiologist. Listed below, according to body region, are the radiographic examinations performed and a few comments that will help you with your understanding of the studies.

Skull and Headwork

Radiographic studies of the region above the neck comprise the skull and headwork category. Many of these procedures are performed primarily with computed tomography (CT) or panoramic tomography. Those examinations that may still be performed without CT include the skull, facial bones, nasal bones, mandible, temporomandibular joints (TMJs), and sinuses. These examinations require multiple views, and some are rather difficult to perform. Headwork usually is performed to evaluate possible fractures, locate foreign bodies, or examine abnormalities. Areas such as the sella turcica, zygomatic arches, mastoids, and orbits are increasingly imaged using CT. The mandible and TMJs are primarily imaged using panoramic tomography.

Thoracic Cavity

The thoracic cavity includes the bones and tissues of the chest region, and this is the most commonly radiographed region of the body. Exact positioning and careful exposure techniques are essential for proper imaging. Other studies of the thoracic cavity include the ribs, the sternoclavicular joints, the sternum, and the heart. A heart examination may include introducing barium into the esophagus to see if the heart is enlarged and pressing on and displacing the esophagus.

Thoracic studies may be performed to evaluate fluid in the lungs, overexpansion, collapsed lungs, tumors, heart enlargement, other heart and lung abnormalities, as well as fractures of the ribs, sternoclavicular joints, and sternum.

Extremities

This category is generally divided into the upper and lower extremities, and it also includes the shoulder and pelvic regions. Upper extremity studies are done of the fingers, the hands, the wrists, the forearms, the elbows, the humeri, the shoulders, the clavicles, the acromioclavicular joints, and the scapulas. The lower extremity studies include radiographs of the toes, the feet, the heels, the ankles, the lower legs, the knees, the patellae, the femurs, the hips, and the pelvis. Bone studies always require at least two views that are to be taken at right angles to one another; joint studies may also include an oblique view. Care must be taken when performing bone and joint studies because of the possibility of broken bones (fractures). Studies in patient care explain how injured patients are properly handled. Radiologic examinations of the extremities are performed to evaluate bone fractures, dislocations, arthritis, osteoporosis, and tumors.

Spine

This category includes studies of the cervical spine, the thoracic (dorsal) spine, the lumbar spine, the sacroiliac joints, the sacrum, and the coccyx. Also included are examinations such as scoliosis evaluation and bone age determination. Spinal injury patients must be handled carefully, because further injury can result if the nerves are damaged. Spinal injuries are painful, and the radiographer must make the patient as comfortable as possible while obtaining as many diagnostic radiographs as necessary for the physician's evaluation. In addition to evaluating severe trauma, spinal studies are performed to evaluate the extent of arthritis of the spine, abnormal curvatures, muscle spasms that may be causing the spine to curve, and slipped vertebrae.

Abdomen

Many of the studies involving the abdomen require the use of fluoroscopy and are discussed more fully in the next section. However, some radiographic surveys are made of the abdomen without the use of contrast agents and fluoroscopy. Careful patient handling is important, because many patients who are having abdomen examinations are quite ill and in pain. Again, it is your responsibility to properly care for the patient in the radiology department. Abdominal studies often determine the presence of foreign masses, calcifications, the distribution of air in the intestines, the size, shape, and location of major organs, such as the liver, kidney, and spleen, and bony and soft tissue damage. They are also used to evaluate individual organs, though most such studies are performed using CT.

Radiographic studies of the urinary system called **excretory urography** (sometimes also called *intravenous urography* or *intravenous pyelograms [IVP]*) are often performed. These involve the use of an iodinated contrast agent injected into the bloodstream through a vein in the arm. Radiographs are obtained at intervals of several minutes during the time that the kidneys, the ureters, and the bladder are highlighted by the contrast material. Intravenous urography helps to visualize stones in the urinary system and to evaluate kidney function. Examination of the urinary system is increasingly being performed using CT.

FLUOROSCOPIC EXAMINATIONS

Fluoroscopic studies require a radiologist or radiologist assistant (RA) to perform and monitor the examination in most circumstances. There is a need to view the study "live." The following discussion highlights the most commonly performed examinations. Digital images or spot films are obtained by the radiologist during the fluoroscopy. Non-digital fluoroscopic studies are followed by radiography of the body part and region on larger radiographic film. Digital studies involve postprocessing of the digital fluoroscopic image.

Esophagram

The **esophagram**, which is a study of the esophagus, requires the patient to swallow a barium sulfate preparation. The radiologist or RA obtains digital images or spot films. Often the patient has difficulty swallowing the barium because it is a thick, paste-like mixture that lingers in the esophagus. Esophagrams may visualize tumors, constrictions, and spasms.

Upper Gastrointestinal Series

Studies of the stomach, often called an **upper gastrointestinal (GI) series**, are performed with the use of barium sulfate. The patient must drink the solution while fluoroscopically controlled images are obtained (Fig. 10-2). The upper GI series is performed to evaluate hiatal hernias, peptic ulcers, and other stomach disorders. If the small intestine must be evaluated, a small bowel examination is performed; this involves radiographing the abdomen every hour to watch the progress of the barium meal through the small intestine. It is important to advise the patient ahead of time that this study takes several hours to perform. Small bowel studies are performed to investigate tumors, inflammation, obstructions, and the malabsorption of nutrients. Fiber-optic endoscopy is also used to examine the stomach.

Barium Enema

The radiographic examination of the colon, which is called a **barium enema**, involves introducing a barium solution into the colon. Although this study is not unduly painful, it is often considered uncomfortable. Because the barium solution may cause cramping and discomfort, it is imperative that the radiologist and radiographer work rapidly and accurately so that the barium solution can be excreted as soon as possible. Glucagon is often used in air contrast studies of the colon to reduce cramping and peristalsis. Barium studies may indicate tumors, bowel obstructions, diverticula, and inflammation. A study called the air-contrast barium enema is performed by introducing air in addition to the barium to provide a double contrast; this allows for better visualization of such abnormalities in the colon as diverticula and polyps. Colonoscopy using an endoscope is proving to be a more effective tool in visualizing the colon and has the advantage of being able to obtain a biopsy at the same time. It is gradually replacing the barium enema, as is virtual colonoscopy, a CT procedure used to reconstruct the colon using computer images.

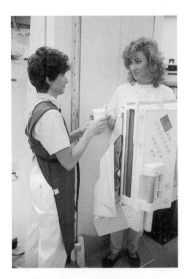

Fig. 10-2

The radiographer provides patient care during an upper GI series and explains the use of the contrast agent barium sulfate.

Urinary System Studies

In addition to the previously described IVP, there are studies of the urinary system that may be done under fluoroscopic control. For example, the **cystogram**, which is a study of the urinary bladder, involves filling the bladder with a contrast agent and then taking spot films and radiographs. A **voiding cystourethrogram**, which evaluates urination, is similar except that the patient empties the bladder while under fluoroscopic observation.

Endoscopic Retrograde Cholangiopancreatography

An endoscopic retrograde cholangiopancreatography (ERCP) is performed to diagnose anomalies in the biliary system or the pancreas. A contrast medium is injected into the common bile duct after it is located with a fiberoptic scope passed down the esophagus, through the stomach, and into the small intestine. Radiographs are then taken with a digital fluoroscope or spot-film device.

SPECIAL RADIOGRAPHIC PROCEDURES

Special radiographic procedures are studies that require special equipment or that are not performed routinely. The studies listed here require the use of x-rays and do not include special imaging modalities, which are included in Chapter 9.

Arteriogram (Angiogram)

The **arteriogram** is a study that visualizes the arteries of a particular body region. An iodine-based contrast material is injected, and a very rapid sequence of images is made; this allows for the viewing of the blood flow through the artery and evaluation of the shape and condition of the artery itself. Performing arteriography involves the use of digital fluoroscopy, automatic injectors, and a sterile field (Fig. 10-3, *A*).

Arthrogram

The **arthrogram** is used to evaluate the structures in and around a joint space; the most common joints involved are the knee and shoulder. An iodinated contrast medium is injected directly into the joint space. Fluoroscopy is used and, if digital, images are obtained by the radiologist. Spot films obtained by the radiographer may be taken following routine fluoroscopy. Arthrography is gradually being replaced by magnetic resonance imaging (MRI).

Hysterosalpingogram

The **hysterosalpingogram** is an examination of the uterus and fallopian tubes. This examination allows for the evaluation of the shape of the

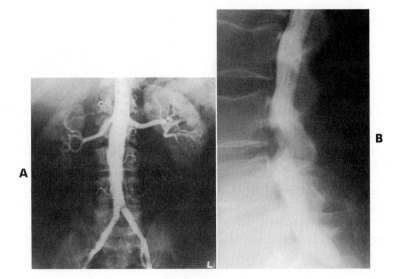

Fig. 10-3

A, An arteriogram. **B**, A myelogram.

uterus and the patency of the oviducts. Usually an oil-based iodinated contrast medium is used to fill those structures. Fluoroscopy is used, and conventional radiographs may also be obtained.

Lithotripsy

The radiographer may also be involved in a lithotripsy procedure, which destroys stones in the kidney or ureter by using sonic shock waves. The patient is placed in a tub of water against a special probe. The shock wave passes into the body and destroys the stone. The radiographer's role may include taking localizing radiographs and assisting with fluoroscopy, which is necessary for the proper placement of equipment both inside and around the patient.

Mammogram

A **mammogram** is a radiographic study of the breast. Because breast tissue has very little inherent contrast, high-contrast radiographic film and specially designed cassettes are used. The breast is compressed to allow for maximum visualization. Modern imaging equipment provides the detail that is of critical importance in the early detection of breast cancer.

Myelogram

The **myelogram** is an examination of the subarachnoid space of the spinal cord. After removal of some of the spinal fluid, a water-soluble iodine-based contrast agent is injected into the space through the patient's back or neck. Fluoroscopy is used to guide the flow of the contrast agent and to obtain radiographs of the region. The patient may be given a sedative, and this causes drowsiness; therefore, patient care must be at its best (Fig. 10-3, B). Myelography is gradually being replaced by MRI.

Sialogram

A **sialogram** is a study of the salivary glands after they have been injected with a contrast agent. Both fluoroscopy and routine radiography of the mandible may be used, usually to detect blockages caused by stones.

Tomography

Tomography, which is also called body-section radiography, is a procedure that puts the x-ray tube and film in motion during exposure to blur structures above and below the body part of interest. This is a means to radiographically "cut through" sections of tissue in the body. Though used less often because of the availability of other imaging modalities, a basic understanding of tomography is still quite necessary as a result of its continued use in urography. During tomography, the x-ray tube and the tray holding the cassette are connected so that they travel in opposite directions during exposure. The tube travel length can be set in relation to the cassette travel length by adjusting the pivot level. The tissue section of the body at the level of the pivot point will be in focus while the other tissue layers will blur.

Venogram

A **venogram** is a study used to evaluate the veins in a particular area of the body. Contrast medium is injected into the veins, and radiographs are made. Fluoroscopy is not usually used when only a venogram is performed. Venograms of the lower extremities may be performed with a device that allows for visualization from the pelvis to the feet on one film. Venograms of other body parts are performed with cassettes sized to match the body part. Venography is supplemented with, and gradually being replaced by, sonography.

CONCLUSION

The preceding discussion of radiographic, fluoroscopic, and special radiographic examinations is not meant to be all-inclusive; the studies described are the ones that you will most likely see in average and large departments. Smaller departments may never perform some of the procedures, whereas others are involved with even more specialized studies. The step-by-step procedures for performing these examinations will be presented in your course about radiographic procedures. However, you may soon be observing these procedures or hearing discussions about them. This basic knowledge of examinations will help you become oriented to the clinical environment.

Review Questions

1. For what reason must clothing and jewelry be removed from the area to be radiographed?
   a. They will become radioactive when the x-rays strike them.
   b. They may obscure the area of interest.
   c. They may become hot.
   d. They may be ruined, and the patient will be upset.

2. Preparation of the patient for a radiographic examination is the responsibility of the:
   a. physician who orders the procedure.
   b. nurse.
   c. radiographer.
   d. All of the above

3. Which of the following contrast agents is used in chest radiography?
   a. Barium sulfate
   b. Dye
   c. Iodine
   d. Air

4. Which of the following is the contrast agent that may cause an adverse reaction?
   a. Air
   b. Iodine
   c. Barium
   d. Dye

5. Portions of the circulatory system may be imaged during a procedure called a(n):
   a. cholangiogram.
   b. voiding cystourethrogram.
   c. esophagogram.
   d. arteriogram.

6. An x-ray study of the female reproductive system is called a(n):
   a. lithotripsy.
   b. mammogram.
   c. hysterosalpingogram.
   d. myelogram.

7. A radiographic examination of the salivary glands is called a(n):
   a. sialogram.
   b. cystogram.
   c. hysterosalpingogram.
   d. myelogram.

8. The IVP images the:
   a. urinary system.
   b. colon.

   c. gall bladder.

   d. joints.

9. Arthrograms are performed to visualize which of the following areas?

   a. Urinary system

   b. Colon

   c. Gallbladder

   d. Joints

10. Preparation of the patient should include which of the following skills?

   a. Visual

   b. Verbal

   c. Tactile

   d. All of the above

BIBLIOGRAPHY

Callaway W: *Mosby's comprehensive review of radiography*, ed. 4, St. Louis, 2006, Mosby.

Ehrlich R, McCloskey E, Daly J: *Patient care in radiography: with an introduction to medical imaging*, ed. 6, St. Louis, 2004, Mosby.

Eisenberg R, Dennis C: *Comprehensive radiographic pathology*, ed. 3, St. Louis, 2003, Mosby.

Snopek A: *Fundamentals of special radiographic procedures*, ed. 5, St. Louis, 2006 Saunders.

Torres L: *Basic medical techniques and patient care for radiographers*, ed. 6, Philadelphia, 2003, Lippincott Williams and Wilkins.

Imaging: Life Cycle and Quality

LaVerne Tolley Gurley

OBJECTIVES

On completion of this chapter, you should be able to:

- **Explain the function of the film processor.**

- **List radiographic factors that affect film density.**

- **List radiographic factors that affect contrast.**

- **Explain what is meant by radiographic distortion and magnification.**

- **List radiographic factors that affect distortion and magnification.**

- **Explain radiographic details.**

- **List radiographic factors that affect image detail.**

- **Discuss the radiologic technologist's role in image production and evaluation.**

LIFE CYCLE OF A RADIOGRAPH

By carefully examining the route that a radiograph travels from the time it is ordered until it is placed in the patient's file, it is possible to follow what might be called its "life cycle." This chapter traces this progression in an attempt to outline several of the factors that go into the production and use of radiographs. For every concept briefly presented here, there is a substantial amount of theory and practical application that will be presented in the classroom and in clinical experience.

KEY TERMS

collimators
contrast
density
detail
distortion
filters
focal spot
grid
kilovoltage
milliamperage
milliampere-seconds
  (mAs)
processing
subject contrast

CHAPTER OUTLINE

Life cycle of a radiograph
    Conception in the mind
        of the physician
    Growth in the hands of
        the radiologic
        technologist
    Birth in the processor
    Useful life
Factors affecting
    radiographic quality
    Density
    Contrast
    Distortion and
        magnification
    Detail
Conclusion

Conception in the Mind of the Physician

The cycle begins as a concept in the mind of the physician when he or she is considering the best method of diagnosis for a disease process or injury; frequently the use of radiographic studies is the course of action. The physician decides that, by studying a particular region of the patient's body with the use of radiographs, it may be possible to identify the patient's problem. The examinations ordered usually cover the area of interest as well as the surrounding tissues.

Growth in the Hands of the Radiologic Technologist

The radiologic technologist excels in the art and science of making radiographs. Once the physician has determined the need for radiographic studies, it is up to the radiologic technologist to obtain the best possible diagnostic radiographs. The growth of the radiograph begins when the radiologic technologist evaluates the orders from the physician and greets the patient in the imaging department. Establishing a cordial relationship with the patient aids the radiologic technologist in obtaining the needed radiographs.

The radiograph continues in its cycle with the positioning of the patient. Next, the radiologic technologist determines the appropriate exposure factors to be used to place the image on the film. On measuring the thickness of the patient and determining the overall tissue density, the radiologic technologist may consult a technique chart for the proper exposure factors. The exposure is made when the radiation passes through the patient and strikes the film/screen system. Factors that affect radiographic quality are discussed later in this chapter.

This is a greatly simplified account of what transpires in the production of the image. At this point, a diagnostic radiograph still does not exist. The image of the patient is contained in the emulsion of the radiographic film and is called the latent image; it is not visible to the human eye and thus needs to undergo **processing**, which is a series of steps that converts the latent image to a visible image.

Birth in the Processor

An automatic film processor is used to make the latent image visible. The birth of the radiograph occurs at this stage. Film processors are now automatic and perform the functions that were once done by hand. Mechanization and computerization of this procedure has led to excellent quality control and consistency from one film to the next.

The automatic processor contains four compartments through which a series of rollers transports the film. As the film is fed into the processor, it goes directly into a solution called the *developer*. The developer causes the film to swell slightly so that the chemicals can act on the image. These chemicals cause the crystals in the film that were struck by x-rays to become black metallic silver; this is what causes parts of the image to appear black. The film is in the developer about 20 seconds, and it is then transported into the next solution, which is called the *fixer*. The fixer acts on the unexposed crystals, removes them from the film, and stops further development. The unexposed areas become the transparent regions on the film.

After development and fixation, the film is moved into a tank of wash water to remove any remaining chemicals from its surface. The last step is passage through the dryer compartment, where the film is completely dried. When it emerges from the processor, the radiograph is completely prepared for viewing.

Useful Life

The radiograph is examined by the radiologic technologist or quality control technologist for proper positioning and exposure. It is then taken to the radiologist to be interpreted, and a diagnosis may then be given. The physician who ordered the studies may visit the imaging department for a consultation with the radiologist. The radiographs have come through a long routine, and, at this point, they have reached their useful life; the entire reason for their formation is the diagnosis of a condition. After the radiographs have been interpreted, they are assembled into the patient's file, along with a typewritten copy of the radiologist's report. Radiographs are kept on file for several years so that returning patients may have previous radiographs compared with recent ones.

When sufficient time has elapsed, old radiographs may be microfilmed and/or discarded. This is the end of the life cycle. Because of the high cost of film and the availability of certain raw materials, discarded film may be sold. The old film may be treated to remove the silver, which may then be reused. It is also possible to reuse the plastic base of the film. Thus, even at the end of the life cycle, the radiograph lives on by being recycled.

This discussion demonstrates that radiography is a long and involved process. There are numerous opportunities for error that must be avoided to produce an acceptable radiograph. Much of your course work will be involved with the individual stages in the life cycle of the radiograph, and Fig. 11-1 is a representation of the entire process.

FACTORS AFFECTING RADIOGRAPHIC QUALITY

Before discussing the factors that affect the radiograph, we should look at the control panel of a radiographic machine to know what controls are available for setting up a technique for obtaining optimal diagnostic quality.

The purpose of this text is not to examine in detail the physics involved in the production of x-rays but to provide an overview that will be helpful in the discussion of technical radiographic factors.

With the typical radiographic machine, the controls to be adjusted are (1) time, (2) voltage, and (3) amperage. Because x-rays are not produced

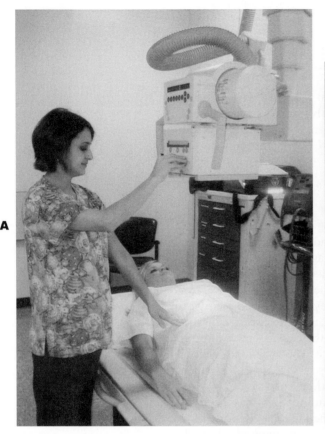
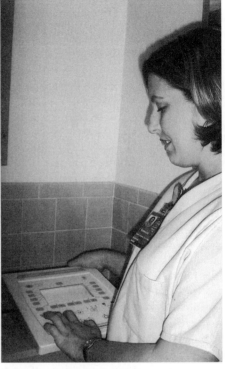

A   **B**

Fig. 11-1

A, The positioning of the patient is critical; the anatomy of interest must be imaged for diagnostic interpretation. (Courtesy of Amy Justice Hill, University of Mississippi Medical Center.) **B,** Exposure factors that affect the radiograph's diagnostic quality are selected at the control panel. (Courtesy of technologist Tamara Rodriguez, University of Mississippi Medical Center.)

unless the voltage is very high (i.e., thousands of volts), the term kilovolts is used. However, with the very high voltage, low amperage must be used, and thus we usually speak in terms of **milliamperage**; a milliampere is one thousandth of one ampere.

The timer is set simply to limit the time that x-rays will exit from the tube. For example, for a very thick body part, more radiation is needed than for a thinner part, and, generally, the time will be longer. Selecting the voltage setting is a more complicated procedure. Think of voltage as a "force" and as the factor that determines the penetrating ability of the radiation; it also affects the amount of radiation to a considerable extent, but mainly we think of voltage as a force that affects the energy of the x-rays. The higher the voltage setting, the more penetrating the radiation; thus more of the radiation will go deep into the tissues and

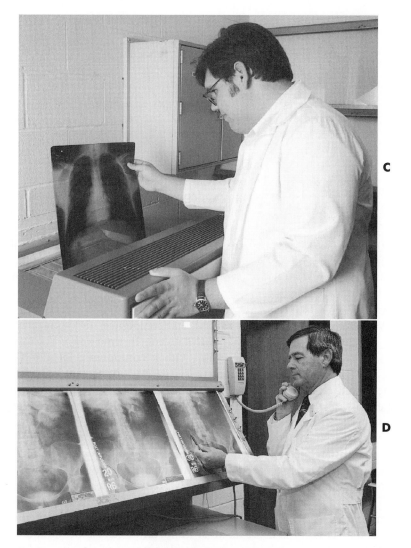

Fig. 11-1, cont'd

C, Checking the radiograph for diagnostic quality at the processor. (Courtesy of Kristopher Gurley; Morgan Murrell, photographer.) **D**, Interpreting the radiograph and making a diagnosis ends the radiographic cycle. (Courtesy of A. Glenn Swinny; Morgan Murrell, photographer.)

through the patient to darken the film. Radiation produced at low voltage settings is weak in energy and may be stopped or absorbed in the first few centimeters of tissue (Fig. 11-2).

Amperage can be thought of as the "amount" of radiation per unit time, and the quantity of amperage controls the darkness or density of the film. For example, at 100 **milliampere-seconds (mAs)** you would have twice the amount of radiation that you would have at 50 mAs. At 200 mAs, you would have twice the amount of radiation that you would have

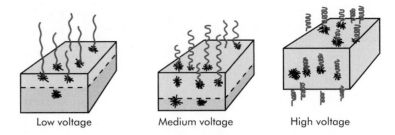

| Low voltage | Medium voltage | High voltage |

Fig. 11-2

The ability of radiation to penetrate solid matter increases
with increasing voltage.

at 100 mAs. Because amperage is "amount" per unit time, it is reasonable
to think of amperage per second or mA/seconds. For example, 100 mA
for 1 second equals 100 mA seconds, usually written "100 mAs"; 200 mA
for 1 second equals 200 mAs, or 200 mA multiplied by 1 half-second,
which also equals 100 mAs.

With these three factors in mind—time, amperage, and voltage—you
can then identify them on the control panel. In time you will learn to
adjust them for the desired results. Other components of the x-ray
machine that make up the control panel are voltage and amperage
meters, an on-off switch, circuit breakers, and other components,
depending on the complexity of the unit. Basically, however, voltage,
amperage, and time factors control the amount and quality of radiation
generated by the machine.

Many other factors affect the amount and quality of radiation the
film receives, and many other conditions and adjustments affect the quality of a radiograph.

The four factors that affect the quality of a radiograph, listed in order
of importance, are density, contrast, distortion or uneven magnification,
and detail. Density is listed as most important because detail and contrast are nonexistent without a perceptible amount of density, and more
radiographic examinations are repeated because of improper density
than because of all other factors combined.

Density

Density is defined as the logarithm of opacity (blackness). The *opacity* of
a film is the ratio of the amount of light incident on the film to the amount
transmitted by the film. In medical radiography, the x-rays responsible for
darkening the film represent *remnant* radiation; that is, the radiation
remaining in the beam after it has traversed the various thicknesses and
densities of tissue interposed between the tube and the film. Density, or
opacity, is mainly a measure of black metallic silver on the film.

Many factors affect the amount of remnant radiation available to
produce the darkening effect of the radiograph. There are also methods

of intensifying to enhance the effectiveness of the remnant radiation, all of which relate to radiographic density.

The factors that affect radiographic density include the following:
- Subject thickness and tissue density
- Kilovoltage
- Milliamperage
- Time
- Distance
- Film
- Intensifying screens
- Fog
- Cones and collimators
- Processing
- Grids
- Filters

Subject Thickness and Tissue Density

The subject or anatomic part is made up of several densities; for example, bone is denser than the surrounding soft tissue. The skull, with a high ratio of bone to soft tissue, will require more radiation than another body part of the same thickness for adequate density.

The density of tissues is mainly a matter of atomic number of the elements making up the tissues. Bone, which is made up of calcium (atomic number 20), phosphorus (atomic number 15), and other elements, has an average atomic number of approximately 14. However, soft tissue, which is mostly water, has an average atomic number of 7.5. The atomic number, however, does not tell the whole story, because the average atomic number of air and soft tissue is about the same. Yet, because air is a gas, it obeys the law of gases and fills a container; thus air molecules are not as tightly packed as water molecules. Another example is ice, which is frozen water with the same atomic number as water; however, it is about 9% less dense than water because of the molecular arrangement (Fig. 11-3).

The human body consists of four radiographic densities. They are listed here in order of the least dense to the most dense:
1. Gas, or air, which is present in such organs as the lungs, stomach, and intestines
2. Fat, which surrounds the kidneys and is present along the psoas muscle, the abdominal wall, and other organs
3. Muscle, which contains large amounts of water and has approximately the same density as the heart and blood vessels
4. Bone, which is denser than other tissues, with tooth enamel being the densest

A fifth density often encountered in radiography is metal. Metal is encountered in three ways:
1. Foreign bodies (e.g., swallowed articles such as gunshot pellets)
2. Prostheses such as metallic nails, screws, pins used to align fractured bones, and radium applicators

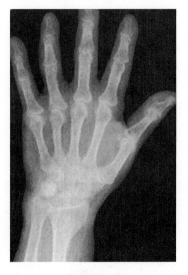

Fig. 11-3

Radiograph of the hand. Note thick wrist as opposed to fingers showing a difference in density.

3. Contrast media such as barium, which is a metallic salt, and media that contains iodine

Each radiographic density presents a difference in the degree of absorption of radiation. Gas is less dense than fat and thus absorbs less radiation. Fat is less dense than muscle and thus absorbs less radiation than muscle but more than air. Bone, being the most dense, absorbs more radiation than muscle, fat, or gas. Fig. 11-4 illustrates various radiographic appearances.

The thickness of the part to be radiographed also influences radiographic density. With all other factors remaining the same, the thicker the part, the greater the radiation absorption; thus the radiograph is less dense.

Kilovoltage

There are two reasons that kilovoltage has a profound effect on density:

1. The amount of x-rays produced is affected by tube kilovoltage.
2. The energy of the x-rays is affected by the kilovoltage. Kilovoltage determines the wavelength of radiation and thus its penetrating power; the greater the penetrating ability of the x-rays, the greater the amount of remnant radiation reaching the film to darken it.

As mentioned earlier, the higher the kilovoltage, the greater the energy of the radiation; hence, more x-rays traverse the patient and exit on the other side to darken the film (Fig. 11-2).

Milliamperage

The x-ray exposure rate is directly proportional to milliamperage; this is because milliamperage determines the amount of x-ray produced per unit of time. With all factors remaining the same, the greater the milliamper-

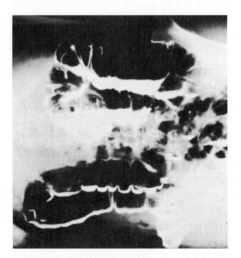

Fig. 11-4

This radiograph shows the radiographic densities of gas (or air), fat, muscle, and bone. The fifth density—the metallic contrast medium barium—is shown in this air-barium double-contrast colon study. NOTE: The heavy barium gravitates to the lower level; the lightweight air rises to the top.

age, the greater the amount of radiation produced. If the milliamperage is halved, the amount of x-rays is reduced by half. Thus the amount of remnant radiation is directly proportional to the milliamperage.

Time

A change in time produces the same effect as a comparable change in milliamperage; double the time and the density is doubled, halve the time and the density is halved. This is because a given exposure rate is allowed to act longer, and therefore more silver bromide crystals in the emulsion are, subsequent to processing, changed to black metallic silver. The term mAs is used to express quantity of radiation and represents the product of time and milliamperage. For example, 200 mA $\times$ $\frac{1}{10}$ sec = 20 mAs.

Distance

Distance as discussed here relates to the distance from the radiation source (the x-ray tube) to the radiographic film. X-rays emerge from the tube, diverge, and proceed in straight paths. Because of the divergence, they cover an increasingly larger area as they travel farther away from the tube. The radiation emitted from the tube remains the same, but because a larger area is covered as the distance increases, the amount of radiation per square inch is reduced.

The intensity of x-rays reaching the film varies inversely with the square of the distance. Therefore, at twice the distance, the density is one fourth its original value; at half the distance, the density is four times greater.

The decrease in density at greater distances is solely a geometric factor relating to the divergent x-ray beam (Fig. 11-5). The absorption of x-rays by intervening air is insignificant and can be totally disregarded.

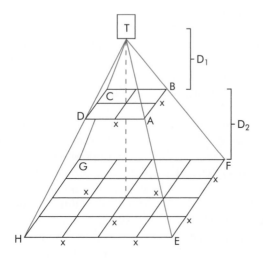

Fig. 11-5

Divergent rays increase the area covered. The diagram shows the lower surface area four times the size of the upper surface area because it is twice the distance from the x-ray source.

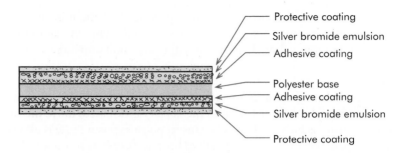

Fig. 11-6

Cross-section of a double-emulsion film.

Film

Radiographic film is composed of emulsion spread on a thin transparent sheet of polyester plastic. Except for special usage such as mammography, the emulsion is spread on both sides of the polyester base sheet. The emulsion is the "image" component of the film and consists of microscopic silver bromide crystals in a gelatin suspension (Fig. 11-6).

The characteristics of the emulsion determine the density of the radiograph. Some emulsions respond to radiation such as light and x-rays more readily than others do, and so film is roughly categorized as fast, medium, and slow film. Generally speaking, the thicker the emulsion—that is, the more silver bromide crystals present—the faster the film. The film speed (sensitivity) is the relative ability of an emulsion to respond to light and x-rays. High speed (fast film) will increase density as compared with low speed (slow film) when employing the same dosage of radiation.

Intensifying Screens

The use of intensifying screens may increase the density by 20 to 40 times over nonscreen exposure. This means that with screens, the patient radiation dose can be reduced to a small fraction of the radiation required for the same density without screens. Screens are placed in the front and back of a lightproof film holder called a cassette (Fig. 11-7). The film is loaded in the cassette and sandwiched between the two screens. The intensifying screens are made of crystals that will fluoresce when struck by x-rays. The light emitted from the screen crystals exposes the film (Fig. 11-8). Only about 5% of the radiographic film density is a result of the x-rays; 95% of the density is a result of the light from the screen crystals (Fig. 11-9). Some screens emit more light than others when struck by x-rays, and they, too, like film, can be categorized by speed numbers; for example, a 200-speed screen emits twice the light of a 100-speed, and it is said to be twice as fast. The factors that influence the screen speed are crystal size, thickness, and the type of phosphors used. Use of fast film-screen combinations cuts down on the radiation required and thus the patient dose, but detail on the radiograph is sacrificed significantly.

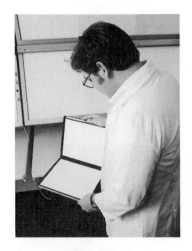

Fig. 11-7

A radiologic technologist examines the intensifying screens mounted inside of a cassette.

Screens are made with phosphors such as gadolinium, lanthanum, and yttrium. These minerals were at one time considered to be rare, and thus the term *rare earth* has been given to these screens. The rare earth screens are very efficient at converting x-ray photon energy to light energy. Although the speed of the screens is greatly increased, detail does not suffer. This obvious advantage has made rare earth screens the screens of choice in the medium kilovoltage range. The higher the screen speed, the greater the density of the radiograph.

Fog

Fog from any source increases the overall density of the radiograph. The density produced by fog does not add to the diagnostic quality of the radiograph; rather, it detracts from the quality, because the overall grayness obliterates small structures that are beneficial to diagnostic quality. Fog increases as the volume of tissue increases. In the case of the skull radiograph shown in Fig. 11-10, *A*, the film is so overcast with fog that its diagnostic quality is unacceptable. There is a dramatic reduction in fog when the field size is reduced to a small volume of tissue (Fig. 11-10, *B*). Whenever possible, fog should be avoided.

Cones and Collimators (X-ray Beam-Limiting Devices)

Beam-limiting devices such as cones and **collimators**, which are devices attached to the x-ray tube to reduce exposure field size, decrease density because they reduce the cross-sectional area of the x-ray beam and thus decrease a proportion of the amount of scatter radiation. Scatter radiation increases as the volume of irradiated tissue increases. A radiograph of the entire skull produces more scatter radiation than a 3-inch-diameter spot film of the sella turcica.

Processing

The method by which a radiograph is processed affects the density of the film. If films are allowed to remain in the developing solution for an excessive length of time, chemical fog results and increases the film density. Chemical fog also results if the solution temperature is too high. Conversely, film density decreases if the processing time is cut too short or if the solution temperature falls below the optimal point. Contaminated, oxidized, or deteriorated developer may also produce chemical fog.

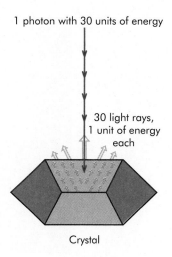

1 photon with 30 units of energy

30 light rays, 1 unit of energy each

Crystal

Fig. 11-8

X-ray energy is converted to light energy, thereby intensifying the effect of the x-rays.

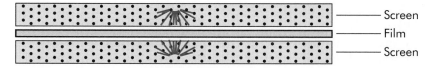

Screen

Film

Screen

Fig. 11-9

Cross-section of film between two screens; light is given off from the screen crystals.

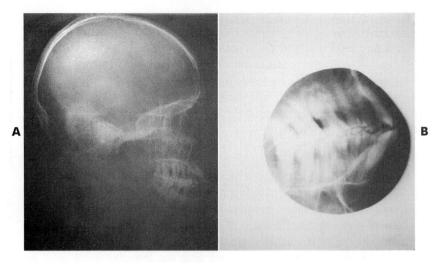

Fig. 11-10
A, Radiograph made without the use of a beam-limiting device.
B, Radiograph made with a beam-lighting device. NOTE: Scatter radiation is reduced with a decrease of tissue volume.

Grids

A **grid** interposed between the patient and film will cause a decrease in film density. There are two reasons for this:

1. The grid may absorb as much as 90% of the scatter or secondary radiation.
2. A significant fraction of the remnant radiation is absorbed; exposure technique charts compensate for this decrease in density.

Scatter radiation occurs when x-rays strike matter and scatter in a multidirectional pattern. These rays may strike the film and give it an overall gray, foggy appearance that detracts from the diagnostic quality of the film. To prevent the loss of radiographic quality, a grid is used. A grid is a device that is placed between the patient and film to trap or absorb the multidirectional scattered rays; however, the useful straight-line rays are allowed to pass through the grid to darken the film (Fig. 11-11). The grid consists of alternating strips of lead and x-ray translucent strips. The x-ray translucent strips allow the straight-line radiation to pass through, whereas the lead strips trap the scattered rays. This greatly improves the radiographic image. However, more radiation is required to produce the required density.

Filters

Any material interposed between the x-ray tube and the film reduces film density; filters are no exception. However, **filters** are used to protect the patient, and because the filter removes relatively more soft rays than hard rays, the film suffers very little reduction in density. Most of the soft rays would otherwise be absorbed by the patient and would not emerge as remnant radiation to darken the film. The exposure rate to the patient is reduced considerably, but there is only a slight reduction in film density.

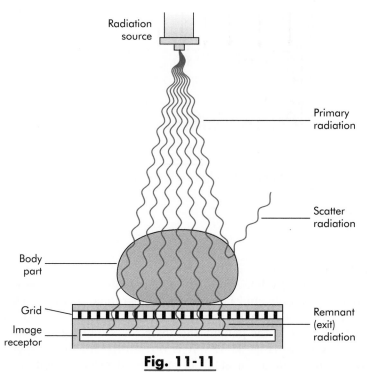

Radiation
source

Primary
radiation

Scatter
radiation

Body
part

Grid

Image
receptor

Remnant
(exit)
radiation

Fig. 11-11

Scatter radiation and absorption of scatter radiation by lead strip in the grid.

Contrast

Radiographic **contrast** may be defined as a variation in density. This definition tells us that contrast is a difference in densities and that at least two density levels must be present. Density and contrast are discussed as if they were separate properties, but the definition of contrast reminds us of the interdependence of the two. Although it is possible to have density without contrast, it is not possible to have contrast without density.

The factors that affect contrast are as follows:
- Subject contrast
- Kilovoltage
- Contrast media
- Type of film
- Intensifying screens
- Fog
- Grids and beam-limiting devices
- Film processing
- Filters
- X-ray beam angle

Subject Contrast
Subject contrast is the contrast inherent in the anatomic part that is being radiographed. If patients were homogeneous in thickness and

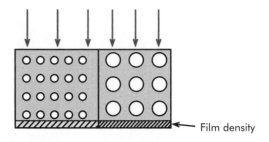

← Film density

Fig. 11-12

Contrast resulting from different tissue densities.

opacity, no contrast would be exhibited on the radiograph. However, as discussed, the body is made up of four radiographic densities: gas (or air), fat, muscle, and bone; each radiographic density presents a difference in the degree of absorption of radiation. These tissue densities are inherent in the patient and therefore are not under the technologist's control (Fig. 11-12). It is obvious, then, that the greatest contrast will be demonstrated between the density of bone and the density of air, because the greater the absorption differences, the greater the contrast.

Conversely, contrast is quite low if the anatomic part is made up of tissues with very little difference in the atomic number of the structures and, consequently, little absorption difference (e.g., breast tissue) (Fig. 11-13).

Also, the condition of the tissue will have a marked effect on the degree of x-ray absorption and hence will affect contrast. The age of the patient, the patient's lifestyle, and the patient's state of health play a part in the texture, structure, and condition of the tissue. For example, a disease may be demonstrated on the radiograph as a denser or less dense area as compared with the adjacent healthy tissue.

There is another factor that must also be considered: the thickness of the subject part. For two objects of equal density that are of unequal thickness, a difference in density will appear on the radiograph. Thus, parts showing a great variation in thickness increase contrast (Fig. 11-14).

Kilovoltage

Kilovoltage determines the penetrating power of radiation. If the kilovoltage is low, radiation with little penetrating power is produced. If the kilovoltage is high, however, radiation with great penetrating power is produced. Because the contrast is greatest when the absorption difference is greatest, it therefore follows that contrast is greatest with a low kilovoltage and that contrast decreases as the kilovoltage increases (Fig. 11-15).

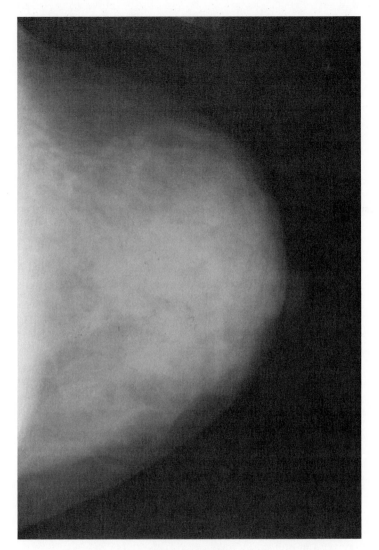

Fig. 11-13

Breast tissue has little contrast because of the small variations in the atomic number of the structures.

Contrast Media

As the name implies, any medium introduced into the anatomic part being radiographed that has a different radiation-absorbing potential increases the contrast. For example, barium, which is a metallic salt of high atomic number, will absorb relatively more radiation than the adjacent tissues and thus increases contrast. Air, which is less dense than tissue and absorbs less radiation than adjacent tissues, also improves contrast, proving again that the absorption differences of structures and material greatly affect contrast (see Fig. 11-4). The scale of contrast in a

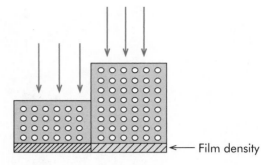

Film density

Fig. 11-14

Tissue density is the same, but there is contrast because of a difference in tissue thickness.

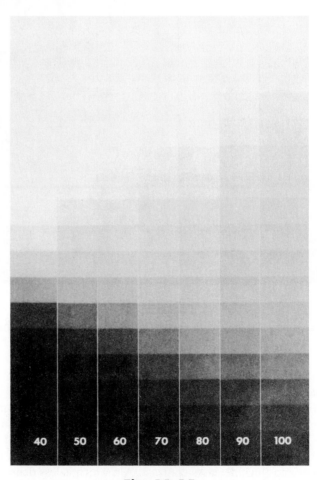

Fig. 11-15

Radiographs of an aluminum step-wedge demonstrating a change in contrast with varying kVp.

radiographic image is determined by the number and tone value of the various densities; this is referred to as short-scale or long-scale contrast. Short-scale contrast is shown in radiographs with a small number of densities; the densities seen in these radiographs exhibit a large tonal difference as compared with their neighbors. Long-scale contrast is demonstrated in images with a wide range and great number of shades of gray with little difference in the adjacent tones. Short-scale contrast is characterized by low kilovoltage; long-scale contrast is characterized by high kilovoltage. The kilovoltage, which determines the penetrating power of the radiation along with the part densities, has a major influence on contrast.

Type of Film
Film contrast is to some degree determined by the manufacturer in that each type of film has an inherent contrast factor. The contrast is determined by the film's ability to accurately record differences in radiation absorption.

Intensifying Screens
Screens increase contrast, and high-speed screens do this even more than medium- or low-speed screens; however, all increase the contrast of a radiograph.

Fog
Fog from any source decreases contrast. Contrast always deteriorates when fog is present, because fog increases the overall density with no differentiation or discrimination of structures.

Grids and Beam-Limiting Devices
Fog is markedly reduced with grids and beam-limiting devices, and for this reason contrast is improved.

Film Processing
Proper film processing methods do not increase contrast, but improper processing can destroy the inherent contrast of the latent image. As was discussed earlier, improper processing may result in chemical fog or inadequate density, either of which reduces contrast.

Filters
Filters reduce contrast only insofar as filters change the quality of the x-ray beam. As the quality of the x-ray beam changes, the contrast is affected in the same way as a change in kilovoltage affects contrast.

X-Ray Beam Angle
The position of the x-ray beam does affect contrast; this aspect is not usually discussed under the topic of film contrast. However, a simple experiment will demonstrate that the angle of the beam has a very definite effect on contrast.

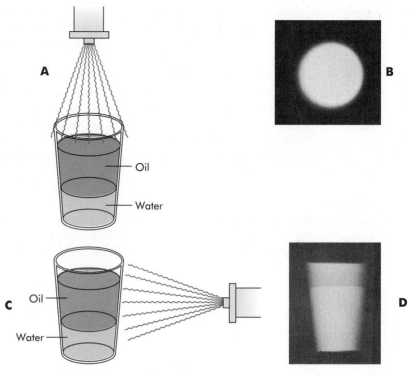

Fig. 11-16

A, Drawing of oil on water with x-ray beam directed vertically. **B**, Radiograph of oil on water with x-ray beam directed vertically. **C**, Drawing of oil on water with x-ray beam directed horizontally. **D**, Radiograph of oil on water with x-ray beam directed horizontally.

If the x-ray beam is directed in such a manner that one density is superimposed over another density, a differentiation of the two densities cannot always be made. If, however, the x-ray beam is perpendicular to the two densities, they can be differentiated, and, thus, contrast is present (Fig. 11-16).

Distortion and Magnification

Radiographic **distortion** is a false representation of the true shape of an object. Radiographic magnification is the enlargement of the object.

The factors that contribute to magnification and distortion are as follows:
- Beam alignment
- Object-to-image distance (OID)
- Source-to-image receptor distance (SID)

Beam Alignment

The alignment of the object in relation to the x-ray tube and film will determine the shape as imaged on the radiograph. The radiograph is a two-dimensional picture; the third dimension is needed to accurately identify the object. In three-dimensional structures, some parts will overlay others and thus prevent the true shape from being shown. For example, an oval object will be imaged on the radiograph as a circle (Fig. 11-17, A), and a rectangular object will be imaged as a square (Fig. 11-17, B). The oil on water in Figure 11-16 with the x-ray beam directed downward is not discernible. Only when the tube is directed to be horizontal to the object can the difference in densities be seen.

If the long axes of these objects are placed at right angles to the direction of the beam and parallel to the film, the images will be shown in another perspective. They can then be identified by their actual geometric shape.

Object-to-Image Distance (OID)

Distortion and magnification result when the object or subject of interest is located at some distance away from the film; this is because x-rays travel in straight lines that diverge from the x-ray tube. The radiograph is an x-ray shadow similar to shadows produced by visible light (Fig. 11-18, A). Just as shadows produced by light are magnified more as the object moves closer to the source of light, shadows imaged on the film are magnified as the object is placed farther from the film (Fig. 11-18, B).

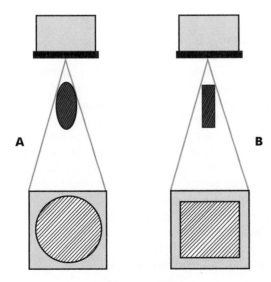

Fig. 11-17

A, The oval object radiographed may appear as a circle. B, The rectangular object radiographed may appear as a square.

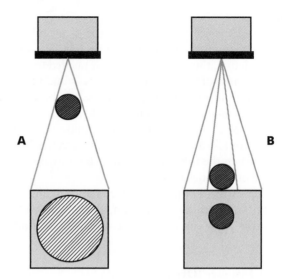

Fig. 11-18

A, The object being radiographed is magnified on the film because of its distance from the film. **B**, The object is near the film, and little magnification is present.

Source-to-Image Receptor Distance (SID)

Magnification can be reduced by increasing the SID. The discussion about OID on page 157 also applies to the SID.

Detail

Radiographic **detail** may be defined as the distinctness with which images of structures are recorded on the radiograph.

The term visibility of detail is often used in reference to the acuity of the eye in differentiating structures on the radiograph. Visibility of detail depends on several factors, including the visual acuity of the individual.

In this discussion, "detail" relates to the ability of the film to record images of structures even though the structures may be microscopic in size and thus visible only with the "aided" eye through magnification.

From the viewpoint of the radiologist who is interpreting the radiograph, detail is the crux of radiographic quality and thus is first in importance. Detail can be thought of as the end result of the interrelation of the other three factors: density, contrast, and distortion and magnification; a discussion of these factors was necessary before attempting to discuss them in relation to detail.

Factors that relate to detail are as follows:
- Density
- Contrast
- Fog
- Film processing

- Patient motion
- X-ray tube focal spot size
- OID
- SID
- Film
- Intensifying screens
- Screen-film contact

Density
As discussed earlier, density must be adequate for structures to be recorded with optimal visibility.

Contrast
Contrast is necessary for the perceptibility of detail. The detail on a radiograph is distinguished by the extent to which it contrasts with its background; a detail becomes perceptible only when its contrast, with respect to its background, possesses a certain minimum value. If the contrast is reduced below this value, the structure will have to be larger to be visible to the "unaided" eye. Conversely, when the contrast is greater, smaller structures can be discerned.

Fog
Fog obliterates detail in that the overall random darkening of the radiograph does not contribute to the formation of a useful image but rather is superimposed over the image.

Film Processing
Processing the film completes what the exposure started: a visible image. Processing cannot bring out more detail than was inherent in the latent image. However, poor processing techniques can have a deleterious effect on detail because of fog or other processing errors that tend to obliterate detail.

Patient Motion
Patient motion is perhaps the greatest factor encountered that affects detail in medical radiography. Movement of the patient causes blurring of the image, and detail is greatly impaired; this arises from the fact that the projection of the structure on the film is moved with respect to the film during exposure so that the image is spread out over a certain area (Fig. 11-19).

X-Ray Tube Focal Spot Size
Geometric unsharpness resulting from x-ray tube focal spot size results because x-rays are not emitted from a point but rather from a source with a finite size. The **focal spot** is the spot or source from which the x-rays originate. With a large focal spot, the edge does not demonstrate a sharp black-white contrast; it becomes indeterminate, from black to gray to white. The width of the half-shadow region on the film, called geometric unsharpness,

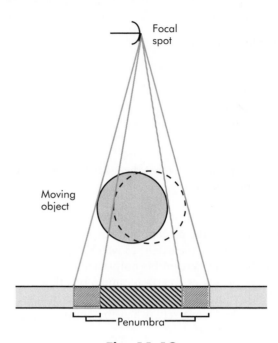

Fig. 11-19

The effects of motion on unsharpness.

is often referred to as *focus unsharpness* or edge gradient. This concept is convincingly demonstrated by comparing the shadows made on a wall with a large light source and those made with a small light source. Geometric unsharpness is directly proportional to the size of the focal spot; the smaller the focus, the sharper the structure lines (Fig. 11-20).

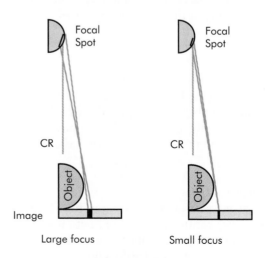

Fig. 11-20

Focus unsharpness or edge gradient caused by the focal spot size.

OID

X-radiation can be compared with visible light in that x-rays follow many of the rules that govern the formation of shadows by light. A familiar observation is the shadow cast on the surface of a plane at some distance from a light source; the nearer a hand to the plane's surface, the sharper the edges of the silhouette. As the hand moves farther away from the plane's surface, the more indistinct the edges of the shadow will become. To improve the sharpness of the image (and thereby enhance detail), the anatomic part of interest should be placed as near to the film as possible (Fig. 11-21).

Focal-Object Distance

Detail in the radiograph is also controlled by the distance from the focus to the object or patient. As this distance decreases, loss of detail occurs; this loss of detail is a result of magnification of the image and blurriness around the edge of the image. When this distance is kept at the maximal practical level, detail in the image remains sharp.

SID

Loss of detail in radiography is also a function of SID. As this distance is increased, the effect is similar to a decrease in focal spot size: detail is increased (Fig. 11-22).

Film

The loss of detail (also called media unsharpness) is a function of the film, the type of intensifying screens used in the procedure, and the closeness of contact between film and screen.

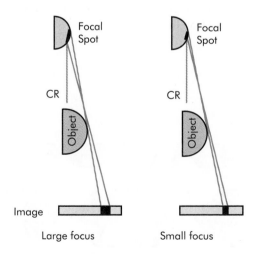

Fig. 11-21

Edge unsharpness due to OID.

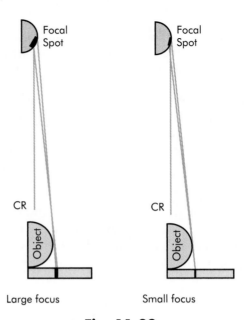

Fig. 11-22

Detail is improved with increased SID.

Intensifying Screens

Intensifying screens contribute far more to unsharpness of detail than does film (Fig. 11-23). Slow, fine-grain screens exhibit less unsharpness than fast, coarse-grain screens.

Screen-Film Contact

One of the most common causes of loss of detail is one that, even though it is well known, is often overlooked: poor screen contact. Screen-film contact is more a function of cassettes than of the screens. Regardless of

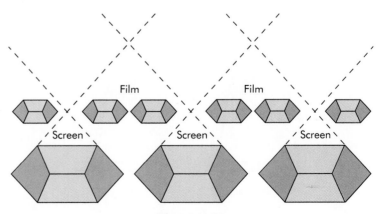

Fig. 11-23

Screen crystals are much larger than film crystals: film crystals are 1.5 microns in size; screen crystals are 4 to 5 microns in size.

the cause, however, a blurred image is produced because of the divergent rays of light emanating from the screen crystal.

Conclusion

The preceding discussions apply to routine or conventional radiography as practiced in all radiology departments; the information presented applies to the vast majority of radiographic examinations. However, new technology has brought about new imaging equipment that may revolutionize the imaging of the human body. Other methods of imaging will be discussed in subsequent chapters.

Review Questions

1. The following radiographic densities are listed from most dense to least dense:
   a. Muscle, bone, fat, air.
   b. Bone, fat, muscle, air.
   c. Fat, bone, air, muscle.
   d. Bone, muscle, fat, air.
2. A change of 100 mA to 200 mA would have the greatest effect on:
   a. Density.
   b. Contrast.
   c. Detail.
   d. Magnification.
3. A change in kilovoltage will have a dramatic effect on:
   a. Density and contrast.
   b. Density and magnification.
   c. Detail and distortion.
   d. Detail and focal spot size.
4. Contrast is influenced by which of the following?
   a. The atomic number of the tissue
   b. The shape of the anatomic part
   c. The energy of the x-ray beam
   d. All of the above
5. The visibility of detail is influenced by which of the following?
   a. Contrast
   b. Magnification
   c. Density
   d. All the above
6. The size of the focal spot has an effect on which of the following?
   a. Density
   b. Detail
   c. Distortion and magnification
   d. Contrast
7. Radiographic grids are used in radiography:
   a. To protect the patient from scatter radiation.
   b. As a substitute for filters.

c. To reduce fog on the radiograph.

d. To reduce patient radiation dose.

8. A radiograph with many shades of gray with little difference between the shades is referred to as which of the following?

    a. Short-scale contrast

    b. High contrast

    c. Long-scale contrast

    d. Low penumbra

9. Of the following, the most effective means of reducing magnification is increasing:

    a. Kilovoltage.

    b. mA.

    c. Time.

    d. Distance.

10. What is the most effective method for reducing the effects of patient motion on the radiograph?

    a. Reduce kilovoltage

    b. Reduce mA

    c. Reduce time

    d. Reduce distance

11. Which of the following has no effect on recorded detail?

    a. Focal-film distance

    b. Focal-spot size

    c. Object-film distance

    d. Heat-units capacity

12. Milliamperage is the technical factor that chiefly influences which of the following?

    a. Contrast

    b. Density

    c. Detail

    d. Distortion

13. Kilovoltage is the technical factor selected to influence all the following except:

    a. Contrast.

    b. Penetrating power of the beam.

    c. Patient dose.

    d. Grid radius.

14. Kilovoltage determines which of the following?

    a. The quantity of radiation

    b. The quality of the radiation beam

    c. Focal spot size

    d. Collimation needed

15. Distortion and magnification can be reduced by which of the following?

    a. Long object-film distance

    b. Short object-film distance

    c. Short focal-film distance

    d. Increased mA

BIBLIOGRAPHY

Bushong S: *Radiologic science for technologists*, ed. 8, St. Louis, 2004, Mosby.

Hiss S: *Understanding radiography*, ed. 3, Springfield, IL, 1993, Charles C Thomas.

Selman J: *The fundamentals of imaging physics and radiobiology*, ed. 9, Springfield, IL, 2000, Charles C Thomas.

Thompson M, Hattaway M, Hall J, Dowd S: *Principles of imaging science and protection*, Philadelphia, 1994, Saunders.

Ethics and Professionalism in Radiologic Technology

James Ohnysty

OBJECTIVES

On completion of this chapter, you should be able to:

- **Interact with patients, peers, and professionals in a civil and considerate manner.**
- **Explain what is meant by professional confidentiality.**
- **Describe effective communication techniques.**
- **Discuss the procedures for protecting patient modesty and self-esteem.**
- **Explain how to project a professional image in attire and conduct.**
- **Discuss personal obligations that radiologic technologists have to their patients, to their profession, and to society at large.**

INITIAL CONSIDERATIONS

By now you have realized that in addition to developing technical knowledge and skills, the foundation of radiologic technology encompasses **standards of conduct** and ideals essential to meeting both the emotional and physical needs of patients (see Chapter 7).

KEY TERMS

attitudes
confidentiality
creed
dignity
modesty
moral
personal obligation
standards of conduct

CHAPTER OUTLINE

Initial considerations
Professional goals
Interpersonal relationships
The patient
    Patient attitudes and
        reactions
    Patient modesty
Communication
Professional
    confidentiality
Professional image
Personal obligations
Professional
    entrepreneurs
Conclusion

Radiologic technology encompasses a variety of specialties and plays an invaluable role in the practice of medicine. This service department provides vital information about structure and function—both normal and abnormal—of the human body, and this information enables physicians to make accurate diagnoses to pursue care and treatment. Practitioners of this art and science play a key role in the total spectrum of health care services.

Those of you entering radiologic or other imaging technologies directly from high school may find that your age (youth) presents some problems. Typically the general public questions the character and competence of anyone to whom they must entrust their care and treatment. With each new patient, your abilities and purposes may be on trial simply because of your age. A majority of patients may likely be senior citizens. To understand their opinions and standards, you must realize that, when they were young people, the people, experiences, and events of several decades ago influenced them. External influences temper attitudes from generation to generation. The degree of social freedom has changed considerably over the last few decades, and older generations may have difficulty believing that today's youth could measure up to the ethical and moral standards associated with the medical professions over the years. Your work and your conduct will prove them right or wrong.

Individuals who are entering this profession must ask themselves questions such as "What do I expect from this field as a professional career?" and "What do I have to contribute?" in order to conduct a thorough self-analysis. Diagnostic imaging, whatever the chosen modality, is a service profession. Do you have a service-oriented personality? Will you be able to work with people who may be experiencing some of the worst situations in their lives, and can you do so with empathy? You need to consider the extremes that can occur. Unfortunately, through television and the many programs associated with medicine, dramatic license has taken over, and reality becomes overshadowed and somewhat glamorized. If you are expecting glamour and high drama, you may need to reconsider. The work will be demanding both physically and emotionally, and it entails a serious responsibility. If you are choosing correctly, the work will be immensely rewarding through the many people that you will help during their pain and illness.

PROFESSIONAL GOALS

In establishing a worthwhile goal, you must first view your chosen profession as more than a job. You should not pursue a simple goal of just passing a series of examinations and eventually becoming certified by the Registry or just earning a degree; you should set a goal that will establish you as a first-rate professional. Radiologic/imaging technology does not need dropouts or those unable to cope with advances in the profession. What caliber of radiologic technologist would you prefer to care for you or your family? Certainly you would want the services of a professional radiologic technologist—a combination of superior technical knowledge and skills applied in an understanding, caring, and compassionate manner—who works in harmony and cooperation with peers, physicians, radiologists, and all other hospital personnel.

Suppose that you, like many others, plan to use radiologic technology as a stepping-stone in your long-range career plans to achieve some higher vocational goal. Does this mean that you need not apply yourself with as much dedication and effort as if radiologic technology were your ultimate professional goal? Definitely not. The needs are still the same. Whether you plan to pursue this profession for a temporary or indefinite length of time, respect it and respect yourself by excelling at all times.

INTERPERSONAL RELATIONSHIPS

Should you enter the field of radiologic technology, you will encounter many individuals who will influence your education and training. First are the didactic and clinical instructors, who are knowledgeable and skilled professionals; they are dedicated to assisting and guiding you to become a first-rate radiologic technologist, but the rest is up to you. The success of your learning experience depends primarily on your own incentive, dedication, and personal application.

As you contemplate entering this profession, you need to consider both your short-term and long-term plans. Medical imaging has and will continue to develop very rapidly in its complexity. Are you interested in staying with and developing your knowledge and skills in keeping with these changes to excel in this field? The goal of health care does not change except to become more efficient in its delivery and successful in diagnosis and treatment. If this excellence in knowledge and skill is accompanied by an underlying desire to provide care and empathy for patients, the goal of service is being well served. Consider if this is the reason that a career in medical imaging appeals to you.

If you are viewing this profession as a short-term goal, you may be shortchanging both yourself and the field. You will limit yourself in the heights that you could achieve and what you would contribute to the field. If you are using this field as a stepping-stone to go on to a more advanced medical profession, you must apply yourself to learn everything you can in your academic and clinical experience to serve as a basis. However, those of us who have spent many decades as technologists and grown with the field would hope that your plans and sense of dedication would become long-range; strive to excel beyond the basic requirements, and become one of the building blocks of this profession.

You need to understand your instructors and their motivations. They may seem regimented in committing you to unmerciful schedules of study and practice, but they have a goal to achieve. Within the 2 or 4 years that seem so long to you, they must teach you a large body of knowledge and assist you in developing your skills simply to meet the minimum standards. They also try to motivate you to take part in additional studies, research, writing, and practice on your own. Their goal is to have you develop into a professional radiologic technologist; thus, your association with your instructors should be one of mutual understanding and cooperative efforts in developing your professional education and training. You may find some comfort in knowing that your instructors—registered technologists, physicians, and radiologists—are all caught up in a process similar to yours; that is, they are constantly striving to keep abreast of continual advances in the field of medicine and related health services. All of these professional individuals represent your sources of information and learning. Obtain their assistance at every available opportunity.

Attending physicians and radiologists you encounter may appear to be distant, preoccupied, and generally indifferent to your presence in the department. Some you will find to be exactly that; others will be a tremendous source of information and assistance with a friendly interest in your progress (Fig. 12-1). Unfortunately, the wide gap between professional standings of the medical and technical fields continues; however, this gap can be bridged as each succeeding generation of radiologic technologists exhibits increasingly higher levels of knowledge, skill, and personal professionalism. Radiologic technologists need to assert themselves as essential members of the total health service team.

Success in the health care industry and in the treatment of patients depends not only on the physicians but also on the total team effort of health care professionals; this includes radiologic technologists, other imaging specialists, and nurses to provide the total information needed for a diagnosis and proper course of treatment for the patient. In the past, physicians were at the top of the pyramid. Although the physician still makes the final decision about the course of treatment, this determi-

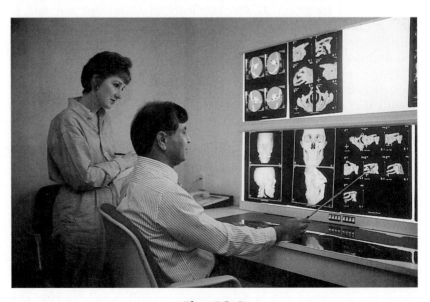

Fig. 12-1

Physicians can be a source of information and learning.

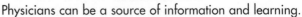

nation is based on findings of the associated professions working as a team. Always keep in mind that your work as an imaging professional is an important contribution to the team effort; you can take pride in carrying out such a serious responsibility. Without imaging technology services, diagnoses and effective patient care and treatment would be extremely difficult and in many instances impossible.

THE PATIENT

When continuing to consider the individuals involved in the course of education and training, we must discuss the patients. Just how important are they and why? Suppose somebody built a hospital, furnished it with the most advanced equipment, and staffed it with a full complement of all professionals—and then no patients came. Now the picture comes into focus! First comes the patient, and then come the physician, the nurse, and the hospital. The patient is the object of all of the attentions and efforts to detect injuries, diagnose diseases, and effect treatments.

Who becomes a patient? Each and every member of the human race is a potential patient. Patients come in various shapes, sizes, ages, colors, creeds, religions, and politics. Illness, injury, and disease play no favorites and make no exceptions. The patient is someone's child, sibling, parent, friend, or mate. Each patient is important to someone, and all patients are important; their physical comfort, emotional security, and confidence in an individual who can help them all need to be considered equally.

Your focus must always be on what you can contribute to help this individual who needs your particular service. Your personal attitude towards your patient, your work, and your work environment must be a desire to make your contribution the very best within your responsibilities. In working with students during the past decades, I found that one of the fundamental issues was the attitude of the student and that this attitude would or would not propel that student to excel in their work. The patient senses this attitude, and so do colleagues, instructors, and others. A person with a positive, energetic, and caring attitude will always be a winner; all other issues can be overcome through study, experience, and continuing education.

Patient Attitudes and Reactions

What circumstances influence the **attitudes** (feeling and emotions) and actions of a patient who is entering a hospital? Except when it is for childbirth, entering the hospital is not usually a happy occasion. Hospitalization usually involves pain and fear caused by an injury, illness, or disease; the prognosis can be questionable or hopeless. Emotional reactions may appear magnified or even irrational, and you need to deal with them in an appropriate manner. Fears can be alleviated by a caring, positive approach and an understanding of your patients' concerns. Health care workers who are positive and encouraging, who can deal with negative or defeatist patients, and who are able to elevate their level of stability and comfort are exceptional.

A patient may react by reaffirming or intensifying religious beliefs and practices. Religion is a private, personal matter. You must respect each patient's choice of worship. Religion may be a patient's bid for security or a last hope and source of strength to endure whatever lies ahead. You are not to judge the merits of anyone's religion or to promote the merits of your own; simply respect the right of choice. Sometimes life throws us a curve, making the ability to remain neutral a challenge. Unfortunately, the catastrophic events of 9/11, when our personal/national sense of security was compromised, have created additional personal stresses. History forever repeats itself, and religion has become an issue of conflict in the minds of some. We are faced with the challenge to avoid racial/religious profiling in dealing with the public in general. Dealing with patients is much more critical and can be very stressful especially if the events of 9/11 and in the interim have impacted your family directly. Thus, you are reminded that radiologic imaging is a service profession and one cannot choose one's patients. As a true professional, you must be able to interact with any and all persons without prejudice.

Just as you should not become involved in religious differences, you should also be impartial when encountering patients of a different race, color, or nationality. Each patient is entitled to the highest degree of care and concern that you are able to provide. As a health service practitioner dedicated to saving lives, how could you do otherwise?

Unfortunately, societies' problems, prejudices, and attitudes can be brought into the hospital or clinic by our patients; these can be diminished or amplified by our response to the patients and their particular needs. Outside of the hospital walls, people are generally focused on daily activities and pleasures within their own personal spheres. However, when pain, illness, and trauma enter our lives, we all become equal. Thus, as a medical professional, you will need to recognize and be able to deal with many socioeconomic, ethnic, and religious differences and to treat all patients with equal respect. In summary, you should serve each patient with equal care and dedication, regardless of religion, race, **creed** (a set of fundamental beliefs), color, politics, or economic background.

Patient Modesty

As we continue to consider the patient, we come to the important responsibility of respecting and preserving the patient's **modesty**. All people value their bodies as part of their total person and deserve to have them handled in a respectful manner. The degree of modesty exhibited by a patient may vary from extreme modesty to a total lack of it. You must observe the rules of draping and covering the patient to the greatest extent possible, depending on the examination. As a professional, you may find yourself in a delicate situation that requires you to decide whether you are the most suitable technologist to perform an examination on a certain patient. If an examination requires a position that could be embarrassing to patients of the opposite sex, you should use considerable tact with these patients to preserve modesty and personal **dignity**.

Traditionally, older generations seem to find some of the actions, dress (or lack of dress), and attitudes of the younger generations alarming and possibly distasteful; you can probably expect to encounter many such people during your training. Take into account that singers, entertainers, and actors have made partial nudity an almost acceptable standard in public and continue to push the envelope. Still, patients who would find it comfortable at the beach or at a social event may shun having their bodies touched or exposed by a stranger, even one who is a medical professional. As compared with these other, more regular activities, the issue here is one of loss of choice or control. Therefore, treat every patient as if he or she was modest. This consideration is the patient's right and your responsibility. If you do this, patients will be most appreciative, and they will recognize that you are truly a professional to be trusted.

COMMUNICATION

Effective communication is a technique that you need to master, and you need to recognize that it includes verbal communication, facial expression, and other body language. Your attitude, the tone of your voice, your appearance and dress, and your facial expression combine to present a first impression to the patient. The impression can be positive or negative and can either increase their anxieties or instill confidence that they can expect high-quality, efficient, and caring service from you. As a health care service provider, you must always endeavor to first build the patient's trust in your abilities. Patients must be able to sense your professionalism, and they will respond positively and with confidence to your care.

How you divulge information and what information you share—whether fact or opinion, intentionally or inadvertently—could cause a patient considerable anguish. Your first responsibility is to converse with the patient in an intelligent, professional manner that is pleasant and courteous (Fig. 12-2). A patient who is under stress may be decidedly unpleasant to you at times. However, you must maintain control over your emotions, remain pleasant, and try to alleviate the patient's apprehensions, which may be causing or contributing to the unpleasant behavior. You must be able to determine during your initial contact with the patient just what would be the most appropriate manner in which to handle a particular patient. The patient should leave your care feeling that you were interested and had performed your best service at all time.

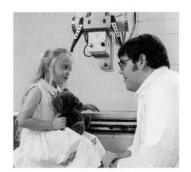

Fig. 12-2

Communication with the patient is vital to alleviating fear and gaining cooperation.

PROFESSIONAL CONFIDENTIALITY

One of the major restrictions that a health care profession imposes on you is the need to maintain strict **confidentiality** of medical and personal information about a patient. The patient may ask the technologist about his or her condition; however, this information cannot be revealed to the patient, the patient's family, or others outside the department without the direct consent of the patient's physician. Breach of confidence is one of the major problems encountered when providing patient care and can result in legal problems for the department and hospital. Information should not be discussed throughout the hospital with other department personnel except in the direct line of duty when requested from one ancillary department to another or with nursing service to meet specific medical needs. Information should never be discussed with your own family or friends in even the most general terms, because you would still be violating the patient's rights and damaging both the department and the hospital's reputation. Your instructors will emphasize and reiterate the need to maintain strict confidence of information about patients, the department, and the hospital. Consider how you would feel if you were the patient and your private information were the topic of a conversation down the hall, during a coffee break in the cafeteria, or anywhere in public (Fig. 12-3).

Because of recent changes in the laws, patients now have the right to access their charts, and you are responsible for knowing all of the rules and regulations concerning patient rights involved in the provision of health care services. Preservation of patient confidentiality is still a vital issue and is challenged in court virtually every day in some part of the country. The patient's condition or any personal information, including whether they have had a particular diagnostic examination, must be held in strictest confidence; this right also applies to any public figures or officials. You need to discuss with your instructors any changes that involve providing medical services so you do not inadvertently violate a public trust.

PROFESSIONAL IMAGE

In developing your professional image, you need to consider another area that is often contested: specific standards for dress and grooming. You should keep in mind that the patient's first impression of you is strongly influenced by your personal appearance, including your facial expressions. Before the first word is spoken, patients begin to formulate an opinion of you, the person to whom they must entrust themselves during the course of radiography or other procedures that you may perform. The dress and grooming of the staff and the appearance of the department and the hospital influence an immediate opinion. For example, in society today, we are exposed to visible body piercing jewelry (e.g., in the nose, tongue, lips, and eyebrows). Although such extremes may be acceptable during high school and college, they are not readily acceptable in professional medical circles. A very high percentage of your patients will be of much older generations or of certain ethnic or religious persuasions that may find extremes in dress and jewelry unacceptable or even offensive. Regardless of the sterling character of the radiologic technologist, professional image is essential.

We are dealing with the individual rights of both the patient and the health care worker. In this instance, the patient will have a preconceived

Lincoln Land Community College Radiography Program

Confidentiality of Record/Patient Information

The Joint Commission on Accreditation of Healthcare Organizations (JCAHO) states that: Medical records shall be confidential, secure, current, authenticated, legible, and complete.

The medical record (including radiographs and all diagnostic images produced in any medium) is the property of the hospital and is maintained for the benefit of the patient, the medical staff, and the hospital. It is everyone's responsibility to safeguard both the record and its informational content against loss, defacement, tampering, and from use by unauthorized individuals while the patient is in the hospital.

A patient record is not to be removed without authorization from the appropriate person in charge.

The release of information form must be signed by a patient before any copies of medical records may be made. This must always be done in accordance with policies established by the hospital. Under no circumstances may a student remove any portion of the patient's medical record without direct authorization of an appropriate department supervisor.

The only medical information or patient history to be discussed with the patient is that which is needed to completely and accurately treat the patient.

Conversation with other healthcare workers must take place outside of the hearing range of any patient, their family or any visitors. Never converse about patients, cases, or make reference in the hallways, lounges, cafeteria, and especially away from the hospital.

Patient information is not allowed to be given to any family member or friend unless authorized by the patient.

Do not discuss hospital incidents.

Refer any inquiries about medical information to the supervisor in charge.

Student Signature	*Witness/Program Director*	*Date*

Fig. 12-3

Patient confidentiality form.

idea of how the health care worker should look and act, and as the patient/customer, his or her right is paramount. The total picture of the radiologic technologist should be one of neatness, cleanliness, and friendly efficiency if the patient is to feel any confidence in the type of treatment that can be expected.

As social attitudes have changed and the manner of dress and grooming have become more casual, these attitudes have carried over into the hospital environment with uniform and grooming codes becoming more lenient. However, no argument is going to change the fact that a casual appearance does not epitomize a technically skilled, highly motivated, and competent radiologic technologist—a professional health care specialist. A professional image of hospital personnel has been perpetuated in the public mind over the years, and changes in ideals of this nature are not readily accepted. The hospital establishes dress and grooming codes appropriate to the hospital environment, and you are expected to adhere to these codes regardless of personal tastes.

In the last few years, when casual Friday was introduced in the business community, the same was soon introduced into the hospital environment. Although widely accepted in other fields, casual wear in the hospital gives the impression of a casual attitude and a lessening in professionalism in the eyes of older-generation patients and patients of various ethnic and religious groups. Patients' concerns are not casual, and they could be discouraged about the quality of service and care that they may receive if hospital personnel are not dressed to the professional level that patients have come to expect. I concur that this may seem unfair, but it is reality, and the patients' needs come first. The rationale is sound and in the best interest of good rapport between the patient and working professionals. You must be willing to accept it.

PERSONAL OBLIGATIONS

What are your personal, professional, and ethical obligations to the art and science of radiologic technology? You are legally responsible for your actions, even as a student. Chapter 14 discusses legal aspects in greater detail. You are protected in part by being limited to basic responsibilities under supervision in early training. As your skills and knowledge increase, this degree of supervision will diminish, and personal responsibility will increase. As a graduate, you will become totally responsible, from the **moral** and legal standpoint, to adhere to the rules and standards that you have been taught.

By now, you should realize that radiologic technology must be more than just a job to you. Can you accept the **personal obligation** to pursue continuing education and to grow in the knowledge and skills of a constantly advancing field so that you will not rapidly become obsolete and second-rate? Do you feel motivated to participate in and support the activities of the professional organizations that have student members so that you can master the new advancements in the field?

To become proficient and a leader in your field, you must demand the highest quality in your classes and clinical experience. In this way, you will develop professionally and advance the stature of the profession among the health service fields. Success can be measured by what you have accomplished technically, by the manner in which you interact with your patients and the rest of the health care staff, and by your personal contributions to writings and research.

Each profession has leaders and followers; radiologic technology is no exception. However, many dedicated leaders have developed and nurtured a professional organization that is worthy of your respect and support. The typical leader expends more than the minimal effort required to survive; he or she motivates others to achieve competent, professional performance.

The professional survival rate among radiologic technologists has decreased as they try to outlast the new information, techniques, and equipment that rapidly render them obsolete in the field. To succeed, you must believe in the merits of the profession and its growing importance in health care. For many, radiologic technology has been a short-term career with high attrition because they lacked the incentive, determination, and personal effort to succeed. Radiologic technology is, in fact, one of the most exciting and challenging health care fields today; it is a scientific wonder that allows the structure and function of every cell and organ of the body to be studied by the human eye and mind. A radiologic technologist abreast of the field today must be an exceptional individual—a technologist, a scientist, and a humanitarian.

PROFESSIONAL ENTREPRENEURS

Imaging has proliferated into a multitude of modalities from initial basic radiography and fluoroscopy to some vascular specialties to ultrasound, nuclear medicine, CT, and MRI, some of which have subspecialties. Along with this continued rapid progress in imaging technology, another change has occurred that affects the profession. The enactment of a new law makes it legal for radiologic technologists to own x-ray equipment. In the past, only physicians and hospitals could own x-ray equipment and provide x-ray services. Currently, physicians are developing joint ownership partnerships with allied health professionals. Imaging technologists can now be part owners of imaging equipment and provide services with varying degrees of responsibility; however, the physician remains the authority for ordering services and providing medical direction. In fact, even nonmedical personnel can now own an MRI or CT center provided there is a medical director and the venture complies with all regulatory standards (a physician administers injections, and a medical specialist/radiologist provides diagnostic readings and reports).

CONCLUSION

The objective of radiographic imaging is to produce images that are diagnostically sound and radiation-safe. This requires that image quality be maintained with a balance of density, contrast, detail, distortion, and magnification—electronic quality as it is now in so many imaging specialties.

With the appropriate educational background and the determination to achieve, you can advance to the top of the radiologic technology field. When you practice professionalism and technical excellence, the patient will benefit, health care will benefit, and you personally will benefit. You will be one of many individuals working together to achieve the best possible treatment of injuries and diseases. Radiologic technology holds the key that has opened many doors for medical advancement, and the potential is still unlimited.

People now entering this profession are at the threshold of some of the most rapid advancements; these are almost impossible to comprehend (e.g., teleradiology, satellite transmission of images). Those of us who have been in the profession for several decades are in awe and look forward with great anticipation to what future advancements are in store. Those of you entering into this program are at the cutting edge of technology; you have the prospect for a strong future in this field and the chance to excel beyond your imagination.

Review Questions

1. Ethics is a discipline that deals with:
   a. Medical-legal issues.
   b. Legal codes for the medical profession.
   c. Morals as they relate to behavior.
   d. Laws that govern conduct and behavior.
2. Patients presenting themselves for radiographic examination are first impressed by which of the following?
   a. The technologist's credentials
   b. The technologist's reputation in the community
   c. The friendliness of the technologist
   d. The personal appearance of the technologist
3. When a patient asks the technologist what the radiograph shows about his or her condition, the technologist should:
   a. Give an honest answer.
   b. Tell the patient what the x-ray shows.
   c. Call the chief technologist for answers.
   d. Tell the patient that the referring physician will have the answers.
4. Which of the following behaviors would be considered unethical for a technologist?
   a. Leaving the patient alone on the table
   b. Repeating the examination
   c. Criticizing the physician
   d. Reporting the unethical conduct of others
5. If an instructor is regimental or appears distant, students should:
   a. Withdraw from the course.
   b. Report the attitude to the program director.
   c. Ask the program director to change the schedule.
   d. Take responsibility for their own learning.
6. The technologist's first duty is to:
   a. The institution or hospital.
   b. The physician in charge.
   c. The chief administrative technologist.
   d. The patient.

7. Technologists who examine terminally ill patients should do which of the following?
   a. Attempt to get the patient to accept the technologist's religion
   b. Attempt to get the patient to accept the technologist's moral and ethical code of behavior
   c. Ask the referring physician to counsel the patient
   d. Simply respect the patient's right of choice
8. Some patients require more time and attention than others because:
   a. They are sicker.
   b. They are full-pay, private patients.
   c. Their economic background is a factor.
   d. All patients require the same amount of time.
9. Professional confidentiality means:
   a. Withholding medical and personal information about the patient.
   b. Maintaining the confidence entrusted to you.
   c. Respecting the patient's right to privacy.
   d. All the above.
10. Moral and ethical conduct of individuals who are handling patients for radiographic examinations is a responsibility of:
    a. The radiologist.
    b. The technologist.
    c. The student.
    d. All the above

BIBLIOGRAPHY

Bontrager KL, Lampignano JP: *Textbook of radiographic positioning and related anatomy*, ed. 6, St. Louis, 2005, Mosby.

Bushong S: *Radiologic science for technologists: physics, biology, and protection*, ed. 8, St. Louis, 2004, Mosby.

Thompson MA, et al: *Principles of imaging sciences and protection*, Philadelphia, 1994, WB Saunders.

Patient Care and Management

Penny S. Mays

OBJECTIVES

On completion of this chapter, you should be able to:

- Prevent injury to the patient during a radiographic examination.

- Protect the patient, yourself, and others from contagious diseases by practicing proper isolation, sterile, or aseptic techniques.

- Reassure and comfort, within the limits of your training, the anxious or fearful patient.

- Use proper body mechanics when moving and transferring patients.

- Discuss the importance of maintaining the existing status of indwelling catheters and other patient attachments.

- Explain what is meant by monitoring vital signs and describe the radiologic technologist's role in this aspect of patient care.

- Discuss the significance of requiring clinical information when radiographic service is requested.

- Explain the importance of recording or charting patient information.

KEY TERMS

acquired
    immunodeficiency
    syndrome (AIDS)
antiseptics
body mechanics
cardiac arrest
cardiopulmonary
    resuscitation (CPR)
contagious diseases
convulsions
disinfectants
fainting
gravity line
isolation room
nosocomial infections
pathogens
seizures
shock
sphygmomanometer
sterilization
stethoscope
vital signs

CHAPTER OUTLINE

*Verification of patient
    identification and
    procedures requested
Patient transfer
Isolation techniques
    Sterile or aseptic
    techniques
Conclusion*

Prevention is always better than treatment for the patient with injury or illness, but not one of us is immune to illness, natural disasters, or human error. Care must be taken so that good patient care and management are assured. Although we know that different measures will be required for varying circumstances, the principles of care and protection are constant and cannot be overemphasized. Five items are listed below as requirements for optimal patient care:

1. Practice high-quality radiographic techniques to include radiation safety in a manner that will minimize further injury or complications.
2. Prevent the spread of disease and injury to others.
3. Prevent hazardous or crippling complications of injuries or illnesses.
4. Alleviate suffering by comforting the patient and preventing emotional complications.
5. Provide the service as economically and in as timely a way as possible while maintaining consistent diagnostic quality.

To assure that these five requirements are met, certain policies and procedures are necessary. These may be written in detail in the hospital or departmental policy manual and will serve as the basis for the way you perform certain patient care functions.

VERIFICATION OF PATIENT IDENTIFICATION AND PROCEDURES REQUESTED

It is essential that a verification or match between information on the examination request form and the patient's wristband be made immediately on arrival at the radiographic room. In the event that the patient has not been identified or is unable to give identification, an emergency control number should be assigned with hospital chart verification so that a cross-reference can be made at the time that identification is made.

To further assist with the proper identification of a patient, many imaging departments have as their internal policy a requirement that the name, date of birth, social security number, and date of the examination be photographed on the film.

The radiology physician director, hospital administrator, and radiology administrator share the responsibility for establishing procedures for requesting radiographic service and for maintaining radiographic films, tapes, and other records of the patient's medical history.

The radiology physician director maintains the responsibility and final approval of the examination requested and can cancel or terminate the procedure at any point. Clinical information about pregnancy or possible pregnancy or precautions to be observed because of special conditions such as deafness, blindness, diabetes, heart problems, and allergies are required in most departments.

PATIENT TRANSFER

Often a medical emergency occurs when a patient is in transport to or from the radiographic suite or in the radiographic area. Therefore, it is important that all students on any radiology staff involved in patient care be qualified in **cardiopulmonary resuscitation (CPR)**, which is the restoration of function of the heart and lungs after apparent death. Transport equipment, such as wheelchairs, stretchers, and beds, should be kept in proper working order. Ancillary equipment such as step stools and intravenous stands must also be maintained, and preventive maintenance safety checks should be conducted often. On arrival at the patient area, an assessment of the patient's condition and armband identification should be made. The ability of the patient to help himself or herself, the patient's injury, and the auxiliary equipment necessary to the patient's condition must be observed, as well as any further precautions noted on the requisition.

Patients must be instructed about where they are to be transported, and assistance must be given when necessary to ensure safe and comfortable transport. The responsible unit personnel should be advised of the patient's destination. Care should be taken to ensure safety to both the patient and the employee. Should the transporter need assistance, the patient should not be moved until such time that sufficient trained staff is available.

Proper **body mechanics** (the action of muscles in producing motion or posture) can best be practiced by employees who have been trained in such techniques. Although a detailed discussion is not appropriate in this text, a few salient points may be helpful. The most important point to keep in mind is that, at all times, human action is influenced by gravity. The center of gravity in the standing human being is at the center of the pelvis. Equilibrium or balance is maintained when the gravity line passes through the base support; the **gravity line** is an imaginary vertical line that passes through the center of gravity. Stability of a body is increased by broadening the base support. Therefore, balance is maintained much more easily with the feet spread apart than when they are positioned closer together. When lifting or moving a patient, you will want to use this advantage and spread your feet slightly to maintain your balance and stability. Lowering the center of gravity also increases stability. The amount of muscular effort required to maintain stability is directly related to the height of the center of gravity and to the breadth of the base support; therefore, to conserve energy and reduce the strain on muscles when lifting or moving patients, lower your body's center of gravity and broaden the base of support. When lifting an object from the floor, you should bend the knees, because this serves as a shock absorber; do not bend from the waist. When lifting a patient, spread your feet slightly to increase base support, and hold the patient close to your body so that the center of gravity is balanced over both feet. Protect your spine by using your arm and leg muscles (Fig. 13-1).

The U.S. Air Force lists some general principles to follow when moving or lifting patients:

1. Place your body in the correct position before moving or lifting.
2. Place your feet far enough apart to maintain proper balance and provide a basis of support.
3. Hold the patient as close to your body as possible to eliminate all unnecessary strain by centralizing the total weight within your grasp.
4. Stoop to the working level, and keep the back straight.
5. Slide rather than lift whenever possible.
6. When a patient is too heavy for you to move alone, get help.
7. When two or more people are moving or lifting, give a signal, and move or lift in unison.

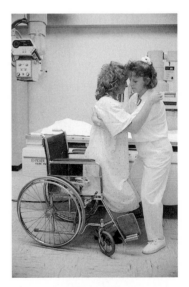

Fig. 13-1

Spreading the feet slightly and holding the patient close to your body so that the center of gravity is balanced over both feet increases stability and protects the back muscles.

The patient should be encouraged to help with the move if he or she is able. Because patients will most likely be slow in their response to your instructions, patience may be required. Allowing the patients to help themselves preserves their sense of independence and control over illness.

The transporter and all radiology staff in patient care should be thoroughly comfortable with the use, identification, and operation of equipment and attachments such as catheters, oxygen masks, drainage tubes, and electrocardiogram (ECG) electrodes. Proper attention must be given so that tubes and catheters remain intact and free of contamination. The hospital department of radiology manual may contain policies and procedures for the care of patients who have equipment attached. The responsibility of the radiologic technologists in monitoring and adjusting the equipment should be stated in the radiology policy and procedures manual. Large departments may employ a technologist with advanced training to adjust and check drainage tubes and other equipment that is attached to the patient. However, regardless of who is assigned the responsibility, you should know some of the most commonly encountered auxiliary equipment and how to care for the patient to whom it is attached; the general rule is to maintain the unit in its present state and prevent contamination. Fainting, shock, seizures, cardiac arrest, convulsions, loss of consciousness, and bleeding are conditions that must be dealt with if and when they occur.* All radiology personnel and students in any patient care area should have the ability to monitor **vital signs**, which include blood pressure, temperature, pulse, and respiration; they should also be able to use a **stethoscope** (an instrument used to hear respiratory and cardiac sounds), thermometer, and **sphygmomanometer** (an instrument that measures blood pressure). Recording vital signs information on the hospital chart, radiology requisition, or incident report form is done in accordance with imaging department policy. It is partially the responsibility of the student to request information about these matters as the need for it arises. Changes from the routine radiographic procedures must be considered. For example, when a patient presents with myelomeningocele or osteogenesis imperfecta, handling with extreme care is essential. When working with a patient with a colostomy or ileostomy, the special guidelines involved in removing and replacing receptor bags must be followed. The intravenous infusion check is an important consideration of care that is needed in the radiology department.

Isolation techniques

Special care must be taken to prevent patients from acquiring a hospital-related disease. These are known as **nosocomial infections**, and they are the cause of thousands of deaths every year.

---

*__Fainting__ is a sudden fall in blood pressure with loss of consciousness; __shock__ is the profound depression of the vital functions with reduced blood volume and pressure, usually caused by severe injuries; __seizures__ are attacks such as convulsions or the sudden onset of a disease; __cardiac arrest__ is a state of complete cessation of the heart's action; __convulsions__ are violent, involuntary muscular contractions or spasms.

Significant research was conducted by Dr. Mary Loritsch of Virginia Western Community College and Sonya Lawson of Virginia Commonwealth University to determine the presence of pathogens on the radiography equipment and accessories. It was found that pathogens could live and even colonize on radiographic equipment, including cassettes. This research is significant, because it points out the importance of cleanliness in the operation of a radiology department. Patients visiting the radiology department should not risk getting another disease in addition to the condition that they already have.

Preventing the spread of diseases is a very important consideration in all hospitals and in any other patient care facilities. **Acquired immunodeficiency syndrome (AIDS)**, a contagious disease contracted through the exchange of contaminated blood or semen, and its devastating sequelae, is one example of a disease that requires special care and treatment.

The Centers for Disease Control and Prevention (CDC) publishes guidelines for isolation precautions in hospitals specifically for AIDS and other communicable diseases. Hospital procedure manuals include these guidelines and make them a part of orientation for new employees and for radiography students.

You may be called upon to do an examination in an isolation ward, so you should be acquainted with the procedures for entering and leaving such a room. When performing radiographic examinations in an isolation unit, special clothing may be required; this will usually consist of a gown, cap, mask, and gloves. The purpose of an **isolation room** is to confine the disease to the patient, to protect the people working with the patient, and to protect other patients; it may also be used to protect the patient from microorganisms carried by people entering the room. All equipment and accessories must be made readily available, but they must not come in contact with the patient until the immediate time of use. Cassettes should be placed in a pillowcase during the examination. The case housing of the radiographic equipment should be wiped with disinfectant solution before leaving the unit. **Disinfectants** are substances that are used to destroy **pathogens** (viruses, microorganisms, or other substances causing disease) or to render them inert. **Antiseptics** are substances that prevent or retard the growth of microorganisms; alcohol is a commonly used antiseptic in hospitals.

Department isolation techniques require very strict procedures if the disease is contagious. **Contagious diseases** such as chickenpox, tuberculosis, herpes zoster, measles, and mumps may be contracted by droplet or airborne routes. Other diseases may be contracted by direct or indirect contact only and thus require a different isolation technique. Typical of these are bacterial and viral infections such as *Salmonella* and *Escherichia coli* and other diseases that affect the bowel with resultant infected feces. Strict isolation techniques are used for patients with diphtheria, eczema vaccinatum, draining lesions, German measles, and smallpox. Protective isolation is used to protect a susceptible patient from becoming infected, as in the case of patients with burns or leukemia. Infants in critical care nurseries and patients with open lesions are also candidates for the isolation ward. For the practice of aseptic techniques, the most important precaution is hand washing, but often, unfortunately, this is the most neglected practice.

Patients with wounds or those in respiratory isolation can be brought into the department of radiology. However, there should be few other patients present, and these patients must be kept separate, examined quickly, and promptly returned to their units. After the examination, the radiographic room, table, and equipment used must be promptly disinfected as protocol specifies. These practices should also be exercised for the patient in protective isolation, with the additional requirement that radiology staff wear face masks when in the presence of the patient.

Sterile or Aseptic Techniques

Operating room aseptic technique is an inherent practice within that unit, and the radiologic technologist must exercise constant watchfulness to avoid the contamination of sterile objects and reserved space on the operative side of the table (Fig. 13-2).

Sterilization implies the complete removal or destruction of microorganisms. It is beyond the scope of this text to describe fully the techniques for providing a sterile field for practicing aseptic techniques. The following items are based on the major principles of the techniques and are offered as a guide to follow (from the *Department of the Air Force Training Manual*):

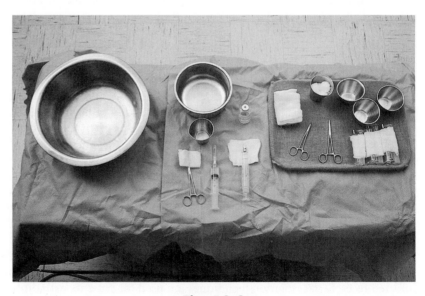

Fig. 13-2

An opened sterile package with sterile items; typical of some used in special radiographic procedures.

1. An article is either sterile or unsterile; there is no in-between. If any doubt exists, you must consider the article to be unsterile.
2. Sterile articles must be kept covered until ready for use.
3. Only the outside of the wrapper or cover is touched when opening a sterile package or container.
4. A sterile article is handled with a sterile instrument or sterile gloves.
5. After an article is removed from a sterile container, it is not to be returned to that container.
6. When removing an article from a sterile container, use the forceps provided. Only that part of the container and the part of the forceps that is covered by disinfecting solution are considered sterile. Always hold the tip of the forceps downward. Remove the cover of the container. Hold the cover in one hand. Remove the article with the forceps in the other hand. Replace the cover. If you must lay down the cover, turn it upside down on a flat surface.
7. When a container becomes contaminated, dispose of it at once. If you cannot do it immediately, turn the cover to show it is contaminated.
8. Avoid reaching over a sterile field.
9. Edges of sterile towels are considered contaminated after contact with an unsterile surface.
10. Keep instrument handles out of sterile fields.
11. Pour sterile solutions so that there is no contact between the bottle and the sides of the container.

Aseptic techniques and special patient consideration must be a part of the department's overall policy routine for preparing syringes; patient prepping; disposal of needles, catheters, and tubes; and cleanup. When medication is administered, great care must be taken. Michael Bloyd, RN, RT, lists "five rights" when medication is given; the right patient, the right drug, the right route, the right amount, and the right time. Charting or recording information about the patient's condition and your role in the patient's examination is an important part of patient care. It is especially so in the case of an accident in which the outcome may be in question. The team concept in isolation or special patient consideration must be exercised at all times. Most departments of imaging have in-service programs available in manual, videotape, or slide presentations for staff and student review.

CONCLUSION

The underlying objective for discussing patient care and management is to provide safety for the patient and for those who work with patients in radiology. Quality radiographic techniques must include those patient-handling tasks that are necessary to prevent injury, the spread of disease, or other hazardous complications.

Review Questions

1. Optimum patient care includes all the following except:
   a. Radiation safety.
   b. Preventing the spread of disease.
   c. Loyalty to the hospital or institution.
   d. Providing economic and timely service.

2. A radiographic examination may be cancelled or approved by:
   a. The administrative technologist.
   b. The nurse.
   c. The radiologist.
   d. Examinations requested cannot be cancelled

3. Knowledge of and competency in cardiopulmonary resuscitation is required of:
   a. Physicians.
   b. Technologists.
   c. Nurses.
   d. All the above

4. When lifting patients or heavy objects, the weight:
   a. Should be held at 10 inches from the center of gravity.
   b. Should be held as close to the body as possible.
   c. Should be distributed equally from the gravity line.
   d. Should be held to the right of the center of gravity.

5. A stethoscope is an instrument that is used to measure which of the following?
   a. Pulse rate
   b. Blood pressure
   c. Microorganisms per cubic centimeter
   d. Chest and heart sounds

6. Pathogens are:
   a. Viruses or microorganisms that cause disease.
   b. Microorganisms that cause fatal disease.
   c. Microorganisms needed to produce vitamin B_{12}.
   d. Benign microorganisms and viruses inherent in the body.

7. Isolation techniques are employed to:
   a. Prevent the patient from spreading a contagious disease.
   b. Prevent the patient from contracting a contagious disease.
   c. Prevent the health care worker from contracting the disease.
   d. All the above

8. The complete removal or destruction of microorganisms is done with the use of which of the following?
   a. Antiseptics
   b. Disinfectants
   c. Sterilization
   d. All the above

9. The most practical precaution one can take to prevent the spread of disease is:
   a. Wearing sterile gloves and a mask.

    b. Using disinfectants to clean the radiographic table.

    c. Thorough hand washing after the handling of each patient.

    d. Isolating diseased patients.

10. Radiographic service can be administered for all the following reasons except:

    a. Protection from lawsuits.

    b. Ruling out pathology.

    c. Diagnosing pathology.

    d. Routine checkup.

BIBLIOGRAPHY

Ballinger P: *Merrill's atlas of radiographic positions and radiologic procedures*, ed. 10, St. Louis, 2003, Mosby.

Capps E: Private communications, compiled for course supplement, Nashville, 1982, S & H X-Ray.

Department of the Air Force training manual, Pueblo, CO, 1974, U.S. Government Printing Office.

Ehrlich RA, McCloskey ED, Daly JA: *Patient care in radiography*, ed. 6, St. Louis, 2004, Mosby.

Hafen B: *First aid for health emergencies*, ed. 4, St. Paul, MN, 1988, West.

Leafer C: Getting it right, writing it down, the technologist's role in charting, *Radiology Today* 5(19):14, Sept. 13, 2004.

Loritsch MB, Lawson SR: Sauer R: Bacterial Survival on radiographic cassettes, Journal of the American Society of Radiologic Technologists 76:507-510, July-August, 2002.

Radiology specialist program #JP90350, Boulder, CO, School of Aviation Medicine, USAF Air University, 1958.

Snopek AM: *Fundamentals of special radiographic procedures*, ed. 4, Saunders, 2006.

Torres LS: *Basic medical techniques and patient care for radiologic technologists*, ed. 5, Philadelphia, 1997, JB Lippincott.

Medicolegal Considerations

Russell A. Tolley

OBJECTIVES

On completion of this chapter, you should be able to:

- Discuss the impact of medical malpractice on society.
- Define tort and explain its several forms in the health profession.
- Discuss patient consent rights and the radiologic technologist's role in assuring the validity of the consent.
- Define respondeat superior and explain its significance in radiology services.
- Define res ipsa loquitur and explain how it may apply in radiology.
- List seven reasons why a radiologic technologist may be named as a defendant in a malpractice case.
- Discuss the steps a radiologic technologist may take to prevent a lawsuit against a health care provider.
- Discuss the importance of maintaining patient privacy.

It has been said that the American society in which we live and work as health care professionals is "a nation ruled by laws, not by men." This quote suggests that law establishes the relationship not only between the individual and the government but also between individuals. The dominant power over our lives is not the authority of a king, junta, or popularly elected president. Rather, political power is embodied in a complex system that we refer to simply as "the law."

Law is not a single entity; it is a composite body of customs, practices, and rules. In our society, these rules and practices come from the federal and state constitutions, the statutes of both state and federal legislatures,

KEY TERMS

case law
civil assault
civil battery
defendant
false imprisonment
negligence
plaintiff
res ipsa loquitur
respondeat superior
torts

CHAPTER OUTLINE

*Medical malpractice
Torts
    Intentional misconduct
    Unintentional
        misconduct
        (negligence)
Patient consent
Respondeat superior
Res ipsa loquitur
Legal considerations of
    the radiologic
    technologist
Conclusion*

regulations issued by the administrative agencies of the executive branch of government, and the interpretations of these constitutions, statutes, and regulations that are rendered by the courts. The law that arises from the courts' interpretations of these constitutions, statutes, and regulations is known as **case law**. Community values generally inform and shape the rules formed by particular administrations, legislatures, and courts; however, any reading of contemporary affairs makes it clear that perceived community values and our laws are not always in agreement. The history of law—in all forms—is a history of accumulating wisdom and experience that is mixed with substantial amounts of give-and-take among all segments of society.

The underlying motivation for all forms of law is to protect people and property, to provide for correcting injustice, and to compensate for injury. The specific area of the law that most concerns health practitioners is known as medical malpractice.

MEDICAL MALPRACTICE

You have probably read of large medical malpractice awards to injured patients. Even large medical institutions can be financially devastated when they are required to pay such amounts. To reduce the risk of such medical malpractice awards, it is important to understand the nature of the legal relationship between the individual patient and health care providers.

The legal rights that exist between the individual patient and those who provide health care to that patient are essentially the same rights that exist between any two individuals, with some significant exceptions. One of these exceptions is that, unlike two individuals who act on roughly equal footing to transact the sale of property or to enter business contracts, the relationship between a patient and a health care provider is rarely that of two equals. Because society has allowed physicians to practice medicine, it also imposes upon them the duty to conduct that practice according to accepted standards. In effect, along with special privilege must go special responsibility. Failure to meet this special responsibility can leave a physician or other health care practitioner open to lawsuits alleging wrongful or negligent acts that result in injury to a patient. The law refers to such wrongful or negligent acts generally as torts.

TORTS

Torts are not easy to define, but a basic distinction is that they are violations of civil, as opposed to criminal, law.* For this discussion we can

---

*However, the same conduct may constitute both a tort and a violation of the criminal law. Intentionally punching someone in the nose without consent or excuse would constitute both a civil battery (a tort) and a crime. If the victim brought a civil tort action against the perpetrator, the perpetrator could be required to pay money damages directly to the victim to compensate for any injury to the victim. If the state brought a criminal action, the perpetrator could suffer a prison sentence or other punishment for that conduct.

also say that tort law is personal injury law. Torts include those conditions where the law allows for compensation to be paid to an individual when that individual is damaged or injured by another.

There are two types of torts: those resulting from intentional action and those resulting from unintentional action.

Intentional Misconduct

There are several situations in which a tort action can be brought against the health professional because of some action that was deliberately taken.

1. A tort of **civil assault** can be filed if a patient is reasonably fearful that he or she was injured by the imprudent conduct of the radiologic technologist. If found liable, the radiologic technologist could be held responsible for providing financial compensation to the patient for damages.

2. A **civil battery** tort would be an appropriate proceeding when actual bodily harm has been inflicted on a patient as a result of intentional physical contact between a health care provider and a patient, again with potential for liability against the radiologic technologist. A health worker cannot touch a patient for any reason unless there is a valid consent by the patient to receive medical care. (The elements that are required for a valid consent will be discussed later.)

3. Other forms of intentional misconduct include invasion of privacy; defamation, whether spoken (slander) or written (libel); and false imprisonment. An example of invasion of privacy is when a radiologic technologist publicly discusses privileged and confidential information obtained from the attending physician or the patient's medical record. An example of **false imprisonment** would be unnecessarily confining or restraining the patient without the patient's permission. If during the performance of a radiographic examination a patient is strapped to the table or similarly confined without having given permission to be so restricted, that patient would have grounds for a charge of false imprisonment.

Unintentional Misconduct (Negligence)

If it is determined that a health care provider acted negligently, he or she may be held liable for those actions that cause injury to patients, even though those actions were unintentional. Negligence can be the basis for tort action because the radiologic technologist, although intending to help, actually caused damage by failure to perform as the patient and the employing hospital had the right to expect that person to perform.

Like the majority of American legal principles, the idea of negligence as a basis for civil liability came from English common law. The concepts of medical negligence and liability have a long history, dating at least to the fourteenth century. We have written records that in 1373 Justice John Cavendish decided the case of *Stratton v Swanlond* with the conclusion that if the patient was harmed as a consequence of the physician's negligence, that physician should be held liable. Justice Cavendish added that if the physician did all he could, he should not be held liable, even if there was no cure. More than 500 years ago, the basic ingredients of negligence and liability were expressed in an English-language court.

Negligence can be defined as a breach or a failure to fulfill an expected standard of care. Generally, the standard of care required is that degree of care that would be used by a "reasonable person" under the circumstances. For health care professionals, however, the standard of care is modified somewhat and is determined by the degree of care or skill that a reasonable health care professional would exercise under the circumstances. This means that the radiologic technologist owes a duty to the patient based on the standard of care that a reasonable radiologic technologist is expected to provide under similar circumstances.[*] Failure to perform to that expected standard of care will constitute negligence and result in liability. For a health care professional to be found negligent in a court and subsequently held liable for damages, the civil proceeding must establish the following elements:

1. What *duty* of care (or standard of care) was owed by the radiologic technologist to the patient
2. That there was a *breach* of that duty by the radiologic technologist
3. That the *cause* of injury was the radiologic technologist's negligence
4. That the *injury* to the patient actually occurred

Each of these elements is discussed below:

1. *The standard of care owed to the injured person.* The radiologic technologist must exercise the care that a reasonable radiologic technologist is expected to exercise under the same circumstances. If a physician instructs radiologic technologist Boswell to radiograph patient Abbott's right leg, Boswell has a duty to properly radiograph Abbott's right leg. If Boswell radiographs Abbott's right leg, Boswell will have performed as a reasonable and prudent radiologic technologist would have acted under similar circumstances. If, however, Boswell radiographs Abbott's *left* leg, Boswell is breaching the standard of care by failing to follow the physician's directions.

Boswell does *not* have a duty to exercise care above and beyond what a reasonable radiologic technologist would exercise. For example, Boswell does not have the responsibility to repair broken bones that are discovered while radiographing patient Abbott.

Evidence about what the standard of care should be usually consists of the testimony of an expert witness such as a competent radiologic technologist or radiologist. Testimony will concentrate on what conduct would be reasonably expected under the circumstances based on customarily accepted standards within the medical community.

---

[*]The "reasonable person" and the "reasonable radiologic technologist" discussed above do not refer to any particular person but rather to a hypothetical reasonable person and reasonable radiologic technologist. Thus, a person described by everyone as "reasonable" will still be liable for negligence if, in a particular situation, he or she fails to act as the hypothetical reasonable person would have acted. For example, if a person exceeds the speed limit and causes an accident, he or she will still be guilty of negligence, even if she finds six very reasonable people to testify that they sometimes exceed the speed limit. The hypothetical reasonable person never exceeds the speed limit. Thus, normal and reasonable people are often found negligent in particular circumstances.

2. Breach of the standard of care. A breach is failure to exercise reasonable care. What if Boswell radiographs the right leg but the quality of that radiograph is not adequate to provide diagnostic information? If a radiologic technologist has the duty to ensure that radiographs are clear and of the highest quality for the physician's diagnosis, then giving the physician an inadequate radiograph is a breach of the radiologic technologist's duty. If a patient's condition deteriorates because the physician could not properly interpret the radiograph, then the patient would have grounds to sue the physician and the radiologic technologist. How inadequate need a radiograph be before a jury would declare the technologist in breach of duty? This is a difficult question that would be resolved in court with the assistance of expert witnesses and by the judgment of a jury on a case-by-case basis.

3. *The radiologic technologist's negligence must be shown to be the direct cause of the patient's injury.* The breach of duty must be the factual cause of the injury. If the radiologic technologist has the duty to make sure that a dizzy or semiconscious patient does not fall from the examination table, it would be a breach of that duty if the radiologic technologist left the room. If, upon the radiologic technologist's leaving the room, the patient fell from the table and sustained injuries, a jury hearing the tort action likely would agree that the radiologic technologist's breach of duty (negligence) *caused* the injuries; this is because leaving the room would be closely related to the patient's falling from the table. Suppose, however, that the radiologic technologist leaves the room and upon return finds that the patient is very upset that the radiologic technologist left the room, although the patient did not fall off the table. Days later, the patient is standing in the hall telling his wife that the radiologic technologist had left him alone while he was semiconscious on the examination table. In describing the incident, the patient becomes upset, faints, and, as a result, fractures an arm. The patient might argue that the radiologic technologist caused the fractured arm. The patient probably would not prevail in court, however, because he or she would have difficulty proving that the radiologic technologist's action was a "proximate cause" of the fractured arm. If the cause of injury is too remote from the breach of duty (the negligence), even though factual cause seems evident, then the negligence is not the proximate cause of injury.

4. *The patient sustains actual injury.* A personal injury case or tort will not be successful in establishing liability if there are no damages. If a patient falls from an examination table because the radiologic technologist leaves the room but does not incur any injuries, the patient cannot expect to receive compensation.

Applying the negligence standard to Boswell's error in radiographing the patient's left leg instead of the right is relatively easy. Obviously, a reasonable radiologic technologist would x-ray the correct limb. In real life, applying the negligence standard is not always as easy, as the following examples demonstrate. These examples are based loosely on real cases. Some facts have been changed to maintain the privacy of those involved.

Case 1

An older adult patient was admitted to the hospital for treatment and tests. She was sent to the radiology department for a routine chest x-ray. While standing at the chest unit, she fell and broke her hip. The patient filed suit against the hospital, the referring physician, the radiologists, and the technologist. In the lawsuit, the patient claimed that these parties acted negligently, that she should have been supported or restrained while being x-rayed, and that the physician should have noted her tendency to become dizzy on the examination request.

In this case, the patient was able to prove that she had a tendency to become dizzy and that the physician knew about it. The evidence in the case also showed that the physician's examination request had no reference to the patient's tendency to become dizzy.

The radiologist and technologist brought forth evidence that the examination and x-ray process were conducted in a manner that was customary, reasonable, and generally accepted in the medical community. They were also able to show that they had no knowledge of the patient's tendency to become dizzy. Accordingly, the radiologist and technologist were able to convince the jury that they were not negligent.

On the other hand, the jury found that the referring physician was negligent for not noting the patient's tendency to become dizzy on the request slip. The jury believed that this breached the physician's standard of care and that this breach caused the patient's injury.

Questions and Comments. By adding facts or slightly changing the facts, the result of this case might be different. For instance, if the physician had noted the patient's tendency to become dizzy on the examination request, the jury probably would have held the radiologist and technologist liable and excused the referring physician. The case also might have been decided differently if the hospital had a policy of restraining all patients during the x-ray process (with the patient's consent) and if the radiologist and technologist had violated that policy.

How do you think the case would have turned out if there were no notations on the examination request but the radiologist or technologist had noticed the patient walking unsteadily prior to the x-ray? Would it matter if this observation occurred 2 days before the x-ray? Five minutes before the x-ray? Why?

Case 2

A hospitalized patient was scheduled for an emergency radiographic examination that required the injection of a contrast medium. The floor nurse inserted the needle into the vein, and the patient was transported to the radiology department. In the radiology department, the contrast medium was injected; however, the needle was not in the vein when the contrast media was injected. This resulted in extravasation and serious damage to the tissue surrounding the vessel. The patient sued, among others, the hospital, the nurse, and the technologist. The suit was settled before trial, and the hospital made a substantial settlement payment to the patient.

Questions and Comments. This case illustrates a real-life example of *res ipsa loquitur.* The circumstances suggest that the injury simply would not have occurred in the absence of negligence by someone. Thus, to avoid liability, each of the defendants must prove that he or she was not the cause of the negligence. Accordingly, if the case were tried, the nurse would attempt to prove that he or she properly inserted the needle in the vein and that the needle became dislodged after the patient left the floor. On the other hand, the technologist would attempt to show that the needle was not inserted correctly in the first place.

The case also raises the question of whether the technologist should have the skill and training to check and determine the proper placement of the needle. Currently, not all schools provide the training for a technologist to make such a determination. Accordingly, the technologist might well be able to show that the required standard of care for a technologist would not include the duty to determine the proper placement of the needle and that this was the duty of the radiologist who injected the contrast media. As was previously discussed, however, the standard of care is subject to evolution and change. It is possible that the patient could have convinced a jury that a reasonably experienced technologist should have a duty to check the proper placement of the needle. If the jury agreed, the standard of care for technologists might well be increased to include the duty to make such determinations. If this happened, educators would have to rethink their curricula.

These comments are not included to suggest what the standard of care for technologists is or ought to be in this situation; rather, they are designed to demonstrate the complexity of the "negligence" concept and to stimulate thinking about how law (i.e., the standard of care) could evolve and influence society (e.g., schools and educators) and vice versa.

Case 3

This case takes a different twist because the technologist is not the defendant—he is the plaintiff. In this case, the technologist sued his employer, alleging that he had developed chronic granulocytic leukemia as a result of overexposure to radiation. The technologist testified that daily he had to support patients while the patients were being x-rayed and that this subjected him to radiation exposure. The technologist stated that he could not use proper restraining devices because of the large number of patients he was required to move through the x-ray process. He also testified that lead aprons, shields, and gloves sometimes were not easily available to him.

In this case, the judge found the hospital negligent and awarded damages to the technologist relating to his leukemia. The judge believed that the hospital did not take reasonable precautions to limit the exposure of technologists to radiation.

Questions and Comments. This case presents a number of interesting issues. It might well have been decided differently by a different judge or jury. For instance, some courts or juries might have determined that the technologist's own negligence (i.e., not insisting on using lead shields, aprons, and gloves) contributed to his disease.

The case also had the potential of presenting causation problems for the technologist. What if the technologist also had a heart condition and such a condition contributed to his injuries? What if the hospital had produced evidence that the leukemia could have been caused by factors other than exposure to radiation?

In any event, this case illustrates the need for technologists to take appropriate precautions to avoid unnecessary exposure to radiation and for hospitals to make appropriate equipment available and to enforce procedures designed to reduce unnecessary exposure.

Case 4

This case involves a staff technologist who was assigned to the gastrointestinal fluoroscopic room. During the examination of a patient, the radiologist asked the technologist to bring the patient's radiographs to the viewing room to determine if another view should be made before discharging the patient. The patient was elderly, and it appeared that restraints were appropriate if the patient was to remain on the table. With the patient securely restrained, the technologist carried the radiographs to the doctor for a quick check for diagnostic reading. The viewing area was several steps away from the patient examination room. While the technologist was in the viewing area, the fire alarm sounded. The technologist rushed back to the patient and found her to be quite frightened and agitated, because she, too, had heard the fire alarm and the commotion of others in the area who were reacting to the alarm. The technologist attempted to calm the patient but did not have much success. Although it turned out to be a false alarm and the all-clear signal immediately followed, the patient sued for false imprisonment.

Questions and Comments. This case presents a troubling situation, because it is routine to restrain patients in some situations. When patients who are unable to control their actions or who are under the influence of drugs or alcohol must remain on the x-ray table for prolonged examinations, it is prudent to restrain them to prevent injury. It is always prudent to get the patient's consent, as this lawsuit points out. However, this is not always possible, and good judgment must prevail. Family members or fellow technologists may be called on to assist. The question here involves how this technologist will defend herself in this case. For example, would the patient have sued if the fire alarm had not gone off? Or would she have sued merely because of the restraints?

PATIENT CONSENT

The general rule is that patients have the right to consent to or refuse anything that is done to them in the hospital. Patient consent can be written, oral, or implied (Fig. 14-1). Implied consent would be used in circumstances where a patient is unconscious in an emergency room; it is assumed that the patient would want to give consent to receive needed care. The patient can revoke consent at any time. Even if the patient has previously granted verbal consent, written consent, or implied consent, at no time can a patient be

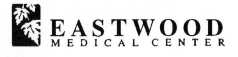

DATE: _____, 20_____

TIME: _____ AM / PM

Patient: _____

1. I consent and authorize Dr. _____ and any associates or assistants or consultants of his choice to perform the following medical/surgical operation, treatment or procedure:

_____ .

(Information to be furnished in layman's language)
and such additional therapeutic operations or procedures as his or their judgement may dictate on the basis of findings during the course of said surgery or procedure including, but not limited to, the transfusion of blood, and the performance of services involving pathology and radiology.

2. The nature and purpose of the operation, treatment and/or procedure, the possible alternative methods, the risks involved and the possibility of complications have been fully explained to me. I acknowledge that no guarantee or assurance has been made as to the results that may be obtained.

3. I consent to the disposal by hospital authorities of any tissue or parts which may be removed.

4. For the purpose of advancing medical education, I consent to the admittance of observers to the operating room and to the photographing, filming or televising of the procedure/operation to be performed, provided my identity is not revealed by the pictures or by descriptive texts accompanying them.

_____   _____

(Signature of patient or person authorized to consent for patient)   Relationship

_____

Witness

Fig. 14-1

Consent and authorization for medical/surgical operations, treatment, or procedure. (Courtesy of Patt Hammer, RT, RDMS, Eastwood Medical Center, Memphis, TN.)

denied the right to withdraw consent. For consent to be valid, three conditions must be met: the patient must be of legal age and mentally competent, the patient must offer consent voluntarily, and the patient must be adequately informed about the medical care being recommended. Because adequate information about treatment is generally known only by the physician or the health care provider, special responsibility is required to ensure that the patient understands the type of care and the potential risks that are being considered. Thus, you should accurately explain to your patients any procedure you will perform and what you expect of that patient.

RESPONDEAT SUPERIOR

The doctrine of *respondeat superior*, which is a Latin phrase that means "let the master answer," requires that an employer pay the victim for the torts committed by its employees. If a radiologic technologist is employed by a hospital, the hospital can be held jointly liable for whatever the radiologic technologist might do in a negligent manner. An injured patient does not have to prove that the hospital was negligent, only that the radiologic technologist was liable. Because the hospital employs the radiologic technologist, the hospital is automatically held jointly liable. Although the employing hospital may be jointly liable with an employee, this does not mean that a radiologic technologist is immune from damage suits or relieved of personal responsibility for breach of duty. All people are responsible for their own injurious conduct.

RES IPSA LOQUITUR

In most tort cases, the **plaintiff** (the injured person bringing the suit) has the responsibility of proving that the **defendant** (the person being sued) should be held liable. There are certain cases of negligence, however, in which the defendant is required to prove innocence. *Res ipsa loquitur* is a Latin phrase that means "the thing speaks for itself." The doctrine of *res ipsa loquitur* applies to a case that is built around evidence that demonstrates that an injury could not have occurred if there had been no negligence. An example of such a case would be one in which it is discovered that a pair of forceps has been left in the patient's abdomen after surgery. They were not in the patient before surgery, and they could be in the patient only as a result of negligence on the part of the surgical team. As another example, a patient's being exposed to radiation sufficient to cause skin lesions could result only from negligence on the part of the radiologic technologist. In these cases, the procedures begin with the facts of evidence and proceed to establish that these facts would not have been true if there had not been negligence on someone's part. In these circumstances, it is incumbent upon the defendants to demonstrate that they were not the party responsible for the negligent act.

Patients may be harmed in ways other than physical, and one way is failure to maintain patient confidentiality. Divulging a patient's condition or other information contained in a patient's medical record could cause financial loss or social embarrassment to the patient. Accordingly, strict laws and policies exist to protect patients' privacy and the confidentiality of their medical records. Maintaining patient privacy is a significant issue not only because failure to do so may harm the patient, but also because such failure will expose the caregiver and employer to embarrassing, time-consuming lawsuits and the risk of financial loss and other sanctions.

Generally speaking, patients' medical records (their radiographs are a part of the medical records) belong to the hospital or institution where their care was given. However, the information contained in the records belongs to the patient. Without the patient's consent, this information *cannot* be divulged or released to anyone else.* A caregiver can be liable for disclosing patient information even if the disclosure is unintentional or inadvertent and even if the caregiver honestly believed the disclosure would not harm the patient. This is an important consideration while working with patients during your clinical practice.

LEGAL CONSIDERATIONS OF THE RADIOLOGIC TECHNOLOGIST

Although the radiologic technologist does not encounter anywhere near the number of malpractice suits that are directed against the physician, there are a number of reasons that a radiologic technologist might be held liable. Saundra Warner, a distinguished radiologic educator and attorney, lists seven reasons why a plaintiff's attorney might choose to name a radiologic technologist as a defendant:

1. To meet the conditions of *res ipsa loquitur*
2. Because the hospital or its physicians are immune from action, or because the radiologic technologist is not directly controlled by the physician
3. Because the hospital and/or physicians cannot be sued as defendants because they are not directly negligent, and proximate causation cannot be applied to the hospital or physicians
4. Because of various trial tactics
5. To secure the radiologic technologist in pretrial testimony and as a witness in subsequent court testimony
6. Because the plaintiff presumes that the radiologic technologist has assets or insurance
7. Because it aids or is essential to the case

It is always prudent to maintain records and documents of any procedure that you think is questionable or about which you might be asked to provide information.

CONCLUSION

You have a duty to give high-quality care to your patients, and this includes not causing them injury. If you professionally apply your knowledge

---

*There are certain exceptions to this rule, such as releasing information in response to a valid court order, but the exceptions are very limited. You should consult the applicable laws of your jurisdiction and the specific policies of your employer before making any patient disclosure.

and training in radiologic technology, thoroughly explain procedures to your patients, work with extreme care, and question any abnormal instructions, you will probably never be involved in a lawsuit.

It will be in your interest to find out about the malpractice insurance policy at any hospital, office, or institution for which you work. In some cases, policies only cover the hospital and staff physicians. Many insurance companies now offer malpractice or liability insurance to allied health professionals. You may wish to consider such insurance coverage.

Review Questions

1. An effective defense for a technologist sued by a patient claiming negligence would be:
   a. The patient willingly submitted to the examination.
   b. The examination was modified slightly for use in a research project.
   c. The examination was performed in a manner that was customary and accepted in the medical community.
   d. The patient did not appear to be seriously hurt and only casually complained.
2. Who is the person who is formally accused in a lawsuit?
   a. Plaintiff
   b. Respondeat
   c. Tort
   d. Defendant
3. *Res ipsa loquitur* is a Latin phrase that means:
   a. "Let the master answer."
   b. "The thing speaks for itself."
   c. "A civil wrong."
   d. "A tort resulting from intentional action."
4. What is the underlying motivation for all forms of law?
   a. To protect people and property
   b. To provide a means for correcting injustice
   c. To compensate for injury
   d. All the above
5. Which of the following conditions would not be a valid consent condition?
   a. Be of legal age and mentally competent
   b. Be a member of the medical profession
   c. Offer consent voluntarily
   d. Be adequately informed about the medical test being recommended
6. Situations in which a tort action may be brought against a technologist are:
   a. Imprudent conduct by the radiologic technologist.
   b. Bodily harm inflicted on a patient.
   c. Invasion of privacy.
   d. All of the above

7. The following conditions would be considered a breach of standard care except:
   a. The radiograph was inadequate for interpretation.
   b. The anatomic part requested for the test was not the part that was radiographed.
   c. The patient's condition did not improve after the test.
   d. The patient falls from the x-ray table and is injured.
8. Law in our society is based on which of the following?
   a. State and federal constitutions
   b. Statutes of state and federal legislatures
   c. Regulations issued by the executive branch of government
   d. All the above
9. Laws are framed and shaped by which of the following?
   a. Conditions of economic need
   b. Population variables
   c. Community values
   d. Individual motives and practices
10. Community values and laws are:
    a. Always in agreement.
    b. Generally in agreement.
    c. Irrelevant entities.
    d. Historically without merit.
11. Patient information may be given without the patient's consent to:
    a. Insurance company
    b. The patient's employer
    c. Medicare
    d. None of the above

BIBLIOGRAPHY

Adler AM, Carlton RR: *Introduction to radiography and patient care*, ed. 2, Philadelphia, 1998, WB Saunders.
American Hospital Association's 1992 Patient's Bill of Rights.
Blaut JM: The medical malpractice crisis: its causes and future, *Ins Couns J* 44:114, 1977.
Bundy A: *Radiology and the law*, Rockville, MD, 1988, Aspen.
Church, EJ: Legal trends in imaging, *Radiol Technol* 76(1):31-45, 2004.
Comment. Medico-legal implications of recent legislation concerning allied health practitioners, *Loy LAL Rev* 11:379, 1978.
Greenberg v Michael Rees Hospital, 83 Ill 2d 282, 415 NE 2d 390 (1981).
Hillcrest Medical Center v Wier, 373 p 2d 45 (Okla 1962).
Hospital Authority v Adams, 110 Ga App 848, 140 SE 2d 139 (1964).
Johnson v Grant Hospital, 31 Ohio App 2d 118, 286 NE 2d 368 (1968).
Keene v Methodist Hospital, 324 F Supp 233 (1971).
Krayse v Bridgeport Hospital, 169 Conn 1, 362 A 2d 802 (1975).
Mulholland HR: The legal status of the hospital medical staff, *St Louis ULJ* 22:485, 1978.
Prosser W: *Handbook of the law of torts*, ed. 4, San Diego, 1971, Harcourt Brace Jovanovich.

Rose v Hakim, 345 F Supp 1300 (1972).

Runyan v Goodrum, 228 SW 397 (Ark 1921).

Simmons v South Shore Hospital, 340 Ill App 153, 91 NE 2d 135 (1950).

Simpson v Sisters of Charity, 284 Or 547, 588 p 2d 4 (1978).

Standefer v United States, 511 F 2d 101 (1975).

Toth v Community Hospital, 22 NY 2d 255, 239 NE 368 (1968).

Tucson General Hospital v Russell, 7 Ariz App 193, 437 P 2d 677 (1968).

Warner SL, former assistant professor of radiology, University of Maryland School of Medicine: Personal communication, 1981.

Washington Hospital Center v Butler, 384 F 2d 331 (1967).

Organization and Operation of the Radiology Department

Penny S. Mays

OBJECTIVES

On completion of this chapter, you should be able to:

- Describe the role of the hospital administrator.
- Describe the role of the radiology administrator.
- Describe the role and function of the policy and procedures manual.
- Construct a radiology organizational chart.
- Describe how requests for radiology services are made and received.
- List essential procedures and policy items included in the procedures manual.
- Describe the rationale for in-service education programs.
- Describe the rationale for a quality assurance program.
- Explain the role of the Joint Commission on Accreditation of Healthcare Organizations (JCAHO).
- List the factors that determine the selection of radiology equipment.

KEY TERMS

compliance evaluations
flowcharts
hospital safety committee
in-service education
Occupational Safety and
    Health Administration
    (OSHA)
organizational charts
personnel monitoring
position description
procedures manual
quality assurance
radiation safety
    committee

CHAPTER OUTLINE

*Administration and staff
    responsibilities
    Radiology staff
        activities
    Effective working
        relationships
    Policies and procedures
    Personnel procedures
    Safety
    Quality assurance
    Equipment
Conclusion*

The characteristics of a radiology department are determined by the roles and functions of the hospital and the needs of the community it serves. If they are part of a large teaching institution, some departments may have teaching and research in addition to patient care responsibilities. In smaller hospitals, the radiology department may be involved only in patient care.

Although there is no typical or average radiology department, certain characteristics are common to most departments. The organization of a radiology department affects its internal structure and the disposition and management of personnel and fiscal resources. Management aims to arrange employees into working groups according to their work functions. Administration directs the efforts and skills of employees toward reaching departmental objectives in a cohesive and satisfying fashion.

Specialized areas within a radiology department may include diagnostic radiology, nuclear medicine, and sonography. In large departments, there may be sections devoted to radiation oncology, radiation biology, and radiation physics.

This chapter is devoted almost exclusively to the diagnostic radiology department, because it is the largest and most often the first clinical affiliation for the student. Currently, the sections of radiology departments that are devoted to diagnostic services only are often called imaging departments, departments of imaging, or diagnostic radiology departments.

ADMINISTRATION AND STAFF RESPONSIBILITIES

The hospital administrator and the medical staff are responsible for the operation of the hospital. The administrator is responsible for planning, developing, and maintaining programs that implement the policies and achieve the goals established by the governing body. This person organizes the administrative functions of the hospital, delegates duties, establishes formal meetings with personnel, and provides the hospital with administrative direction.

The director of radiology and the radiology management staff have the following responsibilities:
1. Participation in medical staff activities as required
2. Establishment of an effective working relationship with the medical staff, the administration, and other departments and services
3. Development and approval of all policies and procedures for the radiology department
4. Verification of the qualifications and capabilities of all radiology staff technical personnel
5. Development of comprehensive safety rules in cooperation with the hospital safety committee
6. Review and evaluation of the quality and appropriateness of radiologic services
7. Advisement of the medical staff and administration of equipment needs, modification, and utilization

Chapters 23 and 24 provide the American Society of Radiologic Technologists (ASRT) **position description**, which is a term that is synonymous with "job description" but that encompasses a broader scope of activities. It should be noted, however, that terminology is not standardized and may vary from institution to institution. A position description similar to the ones listed here may carry a different title and may occupy a different place on an organizational chart.

Radiology Staff Activities

The ultimate objective of the diagnostic radiology department is to aid physicians in their efforts to diagnose and treat disease by providing them with timely and reliable information obtained from radiographic examinations. To ensure the reliability of this diagnostic information, careful attention must be given to the performance of every examination, beginning when the examination is ordered and continuing until the examination results have been returned to the requesting physician. This relentless attention must come from all members of the radiology staff. Diagnostic radiology services should be conveniently available to meet the needs of the patient and should be directed by one or more qualified radiologists and a sufficient number of qualified technical personnel.

Effective Working Relationships

Because patient care is the primary concern of any hospital department and effective patient care depends on cooperation between all of the hospital departments, it is essential for the radiology department to have an effective working relationship with the medical staff, the administration, and other hospital departments and services.

It is also important for members of the radiology department to be familiar with the procedures of the admissions and medical records departments so that the process of patient care runs as smoothly as possible. The radiology staff must interact with the personnel department, which is largely responsible for recruiting personnel and maintaining personnel records. Radiology services are often a substantial part of the patient's hospital expense; therefore, department personnel need to be familiar with business services, which is the department that monitors billing procedures.

Policies and Procedures

It is the responsibility of the radiology administrator to develop and approve all radiology department policies and procedures. When this responsibility is executed thoroughly, the radiology department should function in a smooth and organized manner.

Flowcharts and Organizational Charts
Organizational charts and departmental **flowcharts** establish clear lines of authority, responsibility, and accountability to provide proper spans of control, create appropriate independence of operations, and define administrative

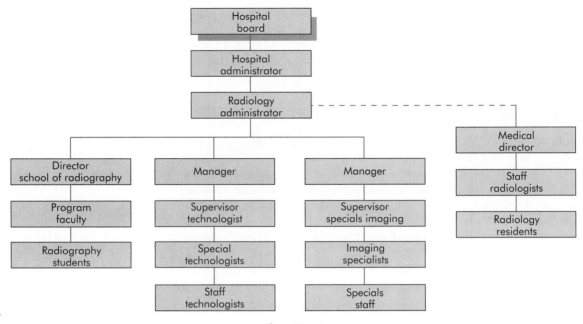

Fig. 15-1

Radiology department flowchart.

record-keeping responsibilities (Figs. 15-1 and 15-2). A plan for internal control should be implemented; this plan establishes the methods and procedures necessary to safeguard assets, monitor the accuracy and reliability of accounting data, promote managerial efficiency, and encourage adherence to managerial policy.

Requesting Radiologic Service

Requests for radiographic examinations are referred to the department of radiology, and each request is reviewed by the radiologic technologist before the examination. Completeness of information pertinent to the patient's condition is important. Precautions regarding infection control and isolation information and detailed instructions on how to move or transport the patient should be indicated on the request form. It is the responsibility of the radiology manager, in conjunction with the radiologist, to see that these examinations are performed promptly and efficiently according to radiation safety criteria and legal codes. The radiology manager is also responsible for seeing that other radiology-related legal codes, quality assurance, and continuing education needs are met to ensure that the patient is given the best quality care in the most effective manner.

Procedures Manual

Many radiology departments develop their own radiology information manuals and make them available to other departments, physicians, or associated institutions. These **procedures manuals** are generally designed

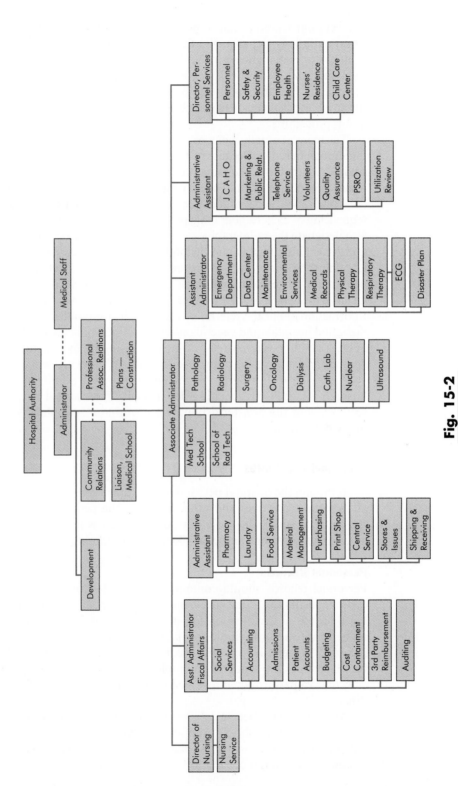

Fig. 15-2

Sample of an organizational chart.

to meet joint accreditation standards, state standards, and hospital codes. Many radiology departments find it helpful to include general instructions for patients who visit the department. The instructions may cover such subjects as appropriate gowning of the patient; transportation of the patient; precautions to be observed in the transport of the very confused, ill, medicated, or feeble patient; and, when indicated, patient isolation procedures.

The manual usually includes samples of authorization forms for various radiographic studies. Because of their potential hazards, many radiographic studies require the authorization or consent of the patient before the study is performed. The manual usually includes a section of instructions about the preparation of a patient for contrast studies. This may include the sequencing of each radiographic procedure that uses contrast agents; it may also designate the radiographic examinations that may be performed on the same day. This information is helpful to students or new personnel who are learning the policies and procedures specific to their particular area. The description of each radiographic examination covered in the manual includes the details of the procedure as well as the preparation for the study. Information about the referral of radiographs from outside clinics, institutions, and hospitals and general radiographic loan policies may be included. Policies about silver recovery, dated film disposal, and microfilmed radiographs and records are often made a part of the departmental manual.

A disaster drill program is implemented by the administrator of the hospital for each participating department. The manual may include a section about the disaster drill program so that it is available to all radiology personnel.

Personnel Procedures

Even though the hospital personnel department maintains records about all hospital employees and often monitors the personnel procedures of the entire hospital, the radiology administrator is responsible for verifying the qualifications and capabilities of all radiology staff personnel.

Personnel Records

Personnel records should contain background information that is adequate to justify the initial employment of an applicant. Applicants requiring a license or certification for employment are usually employed only after verification. Periodic work-performance evaluations should be recorded, and employee health records should be kept on file. Subsequent health services are rendered to employees to ensure that they are physically able to perform their assigned duties and that they are free of active disease.

After they have been established and maintained, these written policies and practices should support optimal achievement and quality patient care. These policies should be provided to employees and discussed in their initial orientation to the department.

Safety

Safety in the health care environment for both the patient and the employee is very important. Equipment safety has become a major concern in many institutions as a result of the proliferation of medical equipment and the increase in the number and complexity of diagnostic tests requested by physicians. Standards set for hospital accreditation require not only initial compliance but also—and more importantly—a continuing program of testing and preventive maintenance.

Radiologic Compliance Evaluations

Compliance evaluations, which include the inspection and testing of x-ray units, should be performed at the recommended intervals. These tests include tabletop exposure rate measurements, half-value layer determinations, scatter radiation surveys, and timer and collimator accuracy checks. All tests and inspections must be documented to satisfy the record-keeping requirements for accreditation.

Shielding Evaluation

Measurements of the adequacy of structural shielding as required by state regulations should be made and documented. Electrical and mechanical safety inspections and tests for compliance with currently accepted safety standards for medical equipment should also be documented.

Personnel Monitoring

Personnel monitoring is the measuring of the radiation exposure received by personnel in the performance of their duties. Exposure reports on personnel should be reviewed on a monthly basis for high exposures or exposures that exceed the maximum permissible dose. The radiation exposure reports should be posted in a highly visible area.

Departmental Safety

The Joint Commission on Accreditation of Healthcare Organizations (JCAHO) recommends that radiation safety precautions be established by the radiologist or **radiation safety committee**, which is a committee responsible for monitoring and maintaining a radiation-safe environment, in cooperation with the **hospital safety committee**, which is a committee responsible for safety in all areas of the hospital. The recommendations of the National Council on Radiation Protection and Measurements are given as a standard that should be known and applied. Some of the radiation safety precautions deal with the monitoring of radiology personnel, including the monthly recording of cumulative radiation exposure to individuals. Equipment calibration and safety maintenance are a part of the function of a radiology department. It is recommended by the accrediting agency that diagnostic and therapeutic equipment be calibrated in accordance with federal, state, and local requirements.

Rules for the safe use, removal, handling, and storage of radioactive elements and their disintegrating products should be established and enforced. In addition to rules for the radiology department, rules should be developed for the protection of nursing personnel who care for patients treated with these substances. Compliance procedures such as swipe surveys, leak tests, radioactive waste disposal, license preparation, and overexposure investigations are scheduled to be performed on a regular basis.

The institution should maintain records that show the radiation exposures of all individuals for whom personnel monitoring is required. These records must be maintained until the state department of health authorizes their disposal. Notices of occupational exposure to personnel should be posted monthly and placed in the employees' personnel files. Institutions also obtain reports of an individual's previously accumulated occupational dose.

Radiation protection devices and accessories should be readily available. Equipment such as gloves, aprons, and radiation beam-restricting devices should be monitored on a 30- to 60-day scheduled basis.

Electrical Safety

Electrical safety is very important in the radiology department because of the high-voltage equipment used. It is also a concern of the entire hospital; thus an electrical safety policy is a hospital-wide program. An awareness of the use of electronic equipment in diagnostic and therapeutic patient support is essential for all personnel. Written policies and procedures about electrical safety are usually available.

Sanitation and Infection Control

Sanitation practices are of great concern to departments of radiology because so many patients are seen in the department daily. Radiologic technologists do not spend a great deal of time with each patient, but they see a large number of patients each day. Maintaining a clean environment is essential; it is important that rooms be kept neat, clean, and orderly. Building and service equipment, such as air conditioning and ventilation systems, must be well maintained. Attention must be given to storage areas, waste disposal, and laundry. Sanitation practices and policies must also be a hospital-wide concern.

Infection control affects the entire hospital as well as the radiology department. The accrediting body for hospitals recommends a hospital-wide infection control program. Some elements of the infection control program are mechanisms for reporting and identifying infections, maintaining records of infections among patients and personnel, and reviewing and evaluating aseptic isolation and sanitation techniques. Written policies about patient isolation procedures and control procedures relating to the hospital environment (which includes central service, housekeeping, laundry, engineering, food, and waste management) are developed for hospital-wide use.

In-Service Education

There would be little use in developing and instituting safety policies unless all employees were familiar with them; therefore, all radiology personnel should receive instruction about safety precautions and about the management of radiation-related accidents and emergencies. Most radiology departments enable radiologic technologists to further their knowledge and skills by providing them with and making them aware of educational opportunities such as **in-service education** (education in knowledge, information, and skills related to specific tasks, policies, and procedures that is provided by the hospital), outside workshops, and institutes. Ideally in-service education programs are developed on the basis of the evaluation of needs and are designed to improve the quality of radiographic service.

Quality Assurance

The radiology administrator and the radiology management staff must maintain **quality assurance**, which is the monitoring and testing of imaging equipment and the control of variables including personnel in the clinical setting to minimize the unnecessary duplication of radiographic examinations and maximize the quality of diagnostic information. They must also review and evaluate the quality and appropriateness of radiologic services.

The JCAHO publishes a manual about hospital accreditation that establishes standards for hospital services. The latest manual is a radical departure from the traditional format of previous manuals; it is reflective of a change in philosophy regarding hospital activities and functions. Departments are no longer viewed as independent units; rather, the hospital in its entirety is viewed as responsible for overseeing, coordinating, and integrating its activities and functions. Therefore, the aggregation of rules and recommendations are integrated with standards and scoring guidelines. It is described by the JCAHO as an important new venture and is based on a new paradigm of integrating activities and functions.

The **Occupational Safety and Health Administration (OSHA)** is a federal agency that is concerned with safety in the workplace, primarily that surrounding radiation-emitting materials and equipment. The safe handling and disposal of radioactive and other hazardous materials is a major concern of OSHA; it establishes standards for safety in the workplace universally, and, unlike some radiation safety guidelines, OSHA's standards are mandated by law.

Equipment

The radiology administrator, the hospital administrator, and the medical director are responsible for the selection of radiology equipment. With costs ranging from $30,000 to well over $1 million, radiology equipment is the most expensive capital item in a hospital.

When purchasing radiology equipment, the radiology administrator must consider the needs of the department, economic factors, and equipment maintenance requirements. Equipment must meet the requirements of the Bureau of Radiologic Health Standards.

CONCLUSION

The radiology department is a complex operation. Every member of the department needs to be aware of the responsibilities and organizational structure of the department. It is this awareness—coupled with the dedicated, cooperative performance of these responsibilities on the part of radiology personnel—that can make patients' visits to the department as pleasant and employees' service to the department as meaningful and satisfying as possible.

Review Questions

1. Performance standards for the radiology department are set by the:
   a. Hospital administration.
   b. Chief technologists.
   c. Board of directors.
   d. Chief radiologist.
2. Hospital standards are set to conform with:
   a. Community values.
   b. Physician values.
   c. The JCAHO guidelines.
   d. Board of directors' mandates.
3. What is the primary concern of a hospital?
   a. Retaining accreditation
   b. Maintaining good community relations
   c. Patient care
   d. Adequate staffing
4. An organization chart is designed to indicate which of the following?
   a. Lines of authority
   b. Positions of personnel
   c. Areas of responsibility
   d. All of the above
5. The hospital-wide committee that functions to maintain safe working conditions is the committee on:
   a. Radiation safety.
   b. Hospital accreditation.
   c. Hospital safety.
   d. Policy and standards.
6. An in-service education program in radiology departments is:
   a. A requirement.
   b. An optional function.

    c. A nursing function.

    d. Instituted if needed.

7. Radiology department policies and procedures are contained in the:

    a. Hospital accreditation manual.

    b. Hospital physician guide.

    c. Personnel management policies.

    d. Department procedures manual.

8. The person responsible for verifying the qualifications of the technical staff is the:

    a. Hospital administrator.

    b. Radiology administrator.

    c. Radiation safety officer.

    d. Hospital safety officer.

9. Radiologic compliance evaluation is a function of the:

    a. Radiation safety committee.

    b. Quality assurance program.

    c. Hospital safety committee.

    d. JCAHO.

10. Standards for hospital services are established by the:

    a. Committee on Allied Health Education.

    b. Medicare government guidelines.

    c. JCAHO.

    d. Commission on health care insurance.

BIBLIOGRAPHY

Bouchard E: *Radiology management: an introduction*, Denver, 1983, Multi-Media Publications.

Britt GC (Manager, Diagnostic Radiology): Personal communication, Sept 8, 1991, Methodist Hospital, Memphis.

Davies PR (Director, Ambulatory Care): Personal communication, Sept 8, 1991, St. Joseph Hospital, Memphis.

Joint Commission on Accreditation of Healthcare Organizations: *Accreditation manual for hospitals*, Oakbrook Terrace, IL, 1995, The Commission.

Joint Commission on Accreditation of HealthCare Organizations: *Accreditation manual for hospitals*, Oakbrook Terrace, IL, 2004, The Commission.

Shams-Avari P: The office of practice issues tackles profession's changes and challenges, *ASRT Scanner* 37(1), October 2004.

Swinny AG (Director, Radiology Education): Personal communication, Sept 8, 1991, Baptist Memorial Hospital, Memphis.

US Congress, S 3290: A bill: "To provide for the protection of the public health (including consumer patients) from unnecessary exposure to radiation," 95th Congress, 2d sess, Washington, DC, 1968.

US Department of Health, Education and Welfare, Food and Drug Administration: *A look at FDA's program to protect the American consumer from radiation*, 77-8032, Washington, DC, April 1977.

US Department of Health, Education and Welfare, Food and Drug Administration: *Regulations for the administration and enforcement of the radiation control for Health and Safety Act of 1968*, 79-8035, Washington, DC, September 1978.

US Environmental Protection Agency: *Federal guidance report No. 9: radiation protection guidance for diagnostic x-rays*, Interagency Working Group on Medical Radiation, 52014-76-019, Washington, DC, October 1976.

Wesolowski CE: Let's put "care" back into health care, *Radiol Manag* 12(3):49-55, 1990.

Economics of Radiology

LaVerne Tolley Gurley

OBJECTIVES

On completion of this chapter, you should be able to:

- **Define certificate of need (CON).**

- **Describe how staffing needs are computed.**

- **Explain the economics of equipment purchasing in radiology.**

- **Calculate the costs of radiographic examinations.**

- **Analyze the type, frequency, and charges of radiographic examinations that make equipment purchases economical.**

- **Discuss ways to reclaim silver from radiographic film.**

- **Identify steps you can take to economize in a department of radiology.**

- **State the revenue contribution of radiology to the hospital budget.**

KEY TERMS

certificate of need (CON)
diagnosis-related groups
   (DRGs)
life cycle cost
Medicaid
Medicare
mobile unit
multiphase generator
prospective payment
   system (PPS)
rare earth phosphors
   screens
retakes
silver reclamation

CHAPTER OUTLINE

Certificate of need
Staffing
Equipment
Radiographic quality
Silver recovery
Prospective
   reimbursement for
   medicare
Conclusion

Radiology, laboratory, and pharmacy are three important revenue-producing departments in a hospital. These departments help support non-revenue areas such as administration, personnel, maintenance, and housekeeping.

It is important that a radiology department operate efficiently and cost-effectively. An imaging department is one of the most expensive hospital departments to operate, supply, and equip. Radiographic film constitutes the largest supply expenditure in the radiology department. Because silver is the main element in this photographic process, film prices are influenced by the silver market; this was especially obvious in 1980, when silver surpassed $40 a troy ounce, and film prices increased by more than 100% from the previous year.

CERTIFICATE OF NEED

Until the early 1970s, the primary concern of both the health care industry and the federal government was to modernize, expand, and purchase new equipment to provide the public with more and better health care. However, during the mid-1970s, the thrust of government and the health care industry changed. The high cost of health care was, in part, the cause of this change. The government responded to public pressure by imposing numerous regulations on hospitals and other health care institutions. Almost all aspects of hospital operations were reached by government regulations. Probably the most far-reaching of the regulations was the certificate of need program.

The **certificate of need (CON)**, which is a certificate issued by a review committee to the purchaser after the need for the equipment or expansion has been established, was designed to provide cost containment of the health care industry by regulating major capital expenditures and changes in service. Major capital investments, such as computed tomography (CT) scanners or magnetic resonance imaging (MRI) units, that cost $1 million or more could not be authorized until the clear need for this expensive equipment had been demonstrated. If hospitals had policed themselves with cost-effective management and needs assessment, many of these regulations would not have been necessary.

Recently, with government deregulation trends, most states have abandoned the certificate of need requirement and revised and altered cost-containment health care programs with other regulations.

It is important that the student radiologic technologist be aware that economics is as important in radiology as are the other aspects of the profession. Mere technical quality is of little consequence if the cost of the service makes it prohibitive for the patient. In this sense, economics becomes a factor in radiologic quality, because quality care means caring for the patient.

STAFFING

The staff of a radiology department represents 3% to 5% of a hospital's labor force and cost. On the technical side, this staff consists of an administrative technologist, a chief technologist, radiologic technologists, clerical staff, and support staff (e.g., darkroom personnel, patient transporters). The medical side consists of the radiologists and the chief radiologist.

The personnel required to staff an imaging department depends on departmental systems and procedures. The number and function of these employees are based on the volume and type of procedures performed. Many hospitals compute staffing needs by "productive hours per procedure." Productive hours are hours actually worked, excluding vacations, holidays, and sick leave. The guideline for all personnel in a radiology department is one productive hour per procedure.

Overstaffing reduces staff use and creates increased labor costs. It is economically necessary to have the appropriate staffing level to provide good patient care with high productivity.

EQUIPMENT

The major equipment in a radiology department is the most expensive capital item in a hospital today. Costs range from $30,000 for a high-output **mobile unit** (an x-ray machine designed for easy movement for radiographing patients outside of the radiology department) to more than $1 million for a sophisticated computed tomographic (CT) scanner to more yet for a magnetic resonance unit (Fig. 16-1). The selection of appropriate radiographic equipment is a complicated procedure; the department administrator must analyze how many radiographic rooms are necessary and what type of equipment is required to perform the procedures efficiently. Each year, 6,500 radiographic procedures should be performed in each radiographic, radiographic/fluoroscopic, and radiographic/tomographic room. Fewer procedures are performed in angiographic rooms; therefore, a department that performs 26,000 procedures per year requires 4 radiographic rooms (26,000 ÷ 6500 = 4). An analysis of the types and frequency of procedures offered should be made. Specialized hospitals, such as children's, veterans', orthopedic, and psychiatric hospitals, do not offer the same services as general hospitals that serve all types of patients. Typically, 30% of the radiology procedures are chest radiographs, 10% are fluoroscopic studies, 9% are pyelographic studies, and most of the remaining 51% are general radiographic procedures such as bone, spine, abdomen, and skull studies.

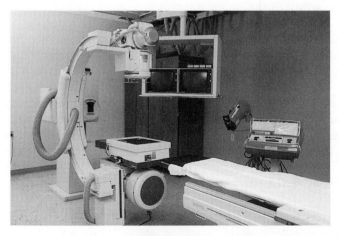

Fig. 16-1

An angiographic suite is another example of a very expensive yet vital component of most imaging departments.

It is not economically sound, then, to spend thousands of dollars for equipment that will not be used effectively. When purchasing new equipment, the availability of maintenance and repair services should be analyzed. It is senseless to spend $50,000, $100,000, or more for a specific unit when there are no local services. Each hour and day a radiographic unit is inoperable, the department and hospital lose revenue. Service, therefore, should be one of the prime considerations in deciding what brand of equipment to purchase.

There are three basic types of equipment maintenance contracts. The first type is a prepaid contract with the original equipment manufacturer (OEM); these contracts are usually long-term and give the choice of including or excluding glassware, such as x-ray tubes, in the contract. Next is the time and materials (T&M) contract, where payment is made to whomever provides the service for only the time and materials used to repair the equipment on a case-by-case basis. The last type is a third-party contract using an independent service organization (ISO). Like the OEM, the ISO provides both prepaid maintenance contracting and T&M.

Using T&M maintenance is the lowest cost option and can be used effectively for less sophisticated pieces of equipment. The more complex the system (e.g., CT scanners, MRI units, angiography equipment), the more costly the T&M will be. For this type of equipment, usually a prepaid maintenance contract with the OEM or an ISO is the method of choice.

It is important to negotiate maintenance contracts with manufacturers before the issuance of a purchase order for the equipment. By doing this, you can negotiate the lowest possible contract price. After the equipment is purchased, any leverage in negotiating the maintenance contract is lost. This is important, because you want all the imaging equipment to have the lowest possible life cycle cost. **Life cycle cost** is defined as the acquisition cost of the equipment plus the cost of maintaining it through its useful life.

Generally, a less sophisticated unit is less expensive than a more complex unit; for example, a single-phase generator is less expensive than a **multiphase generator**. Because of the introduction in the 1970s of high-speed screens that make use of rare earth phosphors, lower-powered generators can be used without sacrificing quality. Unlike the earlier high-speed screens, **rare earth phosphors screens** (screens made from lanthium, gadolinium, lithium, and yttrium) provide excellent detail. The faster the intensifying screen, the less output required from the radiographic unit. With the proper use of this type of screen, the cost of radiographic unit generator replacement can be decreased.

RADIOGRAPHIC QUALITY

Too often when students (and many technologists) think of the cost of a repeat radiographic examination, they think only of the cost of the film itself. Additional chemicals, staff time, equipment usage, and room occupancy are costs that must be considered, in addition to increased radiation exposure to the staff and patients.

How do these factors influence the economics of a radiology department? Table 16-1 shows the expenses for a department with an average repeat rate of 10% that performs 50,000 procedures per year with an average of 4 exposures per examination.

In this case, 50,000 examinations x 4 exposures per examination = 200,000 exposures per year.

As you can see by looking at Table 16-1, the cost of taking a radiograph is $11.30; therefore, the retake rate of 10% of 200,000 exposures is 20,000 retakes. **Retakes** are radiographs that have to be repeated because of inadequate technical quality. These 20,000 retakes cost $11.30 each, for an annual cost of $226,000. A 3% reduction of retakes could save the hospital $158,200 per year.

It behooves the staff and the student radiologic technologist to minimize the number of repeats not only for the economy of the hospital but also to reduce unnecessary radiation exposure to the patient and staff.

SILVER RECOVERY

The source of silver in the radiology department is the x-ray film itself. When film emulsion is exposed to x-ray or light, a photochemical reaction occurs. When the film is processed, the developer darkens the exposed area in proportion to the amount of exposure. To remove the remaining silver to make the image permanent and visible, the film is transported through a fixer bath. The fixer solution is a solvent that washes the undeveloped silver from the film. When the undeveloped silver crystals are removed into the solution, they are not metallic; they are silver ions with a positive charge.

During late 1979 and early 1980, the world became aware of the value of silver when the price surpassed $40 a troy ounce. Although the price of silver is considerably lower today, the hospital pays for the silver

---

TABLE 16-1

RADIOGRAPHY DEPARTMENT EXPENSES

Expense Items	Total Cost	Total No. of Exposures	Cost per Exposure
Personnel	$868,000	200,000	$4.34
Equipment	$788,000	200,000	$3.94
Film and chemistry	$308,000	200,000	$1.54
Screens/cassettes and other supplies	$296,000	200,000	$1.48
Total cost/exposure			$11.30

when the film is purchased; therefore, this silver should never be allowed to go down the drain.

There are a number of methods available for **silver reclamation**, but the best-recognized method to recover free silver from fixer is with an electrolytic recovery unit. This unit has a stainless steel, negatively charged cathode and a carbon, positively charged anode. The positively charged silver ions are propelled by the anode and attracted by the stainless steel cathode, where they are built up into a layer. One gallon of used fixer solution should contain 0.3 troy ounces of recovered silver.

A radiology department that uses 4,000 gallons of fixer solution per year should collect 2,400 troy ounces of silver. Using the average 2005 silver market price of $7.40 per troy ounce, the silver revenue would be $17,760.

Because the radiographic film itself is the source of silver, scrap film should be saved and sold for its silver content.

PROSPECTIVE REIMBURSEMENT FOR MEDICARE

Prospective reimbursement is the federal government's response to the problem of skyrocketing health costs. The hospital inflation rate has grown many times faster than the overall inflation rate of the United States. The principal reason that health care costs have become so inflated is that, in the past, hospitals had no real incentive to control them. Basically, the government reimbursed the hospitals for whatever kind of test or treatment was performed.

To understand how Medicare prospective payment became a reality, we must look back to 1965, when the federal government began offering **Medicare** for older adults and **Medicaid** for the poor; these programs were established with a cost-based system for reimbursing medical treatment. There was no incentive provided to control costs, and this open-ended reimbursement system in effect rewarded excessive admissions and services and inefficient use of high technology.

Other factors that contributed to the rising cost of health care included the malpractice epidemic of the 1970s (which resulted in physicians using more tests) and the more liberal benefit programs of employers and unions. So, in essence, all must share some blame for the rising health care costs. Medicare costs were $3 billion in 1967, $49 billion in 1983, $113 billion in 1990, and an estimated $157 billion in 1995.

The concern and public outcry over runaway health care costs led to the new system of prospective reimbursement for Medicare, a system based on **diagnosis-related groups (DRGs)**. Under this system, payments would be limited to the set amount allocated to the specific diagnosis.

Medicare payment limits were first imposed in the summer of 1982 with the Tax Equity and Fiscal Responsibility Act (TEFRA). In October 1983, which was the beginning of the federal fiscal year, the prospective payment system based on DRGs came into effect.

The DRG program has changed hospital incentives by introducing financial risk. Under cost-based reimbursement, a hospital could spend a dollar and be assured of getting part of it back. Under DRGs, a hospital has the opportunity to make a dollar by saving a dollar.

The radiology department is moving from a profit center to a cost center, and the emphasis is on improving productivity and efficiency.

As far as new radiology equipment is concerned, hospitals look for systems with high-quality workmanship and the capability to perform diagnostic procedures with quality and efficiency. Above all, equipment must be cost-effective. To be cost-effective, the equipment must be fully utilized. The systems must be versatile for a wide variety of procedures. With DRGs in force, hospitals and radiology departments are developing cost accounting methods that accurately reflect the cost of the services rendered.

Because of the **prospective payment system**, which is the government's policy of reimbursing hospitals for tests and treatments for Medicare and Medicaid patients, certain medical services are moving out of the acute care hospital and into less costly facilities. These facilities include free-standing urgent care centers, imaging centers, outreach clinics, physical rehabilitation facilities, sports medicine clinics, and various other health care programs. Hospitals are now contracting with physicians and corporations to provide services at a fixed fee.

CONCLUSION

You have learned that a number of economic factors must be considered in the operation of a radiology department. Radiologic technologists have the opportunity to make a significant difference in the cost-effectiveness of the operation of the department. There are a number of ways that this can be done. Perhaps the most important one, however, is to prevent the need for repeating examinations because of technical errors, which not only reduces costs but also prevents the patient from receiving unnecessary radiation.

Another method of reducing operating costs is to schedule examinations for maximal room, equipment, and personnel use. Consistently practicing conservation in the use of materials and supplies throughout all areas of the department will have a considerable effect over a period of time.

Quality patient care means caring for the patient, and this clearly includes the patient's financial concerns.

Review Questions

1. What was the purpose of the certificate of need requirement?
   a. To limit the number of employees to the number needed
   b. To restrict the patients admitted to only those with medical needs
   c. To restrict the medical services to the needy only
   d. To limit equipment and space to the community needs

2. Staffing needs are computed by:
   a. The number of procedures per year.
   b. The number of radiographic rooms available.
   c. The type of procedures performed.
   d. All of the above.

3. The decision to purchase new radiology equipment is based on which of the following?
   a. The number of operators of the equipment available
   b. The modernization of the department
   c. The number of patients who need radiographic service
   d. The number of radiologists available

4. In the typical general service hospital, _____ of the radiographic examinations will be chest x-rays.
   a. 10%
   b. 20%
   c. 30%
   d. 40%

5. The cost of a radiographic examination includes the cost of:
   a. Labor.
   b. Film and film development.
   c. Equipment.
   d. All of the above.

6. Silver from radiographic film can be reclaimed by:
   a. Recovering free silver from the fixer.
   b. Recovering free silver from the developer.
   c. Recovering free silver from the wash tank.
   d. All of the above

7. The cost of producing a radiograph is highest for:
   a. Equipment.
   b. Film and chemistry.
   c. Personnel.
   d. Screens/cassettes and supplies.

8. The trend to move radiologic services out of hospitals and into clinics was accelerated by the government's:
   a. PPSA and DRGs.
   b. TEFRA.
   c. Medicare payments.
   d. All the above

9. The cost of health care since 1995:
   a. Has remained stable.
   b. Has increased.
   c. Has decreased.
   d. Is not known.

10. The guideline for staffing in a department of radiology is _____ production hour(s) per procedure.
    a. ½
    b. 1
    c. 2
    d. 3

BIBLIOGRAPHY

ASRT Scanner 36(10), July 2004.

Business Perspectives Economic Outlook for 2005, Sparks Bureau of Business and Economic Research Center for Manpower Studies, Fogelman College of Business, University of Memphis, Vol 16, November 4, 2005.

EI Dupont de Nemours and Co., Wilmington, DE.

General Electric Medical Systems, Milwaukee.

Hospital Affiliates International Inc., Nashville.

Radiology Today 5(19), September 2004.

3M X-Ray Products Division, St. Paul, MN.

Quality Assurance in Radiology

LaVerne Tolley Gurley

OBJECTIVES

On completion of this chapter, you should be able to:

- **Define quality assurance.**
- **Explain equipment evaluation and monitoring.**
- **Explain what is involved in developing skills and maintaining competency in radiologic technologists.**
- **Describe the role of the radiologist in quality assurance programs.**
- **Discuss methods for evaluating a quality assurance program.**
- **Explain the significance of a quality assurance program from the standpoint of patient care, economics, and staff development.**

Quality assurance is a term that has emerged in the past few years that is intended to connote a broader sphere of action than was usually assigned to the older term "quality control." Quality assurance, as practiced in hospital radiography departments today, includes equipment, accessories, and radiography personnel. Generally, *quality control* is a term referring to the hardware or equipment in radiology departments.

Every hospital radiology department has a quality assurance program. (This is a requirement by law.) It involves all radiology personnel in how they will perform their tasks as well as the equipment for function and safety. Large departments may designate one person to be responsible for the program; however, currently there is a trend toward making all technologists responsible for quality assurance within their scope of practice.

KEY TERMS

densitometer
developer solution
exposure factors
film processing equipment
fixer solution
sensitometer
troubleshooting

CHAPTER OUTLINE

The administrative
    pyramid
The patient
    Psychologic and
        emotional aspects
    Creating good physical
        conditions
    Administrative
        evaluation
The equipment
    Film processing
        equipment
    Radiographic
        equipment
The radiologic
    technologist
    Orientation
    Developing positioning
        skills
    Selecting exposure
        factors
    Maintaining
        competency
    Administrative
        evaluations

Continued

The radiologist
Acceptance limits
Maintaining personal
standards
Communication
Conclusion

Quality is often defined as a degree of excellence. Everyone who enters a health care facility expects to receive the highest possible quality—or excellence—of service. The radiologic technologist plays an important role in maintaining that quality of service.

Every new radiologic technology student is overwhelmed by the complexity of the equipment and the sophisticated techniques used by staff radiologic technologists. As you spend more time in clinical education, you will soon become accustomed to using complex machines and methods to produce radiographs. However, it is important to remember that radiographic services are very complex and sophisticated, no matter how familiar they may become. In fact, this complexity is the primary problem in maintaining quality radiographic services in today's radiology departments.

Remember that no matter how complex the problem may seem, the solution is usually very simple and obvious. In this chapter you will discover a few simple rules that will assist you in solving some of your early problems and help you to maintain an optimal level in the radiographic services you provide your patients.

THE ADMINISTRATIVE PYRAMID

Most radiology departments operate under a pyramidal administrative structure. As shown in Fig. 17-1, this type of structure allows a few administrators to manage a large number of employees. Generally the tip of the pyramid represents the highest-paid employees and the bottom of the scale the lowest-paid employees. This arrangement is economical in that most employees are on the lower end of the wage scale. Communication from the top down is usually formal, so that when an order is issued from a top administrator, it is passed down to the lower levels of the pyramid without undue difficulty. However, when attempts are made to transmit a message back up the pyramid, a problem much like that which occurs in the telephone game played by children is encountered. In this game, participants try to relay a message from one end of a line of people to the other end by each participant whispering it to the next. In this manner, a statement such as "I'm happy to be here" may exit the telephone line as "I've snapped the beads, dear." Although each participant tried to relay an accurate message, each one introduced a personal perception of the message into the original, thereby changing the real meaning as the message progressed along the telephone line (Fig. 17-2).

A similar process takes place in an imaging department when a problem occurs. As each person in the pyramid relays the problem, a personal perception of the problem and its cause is added to the original message. Thus, what began as a small problem can soon take on the appearance of a monstrous problem.

Fig. 17-3 demonstrates how the production of a radiograph can be described by a pyramid that is, in many ways, very similar to the pyramid in Fig. 17-1. The various administrative levels shown in Fig. 17-1 are replaced by various radiographic equipment and personnel to create Fig. 17-3.

It should become apparent that, as a very simple error in radiographic equipment or method passes through the pyramid of radiograph production, the error could easily become magnified until it appears to be a major problem. In this chapter, you will discover the ways in which radi-

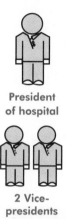

President of hospital

2 Vice-presidents

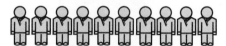

10 Administrators

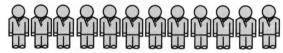

23 Department chiefs

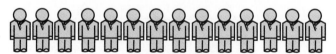

70 Supervisors

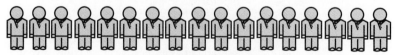

725 Professional workers

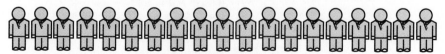

950 Nonprofessional workers

Fig. 17-1

Pyramidal administrative structure.

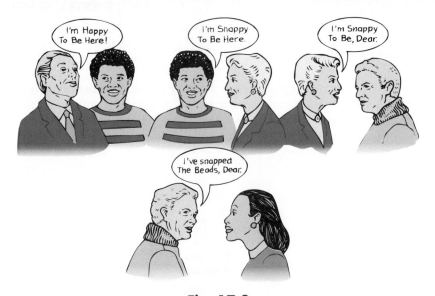

Fig. 17-2

The "telephone line" effect.

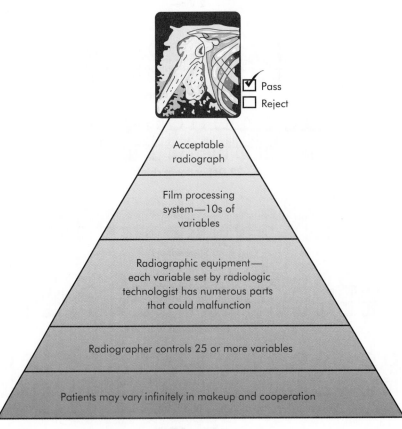

Fig. 17-3

Pyramidal radiograph production.

ologic technologists solve their big problems by working back through the pyramid problem to find the source of the trouble.

THE PATIENT

You will encounter a number of roadblocks in your efforts to achieve an optimal-quality rating. Not only do your patients come in various heights, weights, and widths, but they also arrive for your care with various temperaments and attitudes. You will study in depth the art and science of selecting proper exposure factors; these studies will help you to solve the problem of your patients' various body sizes and conditions. The problem of your patients' psychologic and emotional states, however, is one that you must constantly strive to solve. Many radiologic technologists who enjoy their work profess that it is solving these types of problems that makes their work interesting and rewarding.

Psychologic and Emotional Aspects

You should learn to evaluate your patients before you begin to prepare them for examination. Treat older patients with respect, younger patients with smiles and interesting questions, extremely ill patients with gentleness, and dying patients with compassion but not pity. You will soon learn the best methods for getting on the good side of each of your patients. If you remember that most patients enter the radiology department with some apprehension and uncertainty, you will have a good basis for understanding how to approach their psychologic and emotional problems. You must relieve their apprehensions by demonstrating that they are special to you and that you are competent in your job. You can relieve their uncertainty by explaining exactly what you are going to do before you begin the radiographic examination.

Creating Good Physical Conditions

Creating the proper physical conditions for your patients is one of the most effective methods for alleviating their apprehensions. You can do this in several ways:

1. Read the examination request to learn your patient's name and what radiographic procedure is to be performed.
2. Set up the examination room for the proper procedure by making sure the radiographic tube, table, and other items are in a position that facilitates moving the patient into the room and into position for the examination.
3. Touch your patients gently as you position them.
4. Provide comfort items as necessary, such as sponges to assist in holding uncomfortable positions and pillows and sheets for modesty.

All of these procedures help to create a cooperative and responsive patient.

Administrative Evaluation

The radiology department administration is usually very interested in how staff technologists deal with patient problems. Managers might use any of the following techniques to discover the quality of patient care.

Observation of Technologists at Work

Observing other technologists at their jobs is often a good way to see if patients are comfortable, properly dressed, properly protected from radiation, and treated courteously.

Interviewing Patients

Informal discussions with patients who are waiting for radiographic examination results are an excellent way to discover how they were treated. Formal written comments are also sometimes requested.

Interviewing Technologists

An in-service workshop on patient care or an informal discussion about dealing with patient problems often brings to light particular problems with which radiologic technologists need help.

All of these techniques help managers discover the quality of patient care services in radiology. The patient's optimal rating of the radiology department, as well as successful radiograph production, depend on meeting both the patient's psychologic and physical needs.

THE EQUIPMENT

The radiographic equipment is the first thing that most people think of as the major concern of high-quality radiographic services. In many respects this is justified, because radiographic equipment is indeed the most complex and potentially complicating factor in the entire pyramid. Regardless of the complexity and intricacy of the equipment, tests to identify the problem are well developed, and some are quite simple. During the course of your study, you will learn how to perform many of the tests with a high degree of accuracy.

The equipment is the most likely place to begin a search for the source of a problem. This is especially true when a problem persists throughout a number of different patients and procedures. The most reliable method of attacking equipment problems is the **troubleshooting** technique; this is similar to the process a physician uses in diagnosing a disease. First, begin by thinking of all the possible causes of the problem. Then, one by one, in order of probability, rule out causes. If this procedure does not pinpoint the cause, think of other possible causes. Although time-consuming, this method will lessen the possibility of totally ignoring important facts.

Film Processing Equipment

Most quality assurance technologists (those people charged with solving equipment problems on a full-time basis) agree that problems with **film processing equipment**, which is the equipment used to develop the latent image on a radiograph after exposure to radiation, is the primary problem in most radiology departments. In recent years, the federal government has focused much attention on reducing the amount of radiation exposure patients receive. The temperature of processing solutions should not vary by more than 0.5° F, which makes film processing a critical operation. When other hard-to-control variables are added to this fact (e.g., the age of the processing chemicals, the method in which films are fed through the processor), it is easy to see why the film processing system is difficult to control. Every film must be processed, and a slight variation in the film processing can destroy a perfectly good radiograph.

Sensitometric Monitoring

Quality assurance technologists use a procedure called sensitometry to maintain the quality of the film processing equipment. The basic idea behind sensitometry is that if you have a device that produces films with the same densities, you can compare films processed by the same film processor but at different times during the day. It then becomes possible to compare the functioning of a film processor to the way it was functioning yesterday or even a month ago.

The device that is used to produce these radiographs is called a **sensitometer**. Another piece of equipment, called a **densitometer**, is used to make sure the sensitometer functions consistently (Fig. 17-4). Densitometers measure the exact amount of density on radiographs, and they are used because they can "see" slight variations in density that human eyes cannot perceive. They are calibrated to give the same reading for the same film density time after time.

Quality assurance technologists use the densitometer to measure the density, the fog levels, and the speed of the radiographic film produced daily by the sensitometer. In this manner, it is possible to monitor the performance of the film processing systems on a daily basis.

When the sensitometry readings do not match the previous day's readings, the quality assurance technologist must decide what changes need to be made. At this point, only the technical knowledge of many years of experience will tell the quality assurance technologist whether the problem is with the chemical strength, the temperature, or any of the many other things that can go wrong in these complicated systems.

Maintaining the Chemical Solutions

The most common problem with a film processing system, other than temperature variations, is difficulty in maintaining the proper concentrations of chemicals in the processing solutions. Most students realize that

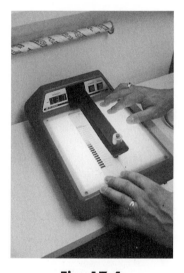

Fig. 17-4

A typical densitometer, which is an instrument used to measure the amount of density on radiographs.

radiographic film processing uses **developer solution**, which is a combination of chemicals in the film processing unit used to develop the latent image of a radiograph into a visible image. **Fixer solution** is also used; it is a combination of chemicals in the processing unit that removes unexposed silver bromide crystals from the film and hardens the film emulsion for preservation of the image. However, many students do not know that most commercial developer solutions contain a delicate balance of eight or more different chemicals. Imagine the pyramidal effect an imbalance of just one chemical could have on the effectiveness of the entire processing system. This becomes an especially important consideration when you realize that each radiograph, as it passes through the solutions in the processor, alters the chemical balance of the system. Each film uses up some of the chemicals in the solution while giving up stray atoms that change the composition of the chemicals. Modern automatic film processors have built-in replenishment systems that add fresh chemicals to each of the solution tanks to help maintain the chemical balance. However, radiologic technologists can misuse this system by improperly feeding films into the processor. For example, most processors are set up to add enough new chemistry for a 14-inch × 17-inch film based on the length of time it takes the 14-inch side of the film to enter the processor. If the film is fed in with the 17-inch side perpendicular to the processor rollers, it will cause the replenishment system to add too many chemicals to the system. If only one or two films are run through the processor in this manner, it is unlikely that any effect could be seen. However, if many films are processed in this manner, the cumulative effect could be disastrous to the chemical balance of each solution.

Maintaining the Equipment

Quality assurance technologists must also deal with malfunctioning microswitches, clogged drains, improperly seated rollers, and many other factors when deciding how to correct deficiencies in the film processor system. Following established departmental routines, such as the proper way to feed films into the processor, will help eliminate problems. Rules and regulations may seem silly and unimportant in the beginning, but as you learn more about the complexities of the radiographic process, you will discover that following simple rules can often eliminate complicated problems.

Radiographic Equipment

As complicated and large a job as maintaining the film-processing systems may seem, it is really the most mundane and ordinary problem faced by most quality assurance technologists. The tough problems come when the radiation-producing equipment itself is monitored for quality performance. When checking equipment problems, quality assurance technologists function in much the same fashion as radiologists do when diagnosing human diseases. Radiologists use all types of equipment to visualize various areas within the human body in an attempt to determine what might be causing a particular symptom. When the radiologist is unsuccessful in determining the cause of the problem, it may become necessary for a surgeon to operate to locate the source of the trouble. In the same way, the quality assurance technologist uses various tools to try to examine the x-ray beam produced by the equipment in an attempt to diagnose the cause of the problem. When the problem cannot be located, someone is called in to perform "surgery" to repair the malfunctioning equipment.

Special tools allow the quality assurance technologist to check the quality of the radiographic equipment kilovoltage settings, milliampere and timer settings, focal spot size, and collimator accuracy. Many of these tests are performed by producing a radiograph with a special tool imaged on the film. Various measurements and calculations of the image allow the technologist to determine the quality of the x-ray beam produced by the particular piece of equipment. In their comprehensive publication for the federal government, Hendee and Rossi recommend that more than a dozen different tests be carried out at intervals ranging from every 2 months to once a year on every piece of equipment used in the production of a radiograph; this includes the intensifying screens in every cassette, the radiographic grids in the tables, and the illuminators on which the radiographs are viewed. Therefore, quality assurance is not only a very important job but also a very large job, even in the smallest departments.

THE RADIOLOGIC TECHNOLOGIST

The radiologic technologist has nearly total control over the quality of radiographic services provided. The radiologic technologist sets the controls for the radiographic density, contrast, and detail and takes care of patient handling tasks. Thus, the radiologic technologist's skill, judgment, and integrity play major roles in maintaining quality.

Orientation

Proper orientation to the equipment and procedures necessary for the operation of x-ray equipment should always be addressed first. Good quality assurance requires all users of new equipment to have a proper orientation to the correct usage of the equipment. Everyone knows of at least one piece of equipment in every department that has several buttons or knobs that no one can recall how to use properly. This is probably because everyone learned the use of the equipment when it was new, but as it grew older proper usage was not passed on to new radiologic technologists; soon, no one could remember the functions. The same thing occurs even with the routine use of equipment. The little things that make a big difference in the quality of the radiograph can easily be forgotten. Exploring the equipment by trying each control without a patient in the radiographic examination area is a good technique for assuring yourself of proper orientation. This is true even in those instances when there is not enough time to become acquainted with new equipment. Taking the time to become familiar with equipment can pay off when you encounter a difficult patient or an unusual examination.

Developing Positioning Skills

Many radiation protection experts agree that the major cause of excessive exposure of patients to radiation is repeated exposures due to positioning errors by the radiologic technologist. Again, the radiologic technologist has total control over this problem. A professional radiologic technologist is a competent positioner. Simply learning the standard and routine procedures for your institution is usually not sufficient to accomplish this goal. To position difficult patients, you must know positioning well enough to be able to adapt a common procedure to an unusual situation and still produce a high-quality radiograph. This can be difficult, especially if the patient is uncooperative because of extreme pain or inability to understand what you are attempting to do.

The best methods of overcoming these problems are, first, practicing routine procedures until you are thoroughly familiar with them, and, second, paying close attention to the techniques used by staff radiologic technologists in unusual situations.

Selecting Exposure Factors

The radiologic technologist has total control over the selection of **exposure factors**; this term refers to the adjustment of voltage, amperage, distance, time, and other factors considered in the production of a diagnostic radiographic study. When the radiologic technologist misjudges the correct amount of kilovoltage, milliamperage, time, or distance, the patient can be exposed to up to twice the amount of radiation necessary because the exposure must be repeated to obtain an acceptable film. Many radiology departments are using automatic exposure devices to help eliminate some of the problems encountered in selecting exposure factors. The photoelectric cell was the first device used to automatically terminate the exposure, and it was called a phototimer; the term is often erroneously applied to all automatic timers, even though the ionization current timer has replaced the photoelectric cell type in most modern equipment. The use of automatic exposure devices requires an extremely fine ability to position the patient; in fact, automatic timing is an art rather than a science.

Some automatic exposure devices function as shown in Fig. 17-5. The ionization chamber, which is located under the tabletop but above (or below) the cassette containing the x-ray film, "waits" until it has received

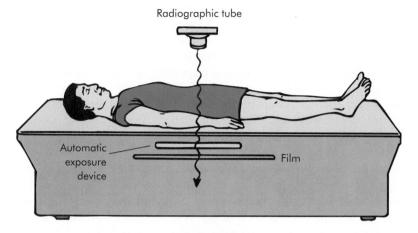

Fig. 17-5

Automatic exposure device may be placed above (as shown) or below the film.

enough radiation to produce an acceptable level of density on the film. It then automatically terminates the exposure. The radiologic technologist must set the kilovoltage, milliamperage, and distance on most machines; the automatic timer controls only the exposure time.

Looking at a frontal view of the automatic timing mechanism and the film as in Fig. 17-6, *A*, it becomes apparent that only a small portion of the film surface is covered by the timer. The timer provides an acceptable amount of density only on that area of the film "covered" by the film. When you position the patient as shown in Fig. 17-6, *B*, an acceptable radiograph of the patient's stomach results. However, when you position

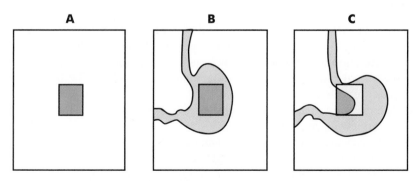

Fig. 17-6

Positioning of an automatic exposure device. **A**, Automatic exposure device location. **B**, Correct positioning of a stomach to the automatic exposure device. **C**, Incorrect positioning of a stomach to the automatic exposure device.

the patient as shown in Fig. 17-6, *C*, the timer provides for a density that is acceptable for the area outside of the stomach but that may be inappropriate for an acceptable radiograph of the stomach.

Many radiologic technologists begin to think of automatic timers as magic exposure-setting devices. It is important to remember that most of these devices control only the exposure time and that only the body part placed between the automatic timer and the x-ray beam determines the amount of radiation reaching the timer.

Automatic timing is not applicable to all radiographic situations. There are many instances (e.g., during portable radiography) when you must select all of the exposure factors to be used for the examination. In these instances, adjustments in exposure factors must be made. Many radiologic technologists tend to use a "guesstimate" when determining these factors; this is never an acceptable method. Working through a complex problem step by step is a scientific approach that nearly always provides you with an acceptable set of exposure factors.

Maintaining Competency

Continuing education provides a means for professionals to keep abreast of advancements in radiologic technology. Because of the rapidly advancing nature of the profession, no individual can afford to rest securely on the knowledge received during the traditional educational program. As new ideas and techniques are introduced into the field, each person must find a way to learn and use this new knowledge. Attending professional society meetings and in-service training programs and reading current professional journal articles help radiologic technologists absorb this wealth of information. Increasingly, states are mandating that health professionals engage in continuing education. Some large departments may have an in-service educator.

Administrative Evaluations

Earlier in this chapter, we discussed how imaging department managers discover the quality of patient care services in their departments. The same techniques may also be applied to determine the effectiveness of the professional radiography staff in overcoming problems. The three techniques are as follows:

1. Observation of radiologic technologists at work
2. Interviewing patients
3. Interviewing radiologic technologists

These three methods are a good way for the department managers to discover which problems should be addressed during in-service educational programs, through individual discussion with radiologic technologists, and through other means. Managers fulfill their duties through these methods as a means of maintaining an optimal rating for the radiographic services in their departments.

THE RADIOLOGIST

Ultimately the radiologist is the most important part of quality control. *The radiologist is the only person in the department who may legally make a diagnosis from a radiograph.* This means that, even though the radiologic technologist is the expert in the *production* of the radiographic image, it is always the eyes of the radiologist that must provide the *diagnosis* of the image. Consequently, it is possible to view the true function of the radiologic technologist as someone who produces images that the brain and eyes of the radiologist can form into meaningful diagnostic information.

Acceptance Limits

Everything you do, from setting the correct exposure factors to positioning the patient, must result in meaningful diagnostic information for the radiologist, or else it becomes necessary to repeat the radiograph. The problems inherent in this process are best demonstrated by the concept of radiologist acceptance limits. If all of the radiographs produced by a particular radiology department are placed on a graph (Fig. 17-7), you can see a profile of the production of the department at a glance. Note that all of the radiographs that are judged to be nearly perfect would be placed at point A on the graph, those that were too light would be placed near point B, and those that were too dark would be placed near point C.

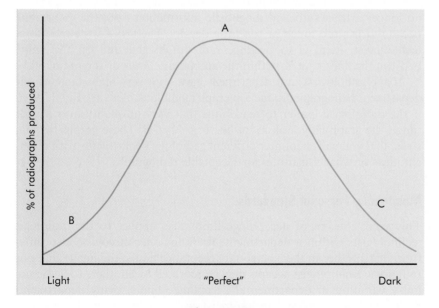

Fig. 17-7

Radiograph production.

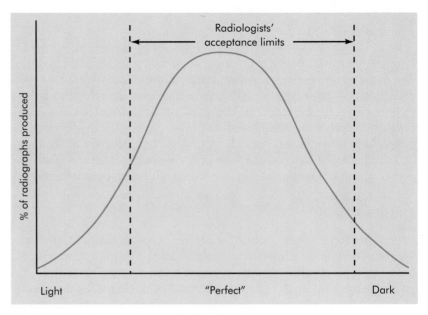

Fig. 17-8

Radiologists' acceptance limits.

The combined acceptance limits of the radiologists in the department may be drawn on the graph (Fig. 17-8). The two dotted lines are drawn at the points where the radiologists' eyes and brains determine that they can no longer extract sufficient diagnostic information from the radiograph because it has too much or too little density. The task of the radiologic technologist, then, is to produce radiographs that fall on the graph between the lines, that is, within the acceptance limits of the radiologists.

If the radiologists in a department have set a very high standard, the department radiograph production graph might look more like Fig. 17-9, *A*; if the radiologists prefer to read films that vary in quality over a wide range, the graph may look more like Fig. 17-9, *B*. These graphs demonstrate that you will encounter different radiology departments with different ideas of what constitutes an acceptable radiograph.

Maintaining Personal Standards

This same concept of acceptance limits also applies to the radiologic technologists within a department. Radiologic technologists also differ from one another in their personal acceptance limits; the image that one radiologic technologist accepts may be repeated by another. To help minimize variation in departmental acceptance limits, many departments designate one radiologic technologist as a quality control person to check the quality of each radiograph as it is produced. This person is often a supervisor who operates near the processors to check each radiograph for quality and to determine whether the film should be repeated.

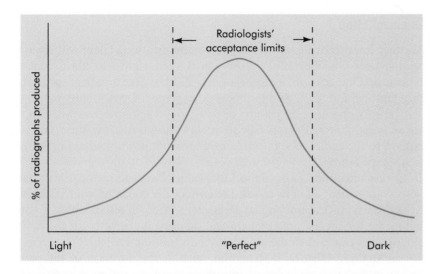

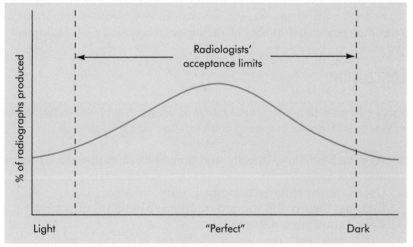

Fig. 17-9

A, Radiology department with high standards of acceptance limits.
B, Radiology department with broad acceptance limits.

In this manner, the supervisor's acceptance level becomes the departmental acceptance level. When this person has a long acquaintance with the acceptance levels of the radiologists in the department, he or she can effectively serve as a screening mechanism for the radiographs the radiologists must read.

Students often have two different standards of radiographic acceptability: one that they use when their clinical instructors are present and another that they use when they work on their own. A true professional must develop personal standards that do not vary, regardless of whether teachers, department managers, or anyone else is present.

Communication

Another important factor is effective communication. There will always be instances when patients refuse—as is their right—to allow repeat exposures. On occasion, a physician may need to take a patient into surgery and will not allow you to repeat an exposure. Occasionally patients may be uncooperative, or trauma or pathology might interfere with making an acceptable radiograph. In all of these situations, it is important to explain to the radiologist the circumstances that prohibited maintaining acceptance limits.

Communication is also important when obtaining medical histories from your patients. Learn to ask the correct questions of your patients. As you learn more about patient assessment, you will discover that if you can locate the precise area of pain and describe it correctly for the radiologist, you can add to the diagnostic information available for reading the radiograph. Historic information, such as the duration of the pain and its intensity or the color of sputum or stool, can affect the accuracy of the radiologic diagnosis. The medical history is just as important as the completeness and quality of the image produced on the radiograph.

CONCLUSION

Finally, to maintain an optimal rating in the quality of the radiographic service provided, the following points should be kept in mind:

1. Approach problems directly, and eliminate causes through a systematic approach.
2. Overcome the pyramid communications problem.
3. Consider the psychologic and emotional conditions of patients.
4. Create good physical conditions.
5. Understand how managers evaluate the care that is given to their patients.
6. Be aware of the importance of the film processor to the quality of the radiographs.
7. Be aware of the complexity of the radiographic equipment, and try to minimize the number of variables included in the quality assurance program.
8. Become familiar with the equipment.
9. Develop good positioning skills.
10. Develop good exposure factor selection skills.
11. Assist managers in determining the rating of the departmental services.
12. Be aware of each radiologist's acceptance limits.
13. Be aware of the department's acceptance limits.
14. Maintain optimal ratings through high personal acceptance limits.
15. Assist the radiologist with good patient histories and explanations of radiographs that fall outside of the acceptance limits.

Review Questions

1. Quality assurance is the responsibility of:
   a. The chief radiologist.
   b. The chief technologist.
   c. Each radiology employee.
   d. All of the above.
2. Quality assurance involves all of the following except:
   a. Monitoring x-ray equipment.
   b. In-service education for employees.
   c. Monitoring film processing units.
   d. The ethnic origin of employees.
3. What is the advantage of the pyramidal arrangement for departmental administration?
   a. Efficiency in two-way communication
   b. Economy in personnel cost
   c. Efficiency in employee work-units production
   d. Employee satisfaction
4. What is the disadvantage of the pyramidal administrative arrangement?
   a. Individual productive efforts decrease
   b. Communication from the base to the upper level is difficult
   c. Individual responsibility is not well defined
   d. It requires most of the highest paid employees to be at the top
5. Evaluating quality in the radiology department may include all of the following except:
   a. Observing the technologist's performance.
   b. Interviewing the patients.
   c. Checking the patient's code of ethics.
   d. Checking the in-service program for technologists.
6. Troubleshooting is an activity for:
   a. Routine daily equipment testing.
   b. Equipment testing on a scheduled basis.
   c. Equipment testing after malfunction occurs.
   d. Preventing future malfunctioning problems.
7. Equipment monitoring is an activity involving:
   a. Periodic routine equipment testing.
   b. Equipment testing after a breakdown.
   c. Testing after complaints of malfunction.
   d. Testing after evidence of poor quality radiographs.
8. Film processing requires which of the following?
   a. Exact combinations of chemicals
   b. Near-constant solution temperature
   c. Controlled replenishment of solutions
   d. All of the above
9. A sensitometer is an instrument used to do which of the following?
   a. Measure the amount of x-ray reaching the film
   b. Provide a controlled amount of light to the film

      c. Provide an exact measurement of the density of the film
      d. Provide a precise measure of the film sensitivity
10. A densitometer is a device for which of the following?
      a. Measuring the radiation that reaches the film
      b. Controlling the amount of x-ray that reaches the film
      (c.) Measuring the blackness or density of the film
      d. Measuring the thickness of the film base

BIBLIOGRAPHY

Bushong SC: *Radiologic science for technologists,* St. Louis, 2004, Mosby.

Carlton R: Establishing a total quality assurance in diagnostic radiology, *Radiolog Technol*, 52(1): 23, 1980.

Curry TS, Dowdy JE, Murry RC: *Christensen's introduction to physics of diagnostic radiology*, ed. 4, Philadelphia, 1990, Lippincott Williams & Wilkins.

Fodor JA III, Malott JC: *Art and science of medical radiography*, ed. 7, St. Louis, 1993, Mosby.

Gray J, et al: *Quality control in diagnostic imaging*, Baltimore, 1983, University Park Press.

Hendee WR, Chaney EL, Rossi, RP: *Radiologic physics, equipment, and quality control, Chicago,* 1977, Yearbook.

McLemore JM: *Quality assurance in diagnostic radiology*, Chicago, 1981, Yearbook.

Price P: Equipment safety and risk management, *Radiol Technol* 75(3), 2004.

Thompson MA, et al: *Principles of imaging sciences and protection*, Philadelphia, 1994, WB Saunders.

Radiation Safety and Protective Measures

LaVerne Tolley Gurley

OBJECTIVES

On completion of this chapter, you should be able to:

- Explain the need for radiation protection efforts by operators of radiation-producing equipment.

- List sources of radiation and explain their significance in dose accumulation.

- Define radiation units of measurement such as roentgen, rad, rem, and curie.

- Describe the role of the National Council on Radiation Protection and Measurements (NCRP).

- Explain what is meant by as low as reasonably achievable (ALARA) for radiation workers and nonradiation workers.

- List and explain the three types of radiation/matter interactions that are significant in radiology.

- List and explain the four possible results that may occur when photons of radiation strike cells.

- List and explain the significance of radiation effects on the total body.

- List and describe the practical radiation protection methods expected of all radiologic technologists on each radiographic test.

- List and describe instruments for monitoring personnel exposure to radiation.

❖❖

KEY TERMS

annihilation reaction
as low as reasonably
    achievable (ALARA)
background radiation
carcinogenic
collimation
Compton scatter
curie (Ci)
deoxyribonucleic acid
    (DNA)
dosimetry
effective dose equivalent
    (EDE)
erythema dose
film badge
gonad
human-made radiation
ionizing radiation
latent period
lymphocytes
pair production
photoelectric effect
rad (radiation absorbed
    dose)
rem (roentgen-equivalent-
    man)
roentgen (R)

CHAPTER OUTLINE

*Need for radiation
    protection
    Radiation measurements
National Council on
    Radiation Protection
    and Measurements*

Continued

Interaction of x-rays with
  matter
  Photoelectric effect
  Compton scatter
  Pair production
Biologic effects of
  ionizing radiation
  Acute radiation
    syndrome
  Long-term effects
Sources of exposure
  X-rays
  Radionuclides
Patient protection
  Exposure factors
  Filtration
  Collimation
  Repeat exposures
  Shielding devices
Personnel protection
  Personnel monitoring
Radiation safety and
  protective measures
Conclusion

It is well known that **ionizing radiation**, which is radiation that has sufficient energy to produce ions (e.g., x-rays), causes damage to living cells—damage that may be repaired, that may be permanent, or that may cause death to the cell. It is imperative, therefore, that everyone involved in the medical application of ionizing radiation have a basic knowledge of the many ways to minimize its lethal and sublethal effects.

NEED FOR RADIATION PROTECTION

There are two sources of ionizing radiation to which everyone is exposed: natural environmental or background radiation and human-made radiation. Examples of natural environmental or **background radiation** include cosmic radiation from the sun and stars; radioactive elements in the earth, such as uranium, radium, and thorium; and radioactive substances such as radiopotassium and radiocarbon, which are found in foods, drinking water, and the air. The amount of radiation that we receive from our natural environment depends, to a great extent, on where we live. In one area of India, there is a high intensity of background radioactivity that gives the population 10 times more radiation than the average background radiation dose in the United States. People who live in high-altitude areas receive more cosmic radiation; for example, the population in and around mile-high Denver receives more radiation than populations in or near sea-level coastal areas. Although background radiation varies from place to place, it accounts for more than half of the exposure that the general public receives. Radiation has existed since time began. Diseases resulting from excessive radiation are not new, either. The same kinds of harmful effects that radiation causes can also be caused by other agents, such as certain chemicals.

Human-made radiation sources are (1) fallout from nuclear weapons testing and effluents from nuclear power plants, (2) radioactive materials used in industry, and (3) medical and dental exposures. The use of medical and dental radiographs and radioactive materials to diagnose and treat disease accounts for 90% of the general public's exposure to human-made radiation.

The possibility of radiation-induced injury was reported shortly after Roentgen's discovery of x-rays in 1895. Since then, research, advanced technology, and the communications media have made society increasingly aware of the possible harmful effects of radiation; this has lead to a belief that patient exposure to ionizing radiation must be kept to a minimum while obtaining optimal diagnostic information for the radiologist. It is the responsibility of the radiologic technologist to understand the characteristics of x-radiation, its biologic effects, and the methods of reducing patient and operator exposure.

Radiation Measurements

As awareness of the possible dangers x-ray use increased, it became necessary to establish a method of measuring its use. In the early days, those who worked with x-rays used a unit of measure called the **erythema dose**; this unit was the amount of x-radiation required to turn the skin red, and its name was derived from the term erythema, which means redness of the skin. However, the erythema dose lacked preciseness and accuracy. A reliable instrument that measured the amount of ionization in gases was later developed, and the accuracy of this instrument allowed for the establishment of the unit of measurement known as the roentgen. This unit is the amount of ionizing radiation that produces, in 1 cubic centimeter of air, ions that carry 1 electrostatic unit of quantity of electricity of either positive or negative charge. The unit was named after the discoverer of x-rays, Wilhelm Conrad Roentgen. In 1938, the roentgen was adopted as the international standard measure of ionization in air. In 1956, another unit, called the **rad (radiation absorbed dose)**, was established to measure the amount of radiation absorbed by a medium.

For introductory purposes, the long history of measurement standards and regulation, a brief overview of the National Council on Radiation Protection and Measurements, and the names and functions of other consumer protection agencies are presented.

Units of measurement are known as the roentgen (R), the rad, the rem, and the curie (Ci); the quantities associated with these units are exposure, absorbed dose, dose equivalent, and activity, respectively. The **roentgen** is a unit of exposure for x-rays and gamma rays. The rad is a unit of absorbed dose of any type of radiation. The **rem (roentgen-equivalent-man)** is a unit that measures the biologic effect of x, alpha, beta, and gamma radiation on humans. The International System of Units (SI) uses *coulomb*[*]/kilogram (C/kg) in place of roentgen, *gray* (Gy) instead of rad, and *sievert* (Sv) rather than rem. For radiation protection from x and gamma radiation, 1 roentgen (C/kg) approximately equals 1 rad (Gy) or 1 rem (Sv). The **curie (Ci)** measures the amount of activity (known as radioactive disintegrations) that a radionuclide gives off. The unit of activity in the SI system is *Becquerel* (Bq); this measure is used in nuclear medicine studies with radionuclides, which are sometimes erroneously referred to as radioactive isotopes (Table 18-1).

National Council on Radiation Protection and Measurements

In 1964, Congress chartered the National Council on Radiation Protection and Measurements (NCRP) as a nonprofit corporation. The NCRP is comprised of scientific committees whose members are experts in their particular field or area of interest, and its primary function is to provide information and recommendations in the public interest about radiation measurements and protection. Another of its functions is to allow a pooling of resources from organizations to facilitate studies in radiation measurements and protection. A third function is to develop basic concepts about radiation protection and measurements and also to develop the applications of these concepts. Last, the council makes a concerted effort

---

*The coulomb is a fundamental unit of electric charge that is equivalent to 6.3×10^{18} electron charges.

TABLE 18-1

UNITS OF MEASUREMENT

Quantity	Traditional Unit		SI Unit	
	Name	Symbol	Name	Symbol
Exposure	roentgen	R	coulomb per kilogram	C/kg
Absorbed dose	rad	rad	gray	Gy
Dose equivalent	rem	rem	sievert	Sv
Activity	curie	Ci	Becquerel	Bq

Multiply the number of "A" by "B" to obtain the number of "C."
Divide the number of "C" by "B" to obtain the number of "A."

A	B	C
R	2.58×10^{-4}	C/kg
rad	0.01	Gy
rem	0.01	Sv
Ci	3.7×10^{10}	Bq

to cooperate with international governmental and private organizations with regard to radiation measurements and protection.

The Radiation Control for Health and Safety Act of 1968 was an attempt to protect consumers from the hazards of radiation-producing electronic products. The Food and Drug Administration's Bureau of Radiological Health is responsible for setting and regulating radiation performance standards that involve the manufacturing and assembly of radiation-producing electronic products, and it conducts ongoing research in an effort to minimize exposure to the patient, radiologic personnel, and the general public. The bureau also has a limited control program for radioactive materials that are not covered under the jurisdiction of the Atomic Energy Commission (AEC). Nuclear power production and the use of certain radioactive materials generally come under the control of the AEC. Environmental radiologic health protection is usually the responsibility of the Environmental Protection Agency.

Effective Absorbed Dose Equivalent Limits

The term **effective dose equivalent (EDE)** (the absorbed dose multiplied by the appropriate quality factor and measured in rems) limit is in adherence to the radiation protection guides. The philosophy underlying the establishment of dose limits is twofold: the first premise is the no-threshold concept, and the second is the risks-versus-benefits relationship. Simply stated, the no-threshold concept is the belief that there exists no known level below which adverse biologic effects may occur. There is much controversy over this theory, because it has not been proven conclusively; it is primarily backed by the observation of clinically induced irradiation to animals and extrapolation of high-dose irradiation received by atomic bomb survivors. If it is assumed that any amount of radiation can possibly cause deleterious effects to humans, then all radiation must be used prudently for the benefit of all concerned. The phrase **as low as reasonably achievable (ALARA)** is the basis for the NCRP's establishment of policies and procedures for radiation exposure.

The NCRP states: "The primary goal is to keep radiation exposure of the individual well below a level at which adverse effects are likely to be observed during his lifetime. Another objective is to minimize the incidence of genetic effects." Whenever physicians order a radiographic procedure, they must weigh the benefits to be obtained against the risk of the exposure.

Although every effort should be exerted to keep the dose of radiation at the lowest possible level for people who are well, this should not be a deterrent for the use of x-radiation for the detection and identification of disease processes in patients who are injured or ill, provided this is performed by physicians and radiologic technologists who are trained and experienced in making such examinations.

Dose limits are categorized into two groups. Radiation workers, who are expected to receive radiation exposure during normal occupational activities, are limited by a maximum EDE of 5 rem per year. The general public is protected by a dose limit of 0.5 rem per year, which is 1/10 of the total body limit for occupationally exposed individuals.

Students who are less than 18 years old and who are exposed to radiation during educational activities should receive no more than 0.1 rem whole-body dose in 1 year. This EDE limit is based on the laws regarding minors. Thus, this limit is the same for students less than 18 years old as it is for the general public. Minors employed in radiation areas are also included in these guidelines. After the age of 18, the student or employee is classified as an occupational worker (Table 18-2).

TABLE 18-2
MAXIMUM EDE FOR OCCUPATIONAL EXPOSURE (ANNUAL)*

Area Affected	Maximum EDE	
	mSv	**rems**
Whole body	50	5
Lens of the eye	150	15
Skin	500	50
Hands	500	50
Forearms	500	50
Other organs	500	50
Long-term accumulation	10 × age (years)	1 rem × age (years)
Dose Limits for the General Public or Occasionally Exposed Persons		
Whole body	5	0.5
Population Dose Limits (Per Month)		
Whole body	0.5	0.05

*The 1987 edition of *NCRP Report No 91* recommends the discontinuance of the MPD formula; it suggests as guidance for protection that the cumulative exposure should not exceed the age of the individual in years ×10 mSv (years ×1 rem).

The total permissible dose to a pregnant woman should be no more than 0.5 rem because of the susceptibility of the developing embryo or fetus to the harmful effects of radiation. It is further suggested that the rate of exposure be controlled by specifying that the dose equivalent should not exceed 0.5 mSv (0.05 rem) in any given month. In fact, it is advisable to postpone any radiation exposure during the entire gestation period or to use another imaging modality, such as ultrasonography, to gather information for diagnosis.

In summary, the radiologic technologist is now aware that there is a standard known as the EDE for occupational workers and that there is a dose limit for the general population. Preventing the embryo or fetus from being exposed to any unnecessary radiation exposure is of primary concern (Fig. 18-1).

The no-threshold concept and risks-versus-benefits relationship should always be kept in mind when considering the use of ionizing radiation in patient diagnosis. The information gained from a diagnostic radiograph should be far more beneficial than the possible risks incurred by exposure of the patient to ionizing radiation.

INTERACTION OF X-RAYS WITH MATTER

An atom is the smallest part of an element and is made up of a nucleus surrounded by electrons. X-rays are packets of energy called photons, which have the ability to knock electrons out of their orbits; this creates

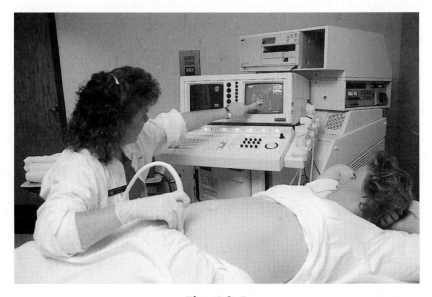

Fig. 18-1

Ultrasonography is often used to obtain diagnostic information about pregnant women. X-radiation can be dangerous to a developing embryo or fetus.

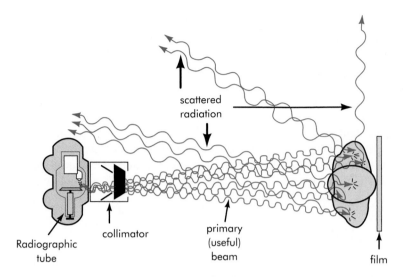

Fig. 18-2

The interaction of x-rays with matter. (From Sherer MA, et al: Radiation protection in medical radiography, ed 4, St. Louis, 2002, Mosby.)

electrically charged ions. When x-rays pass through matter, this process of ionization results in a transfer of energy. The x-ray photons can be absorbed or scattered by the medium with which the photons interact or pass directly through the medium without any interaction taking place (Fig. 18-2).

There are three main types of photon interactions that are important to radiology: (1) photoelectric effect, (2) Compton scatter, and (3) pair production.

Photoelectric Effect

Photoelectric effect is the most common process of energy transfer that occurs when ionizing radiation interacts with matter. The process begins when a photon (packet of energy) knocks an inner-orbit electron out of orbit and transfers all of its energy to the electron. The photon then no longer exists, and the electron becomes a photoelectron that possesses sufficient energy to knock electrons of other atoms from their orbits. The photoelectron and the atom from which it left are known as an "ion pair." Photoelectric effect usually occurs with low-energy photons. The photoelectron may have sufficient energy to cause further ionizing reactions.

Compton Scatter

Compton scatter is characterized by an incoming photon interacting with an orbital electron. In this case, only a portion of the incident photon's energy is transferred to the orbital electron; the orbital electron is then known as the "ejected Compton electron," and it produces secondary ionization in the same manner as the photoelectron. The incident photon then becomes a scattered photon of lower energy, and it moves in a different direction and is capable of interacting with other atoms by Compton or photoelectric effect. The energy of the scattered photon is dependent on the energy of the incident photon and the angle between the incident and scattered photon. There is a type of scattering in which the entering photon changes direction but does not give up any of its energy; this is called *unmodified* or classic scattering. When a collision occurs and the photon gives up part of its energy in removing an electron, it is called *modified* scattering.

Pair Production

In **pair production**, in which a photon of extremely high energy approaches the nucleus of an atom, both a positive electron (called a positron) and a negative electron are formed. In turn, both the electron and the positron ionize other atoms. When the positron reacts with an orbital electron, both particles disappear and create two photons that move in opposite directions; this process is called **annihilation reaction**. Because pair production requires a high-energy photon of greater than 1.02 million electron volts (meV), it does not occur in the normal diagnostic radiography energy range. However, it may occur during radiation therapy.

The major processes by which x-rays interact with matter are responsible for the absorption or scatter of ionizing radiation, which can cause tissue damage and possible adverse health effects. Damage occurs when ionization affects the chemical bonds of molecules that are essential to normal biologic functions. Because orbital electrons are a part of the overall structure of matter, it becomes apparent that any change in their state would be instrumental in creating cellular changes (Fig. 18-3).

BIOLOGIC EFFECTS OF IONIZING RADIATION

The cell is a highly organized structure that is composed of a nucleus that is surrounded by cytoplasm. The cytoplasm contains structures that are responsible for protein synthesis and metabolism essential to normal body functions. The nucleus contains chromosomes, and these chromosomes contain genes. Genes are molecules that contain the genetic material that is responsible for transmitting hereditary information and controlling cytoplasmic activities. The genetic material is called **deoxyribonucleic acid (DNA)**, and it is described as a double-helix structure. This structure is best pictured as a flexible rope ladder that is twisted in a spiral staircase shape. All parts of the cell have an equal chance to be affected by ionization. Because the DNA molecule is less than 1% of the cell, DNA is hit less frequently than water molecules. However, damage to the DNA is more critical than damage to the water molecules.

Photoelectric Effect

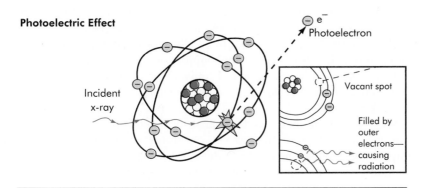

Compton Scatter

Pair Production

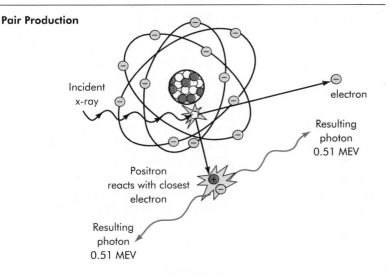

Fig. 18-3

Types of interactions of x-rays and matter.

There are two basic types of cells: (1) germ cells, which are responsible for sexual reproduction, and (2) somatic cells, which perform all other body functions. Germ cells contain 23 chromosomes, and they are able to function with half of the normal number of 46 chromosomes because of their specialization. Somatic cells must carry on many different functions and cannot survive or function normally without maintaining 46 chromosomes.

When radiation hits a cell, there are four possible results: (1) the radiation may pass through the cell without doing any damage; (2) it may temporarily damage the cell, but the cell subsequently regains normal functions; (3) it may damage the cell and no repair takes place; or (4) it may kill the cell.

One theory about radiation exposure to the cell is known as the direct-hit theory. It is hypothesized that when ionizing radiation interacts directly with the DNA molecule, certain breaks can occur in the "rung" of the DNA "ladder." If two direct hits occur to the same rung of the ladder, then a section of the chromosome is deleted. When the division process of mitosis occurs, incorrect amounts of genetic material are given to the new daughter cells. Mitosis is the process of somatic cell division whereby a parent cell divides to make two daughter cells that are replicas of the parent. These new cells either die or function abnormally because of the incorrect amount of genetic material in each cell.

The indirect theory involves radiation reacting with water in the cell. Various ions and free radicals form and may react with the cell or recombine to form a cellular poison. Here the cell is damaged or indirectly destroyed, but it is injured nonetheless.

Because cells differ in their functions, they also differ in their rates of division or mitotic rate. Bergonie and Tribondeau established a law about the sensitivity of cells to ionizing radiation: cells are most sensitive to the effects of ionizing radiation when they are rapidly dividing. Some specific cells that can be categorized by Bergonie and Tribondeau's law are mature white blood cells called **lymphocytes**; these are considered the most radiosensitive cells. Cells that make up the lens of the eye, the ovaries, and the testes are also known to be extremely radiosensitive. Cells that make up skin tissue and that line other body organs such as the bladder, the esophagus, and the rectum are moderately sensitive. Nerve cells are the least sensitive, because they are highly differentiated and do not divide; these cells are said to be radioresistant.

Fortunately, irradiated cells that have been damaged are capable of repair; however, sometimes complete repair is not possible, and often cells are incorrectly repaired. Over a period of time, incomplete or incorrect repair is responsible for the development of adverse effects to the body. The term **latent period** is the time between the initial irradiation and the occurrence of any biologic change. The response of a cell to radiation exposure depends on the radiosensitivity of the cell, the type of radiation (alpha, gamma, x-ray), the rate of radiation, and the total dosage.

Acute Radiation Syndrome

Biologic effects of ionizing radiation that appear in minutes, hours, days, or weeks are known as short-term effects. The signs and symptoms that compose these short-term effects are the acute radiation syndrome (ARS) that occurs when a large dose (larger than 100 R) is received by the entire body over a short period of time.

The important points to remember about acute radiation syndrome are that it is a total-body response to a large dosage received over a short period of time and that it is characterized by short-term biologic effects. It is possible to irradiate a smaller body area with a similar large dosage, but this would produce less critical biologic effects than those exhibited by a total-body response.

Long-Term Effects

Long-term biologic effects of ionizing radiation are divided into two categories: somatic effects and genetic effects. Somatic effects occur in general body cells that are concerned with all body functions except sexual reproduction; these effects include cancer, cataracts, and life-span shortening. Long-term effects may not manifest themselves for periods of 1 to 30 years and therefore are difficult to assess as being specifically radiation-induced. These effects in individuals may be the result of a previous acute high-dose exposure or of chronic low-dose radiation exposures.

Somatic Effects

Birth defects are considered a possible long-term effect of the irradiation of the embryo of a pregnant woman. Some defects manifested at birth may be genetic in nature. Genetic defects are a result of prior damage to the gene cells that participate in the formation of an embryo. Genetic material may be damaged by agents other than radiation, but it is radiation-induced damage that we are concerned with here. Defects induced by radiation in the organism may occur at the genetic, embryonic, or fetal stage. Such effects manifest themselves as forms of mental retardation and skeletal and central nervous system abnormalities. Irradiated embryos also tend to develop childhood leukemia in a greater proportion than do nonirradiated embryos, but the possibility of any effect from diagnostic doses is extremely remote. Because its cells are dividing so rapidly and are still undifferentiated at this stage, the embryo is particularly sensitive to the adverse effects of radiation at extremely low doses.

Radiation has long been accepted as a **carcinogenic** (cancer-causing) agent. Early evidence of its carcinogenic effects was seen in an increase in bone sarcomas of radium dial painters. Paint containing small amounts of radium was ingested by these individuals when they pointed the tips of their brushes with their lips or tongues while painting the luminous dials on watches. Many early radiologists and technicians also exhibited skin carcinomas from occupational exposures. Lung cancer resulting from the inhalation of radioactive materials in the air was present in many uranium mineworkers. Other types of cancers can also be radiation-induced.

Evidence of radiation-induced cataracts came from heavily irradiated A-bomb survivors, a small number of workers accidentally exposed to doses of 100 rads or more, and several nuclear physicists who were working with cyclotrons. Although it was believed that cataracts were formed after exposure to high doses of radiation, it is now generally accepted that the eye lens is one of the most radiosensitive organs.

The first indication of a decreased life span was observed in studies of American radiologists as compared with other physicians. Because there are so many variables involved with this long-term effect, much controversy continues over the assumption that radiation induces a shortened life span; it is, however, based on the fact that there seems to be a smaller differential in each new life-span comparison. This trend tends to reinforce the assumption that early radiologists were exposed to larger amounts of radiation because of the lack of safety precautions and more primitive technology, which created a life-span-shortening effect.

Genetic Effects

Genetic effects are the second category associated with the long-term biologic effects of ionizing radiation. Genetic effects occur in the germ cells, which are responsible for sexual reproduction. The effects that occur within the germ cell are transmitted to future generations and are therefore not evident to the individual in which they initially take place. To transmit genetic information, DNA sends messages in codes. When any part of this code sequence is broken, an incorrect message is transmitted. Any alteration in the structure or amount of DNA is called a mutation. When radiation damages a chromosome of a male sperm or a female egg, the possibility of transmitting a mutation or distorted genetic information to future generations occurs.

Remember that in germ cells genes exist as 23 separate chromosomes and that when a female germ cell unites with a male germ cell, they form a cell (called a zygote) that contains 46 chromosomes. When a genetic mutation develops in a chromosome, it is usually recessive and does not have a correct message to transmit. However, if one recessive gene is found in the sperm and the same recessive gene is present in the ovum, the genetic mutation will express itself in the resulting zygote or mature offspring.

Considerations when assessing the possibility of radiation-induced genetic mutations include the following:

1. Other agents that can cause possible gene mutations are drugs, increased body temperature, chemicals, and viruses.
2. A certain number of spontaneous mutations occur in every generation.
3. The gonads of the individual must have been exposed to ionizing radiation.
4. Mutations may not occur in successive generations because of limited life span, small number of offspring, and unlikelihood of two recessive genes.

5. There appears to be no threshold below which no genetic mutations occur.
6. The increase in society's mobility, number of marriages per person, and crossing of socioeconomic backgrounds increases the probability of recessive genes manifesting themselves in future generations.
7. There is no way to identify whether a chromosome mutation has occurred in an individual's genes.
8. Radiation-induced mutations cannot be distinguished from mutations caused by other mutagens.
9. Mutations are irreversible and inherited.

Ways in which genetic mutations can manifest themselves are miscarriages, physical birth defects, and metabolic or biologic changes causing a predisposition to disease or premature death.

Numerous factors that influence the biologic effects of ionizing radiation on cells, tissues, and organs of humans have been covered. It is important for students to remember that some of the biologic effects are theories established from early unprotected use of radiation and laboratory findings in animals; radiation-induced genetic damage is one such theory that was introduced.

SOURCES OF EXPOSURE

The two sources of medical radiation exposure are x-rays and radionuclides. X-rays are considered an external source, and radionuclides are an internal source.

X-rays

X-rays are produced whenever a stream of high-speed electrons hits the atoms of a metal target in an x-ray tube. A high voltage (also called *kilovoltage*) must be applied to the tube to accelerate the electrons; the kilovoltage controls the quality of the x-ray beam. *Milliamperage (mA)* controls the quantity or amount of radiation produced and functions inside the tube. The resulting x-rays are emitted through a port that is often called a window. The radiographic tube is usually housed above the x-ray table and often is suspended from the ceiling on a movable track; it can, however, have a stationary mounting that is often attached to the table. The x-rays produced from this tube are called *primary* radiation. Easily absorbed, harmful soft x-rays are removed by a filter placed in the port of the x-ray tube housing. When this primary radiation interacts with matter such as the patient, table, or film, it results in two other types of radiation: secondary radiation and scattered radiation. Scattered radiation is not only harmful to the patient, but it also impairs the diagnostic quality of the film.

It is also possible for another radiographic tube, called the *fluoroscopic x-ray tube*, to be under or over the radiographic table. Generally this tube is operated by the radiologist, and it allows for the viewing of an immediate image of the patient or body part. Primary, secondary, and scatter radiations are also emitted from this tube. X-ray tubes produce an external source of radiation.

Radionuclides

An internal source of radiation is produced by radionuclides. This source of radiation is used for the treatment of cancer patients in radiation therapy or oncology; it is also used in the field of nuclear medicine. Radium is a naturally existing radionuclide found in uranium ore. Cobalt-60 is a human-made radionuclide that is artificially produced by changing the ratio of the components found in the nucleus of stable cobalt-59 atoms; the nucleus then releases radiation in an attempt to achieve stability. The value and effectiveness of a radionuclide is related to its half-life. The radioactive half-life of a substance is the time it takes for the activity of that nuclide to be reduced to half of its initial value. More simply, half-life is the time it takes for the disintegration of half of the atoms of the nuclide; therefore, 100 mCi of cobalt-60 would have disintegrated to 50 mCi in 5.2 years, because 5.2 years is its half-life. Remember that activity is related to the number of disintegrations a nuclide gives off per second, which is also called the curie.

The methods of protection from external radiation are time, shielding, and distance. The shorter the period of time a person is exposed to radiation, the less harmful the effects. The greater the distance between the source and the individual, the less harmful the effects. Shielding is an attempt to stop radiation in its path; shielding material absorbs the radiation. The best defense against unnecessary radiation exposure is to use distance and actively employ these methods in your daily work habits.

To inhibit excessive exposure from internal sources of radiation, the radiologic technologist needs to develop good housekeeping practices, because these sources can be ingested, inhaled, and absorbed through the skin. Because of this, eating, smoking, and food preparation or storage should be prohibited in areas where radionuclides are present.

PATIENT PROTECTION

It is the responsibility of the radiologic technologist to learn the philosophy, factors, and methods that minimize ionizing radiation exposure to the patient. Even more essential is the adoption of this responsibility into the everyday work habits and decision-making processes. It is estimated that 65% of the population of the United States receives an x-ray examination each year. A significantly lower total population dose could be received by Americans if all radiologic technologists would use patient protection methods.

Again, the philosophy that governs radiation protection and safety is the no-threshold concept. The acceptance of this approach should minimize the possibility of creating deleterious radiation effects.

Exposure Factors

The exposure factors of kilovoltage, time, and distance are directly related to the amount of radiation exposure a patient receives. Optimum (as high as possible) kV should be used unless it interferes with the study or diagnosis. The result is a decreased skin dose because of a decrease in the number of photoelectric interactions with tissue. The shortest possible time should be employed to decrease patient dose and reduce the chance of motion, unless a breathing technique is warranted for radiographs of the ribs or thoracic spine. In fluoroscopy, the length of exposure to the patient is the key in determining the patient's total dosage. The rate of exposure is directly related to distance as a function of the inverse square law. It is well known that the farther patients are from a source of radiation, the less exposure they receive. With this in mind, the inverse square law states the following:

The intensity of the beam is inversely proportional to the square of the distance.

In other words, as the distance between the patient and the x-ray tube increases, the exposure rate (intensity) decreases. The inverse square law is represented by the following formula:

$$I_1/I_2 = D_2^2/D_1^2$$

For example, at a distance of 15 cm, the intensity of the beam is known to be 100 R/min. What is the intensity at a distance of 30 cm?

$$I_1 = 100 \text{ R/min}$$

$$D_1 = 15 \text{ cm}$$

$$D_2 = 30 \text{ cm}$$

$$100/I_2 = (30)^2/(15)^2$$

$$100/I_2 = 900/225$$

$$900I_2 = 22,500$$

$$I_2 = 25 \text{ R/min}$$

As the distance increases, the area covered by the beam increases. The intensity is less because the same amount of x-ray photons projected from the target have to cover a larger area.

Two correlations derived from the inverse square law have practical application for the radiologic technologist:
1. When the tube distance is doubled, the beam of radiation will have one fourth the exposure rate.
2. Conversely, when the distance is decreased by one half, the resulting exposure rate is increased four times (Fig. 18-4).

Filtration

Filtration is another factor that affects patient exposure. In diagnostic radiology, aluminum is usually the metal used to absorb the harmful soft

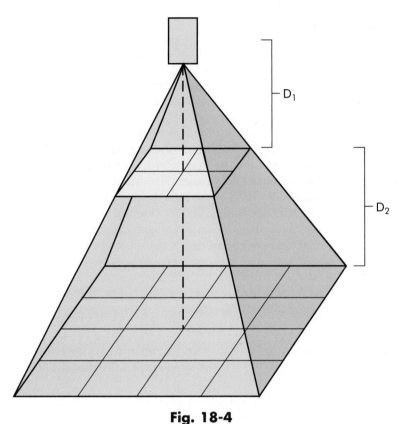

Fig. 18-4

The inverse square law.

radiation. Radiographic tubes are manufactured with an inherent filtration of 0.5- to 0.9-mm aluminum or its equivalent. It is required that a minimum total filtration of the primary x-ray beam be equal to 2.5 mm aluminum or its equivalent whenever the operating kVp* is above 70 kVp. The absorption increases as filtration is added and kVp is decreased.

Grids are used to absorb the scattered radiation that is created by the interaction of primary radiation with matter before this scatter reaches the film. There are several types of grids, but they all employ radiation-absorbing material to remove scattered radiation that would otherwise reach the film and reduce diagnostic quality. Grid use, however, raises the patient dose.

Film-screen combination should also be considered in efforts to reduce patient exposure. A cassette is used to hold the film and protect it until it is exposed to x-radiation. To increase the efficiency of x-radiation to produce a radiographic exposure, intensifying screens envelop the film within the cassette. When x-radiation passes through the patient and reacts with these screens, the screens emit light that ultimately produces an exposure or latent image on the film. When the film is processed, it is the latent

---

*kVp refers to peak kilovolts.

image that becomes visible as the radiograph. Film speed (sensitivity to light) and intensifying screens increase the effectiveness of x-radiation. The greater the speed of the film or screens, the less exposure the patient receives. Consequently, it is advisable for a technologist to use the most effective film-screen combinations without sacrificing diagnostic quality.

Collimation

Collimation is the restriction of the primary radiation to a limited area. For example, if the primary beam is allowed to leave the tube port, it may cover an area that measures 20 cm × 25 cm. If the beam is restricted by the use of collimators, the area covered might be 17 cm × 20 cm. Collimators are located on the tube housing and can be manually adjusted to have the x-radiation cover an area smaller or larger than the film size. In recent years, standards governing the manufacture of x-ray tubes have led to the manufacture of equipment that automatically adjusts the exposure area to the size of the film; usually the radiologic technologist has the option to decrease the area covered even more. Cones and diaphragms are also beam-restricting devices that can be attached to the tube housing. These devices decrease the size of the beam and limit the area of exposure to the patient, thereby reducing the harmful effects of scatter radiation.

Repeat Exposures

Methods can be employed to reduce the number of repeat exposures to the patient; these include restraining devices, technique charts, and a quality control program.

Restraining devices are used to keep the patient from moving during an exposure and thus reduce the necessity of repeat exposures resulting from motion.

Technique charts based on body part size, density, and contrast desired offer guidance about the amount of radiation to use for diagnostic procedures while ensuring optimum kilovoltage usage; they contribute to a quality control program. Many aspects of radiation management and training are incorporated into a quality control program, but processor control and maintenance, film analysis, equipment evaluation, and darkroom procedures can lead to an effective decrease in the number of unnecessary repeat exposures to the patient.

Shielding Devices

There are several types of gonad shields available to protect reproductive cells. A **gonad** is the general term that describes both the male and female reproductive organs. Gonad shields should be used whenever the reproductive organs are in the primary beam if the area shielded is not necessary for the diagnosis (Fig. 18-5). It has been demonstrated that a 95% exposure reduction is possible when the testes have been shielded.

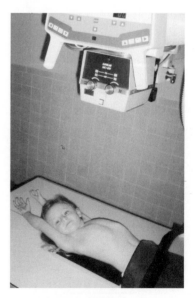

Fig. 18-5

Gonadal shield of flexible lead-impregnated material. (Courtesy Ansley Hill, University of Mississippi Medical Center.)

Because of the location of the ovaries, they are more difficult to shield without compromising the diagnosis.

Metals with high atomic numbers are most efficient in the absorption of scatter radiation; lead has an atomic number of 82 and is the most common material used for this purpose. Lead-impregnated flexible materials are used to make protective aprons, gloves, and gonad shields. The amount of lead (or its equivalent) in these items should be a minimum of 0.25 mm. Many sources suggest that 0.5 mm be used in lead-impregnated aprons for protection during fluoroscopic procedures. The detachable lead skirt, apron, or flaps that absorb scatter radiation emitted from the fluoroscopic unit should be at least 1.5 mm if using up to 100 kVp. When using a range of 100 to 125 kVp, a minimum of 1.8 mm lead should be employed.

There are three types of gonad-shielding devices. The shadow shield is suspended over the patient's gonad area to absorb radiation from the primary beam; these shields can be attached to the x-ray tube housing for easy accessibility. A stand-type shadow shield is made for tabletop use. The shadow shield is most effective for AP and PA projections,* but it is not suited for protection during fluoroscopy. The shadow shield is especially convenient to use on uncooperative patients or in a sterile field. Unlike other types of gonad shields, the shadow shield does not require the radiologic technologist to touch the patient or explain its use. Proper alignment between the x-ray beam and the light beam localizer is essential for correct usage of the shadow shield.

Flat contact shields are strips of lead-impregnated material; these shields are most suitable for AP and PA projections. They are not recommended for use when the patient is standing or during fluoroscopy. Because positioning of the contact shield by the radiologic technologist creates the possibility of embarrassment to both parties, it is suggested that the radiologic technologist explain to the patient the shield's placement and its function.

The third type of gonad shield is the shaped contact shield used by men. This cuplike shield is designed to cover the scrotum and penis, and it affords the male with a maximum amount of protection during AP, PA, lateral, oblique, lying, and standing radiographic and fluoroscopic exposures. The device is usually held in place by special jockey-style briefs or athletic supporters that the patient can put on before the radiographic examination. The disadvantages to the male shield are laundering, replacement costs of cup carriers, and difficult use in sterile fields or with uncooperative patients.

Examinations that give the patient a high-exposure dose to the gonads are the hip, upper femur, lumbar spine, lumbosacral spine, sacrum, coccyx, sacroiliac joints, barium enema, and urography examinations.

Patient exposure can be reduced tremendously when the radiologic technologist employs gonad-shielding devices. The radiologic technologist must take the time and effort to use these shielding devices as an effective means of reducing genetic risks for the whole population (Fig. 18-6).

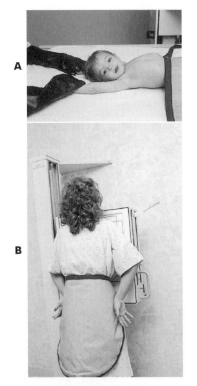

Fig. 18-6

A, Protecting the patient with a simple lead shield reduces exposure to parts of the body that are not being imaged. **B,** A lead apron, placed both in front and in back, protects the patient during chest radiography.

---

*AP is the abbreviation given for "anterior to posterior," which means that the central ray enters from the front and exits through the back. Therefore, in an AP projection, the patient would be lying on his or her back. In the posterior-to-anterior projection, the patient would be lying face down, and the correct terminology would be "PA."

PERSONNEL PROTECTION

Radiologic technologists who receive chronic low doses of radiation are more likely to be affected by its harmful effects if protective measures are not employed. The factors and methods discussed for minimizing patient exposure are equally effective for reducing personnel exposure.

The horizontal opening in the radiographic table, known as the Bucky slot, is a source of scatter radiation when the fluoroscopic tube is in use. Some tables are equipped with a cover for this slot, and this cover should always be in position during fluoroscopic procedures. In addition to gloves and aprons, lead-containing eyeglasses reduce exposure to the lens of the eye, which is a critical organ affected by radiation. These glasses are particularly useful during fluoroscopic procedures or special procedures examinations. It was mentioned that distance could be employed to reduce the amount of exposure an individual receives; this is of particular importance when the technologist is assisting with fluoroscopic procedures or operating a mobile unit. The exposure cord to a mobile radiographic machine should allow the operator to make the exposure from a distance of 6 feet. In both instances, the operator should wear a protective apron and personnel-monitoring device.

The safest place for the operator to stand during any radiographic exposure is in a shielded booth. If unavailable, a portable shield should be used to ensure protection. Just as other shielding devices are, the portable shield is lined with lead. Radiologic technologists should remember to keep their entire bodies within the shielded area, or they have negated its function. Loud, distinct communication and visual contact with the patient can be maintained through the shield's window. Usually the radiographic unit located within a shielded booth has a short exposure cord or a control panel exposure switch to inhibit the technologist from leaning outside the booth's protective confines.

Radiologic technologists should not hold patients or film cassettes for an exposure; there are cassette holders and restraining devices available for this purpose. Less expensive holders can be made by requisitioning the maintenance department to construct homemade devices. The radiologic technologist can also use tape, tongue depressors, sandbags, wood blocks, radiopaque sponges, Plexiglas, and Velcro to eliminate unnecessary patient motion that can cause repeat exposures or the false impression that the patient must be held.

If it becomes apparent, after all techniques and solutions have been exhausted, that a patient must be held, there are certain conditions to be met. First, the person restraining the patient should wear a lead apron, gloves, and protective glasses. A monitoring device should be worn by all radiologic technologists. If a layperson will be holding the patient and does not have a monitoring device, record the date, time, technique, and number of exposures. The restraining individual should stand out of the primary beam of radiation to minimize the scattered radiation exposure received.

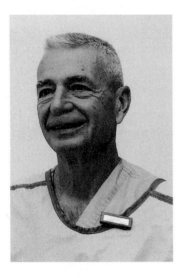

Fig. 18-7

A personal dosimetry device to be worn at collar level outside of the lead apron.

Personnel Monitoring

Although there are many radiation exposure monitoring devices, the **film badge** is the one that is used most often (Fig. 18-7). This device consists of a radiation-sensitive strip of film enclosed in a special plastic holder. The radiologic technologist should wear the film badge at all times during working hours. Depending on departmental policy, the badge may be worn near the neck so that the exposure reading will closely represent the dose received by the eyes. It is imperative that the radiologic technologist wear the film badge in a consistent location.

Generally, the film within the badge is removed monthly to be developed, read, and recorded. A responsible and knowledgeable individual such as a health physicist or radiation safety officer should interpret and record monthly exposure records for each radiologic technologist. Accuracy in interpretation and recording are necessary, because this information becomes a permanent part of the employee's record. Employers are required to maintain exposure dose records that are made available to employees and new employers.

A method of personnel monitoring known as *thermoluminescent dosimetry (TLD)* is highly accurate and more appropriate than the film badge for some radiation monitoring tasks. **Dosimetry** is a measure of radiation dose to an individual. This method uses a material, most often lithium fluoride, that reacts to radiation exposure. When irradiated, this material stores the absorbed energy until it is heated. When heated, the energy is evidenced by the emission of visible light. The temperature can be accurately controlled, and the intensity of the emitted light is a measure of the radiation exposure. The TLD devices can be made quite small, and they are reusable; this characteristic makes them suitable for monitoring small areas, particularly body cavities.

Other types of monitoring devices used for radiation dosimetry include the scintillation counter, the Geiger-Muller counter, the ionization chamber, and the pocket ionization chamber. All of these instruments measure the effects of radiation on matter, but the method used by each device depends on whether the matter being measured is a solid, a liquid, or a gas. Each has advantages that depend on the need to detect the presence of radiation, the type of radiation, or the amount of radiation.

RADIATION SAFETY AND PROTECTIVE MEASURES

Students who aspire to become radiologic technologists should become familiar with the rules, regulations, opportunities, and philosophies that allow them to deliver optimal radiologic health care to patients with a minimum of radiation exposure. The radiation safety officer or radiation protection supervisor is responsible for monitoring exposure rates, designating radiation areas with proper warning signs, and ensuring that equipment monitoring and safety checks are made. The supervisor (or an alternate) must be available at all times for any emergency. Rules, regulations, and protection philosophies are covered in the numerous reports that the National Council on Radiation Protection and Measurements has published. Continued research for increased radiation protection and safety measures affords radiologic technologists the opportunity to become aware of innovative methods, ideas, and products in this area. The Bureau of Radiological Health and independent companies that deal with x-ray products are willing to share information and provide material for in-service educational programs and professional organizations.

CONCLUSION

Radiation safety measures are essential in radiography for the protection of the patient, the technologist, and others who may receive radiation during the course of their duties. Reasonable and achievable safe limits of radiation exposure must be established and practiced. Standards that shape the rules and regulations for radiation protection are based on experience, observations, and scientific research regarding radiation exposure and its effects on living tissue.

Review Questions

1. In diagnostic x-ray, which of the following interactions will occur?
   a. Modified scattering
   b. Unmodified scattering
   c. Photoelectric interaction
   d. All of the above
2. The roentgen unit is a measure of:
   a. The half-life of a nuclide.
   b. The absorbed dose of radiation.
   c. The number of ions created in the air.
   d. rems.
3. What is the filtration manufactured into the x-ray tube called?
   a. Added filtration
   b. A compensating filter
   c. Inherent filtration
   d. Compton filtration
4. What do the letters rad stand for?
   a. Radiation added dose
   b. Radiation absorbed dose
   c. Relative absorbed dose
   d. Relative absorbed disintegration
5. When radiation interacts with matter and changes direction, it is called:
   a. Displaced radiation.
   b. Scatter radiation.
   c. Leakage radiation.
   d. Photoelectric radiation.

6. Which of the following factors will affect patient dose?
   a. Filtration
   b. Distance
   c. Time
   d. All of the above
7. Which examination will give the patient the highest gonadal dose?
   a. Skull series
   b. Chest
   c. Lumbar spine
   d. Abdomen
8. The law of Bergonie and Tribondeau implies that sensitivity is greatest in:
   a. Rapidly dividing cells.
   b. The youngest stage of the organism.
   c. The cells with the shortest life spans.
   d. All of the above.
9. The basis for the NCRP's policies and regulations for personnel and patients is:
   a. ALARA.
   b. rem.
   c. rad.
   d. EDE.
10. The general population is allowed what fraction of the dose allowed for occupationally exposed people?
   a. 1/2
   b. 1/4
   c. 1/5
   d. 1/10
11. The film badge worn by most radiologic technologists measures:
   a. The amount of scatter radiation.
   b. The amount of radiation to the skin only.
   c. The amount of total body radiation.
   d. The ions created in the air.
12. Which of the following are the most sensitive cells of the body?
   a. Nerve cells
   b. Red blood cells
   c. White blood cells
   d. Muscle cells
13. High-speed intensifying screens are used for some examinations because:
   a. The patient dose is reduced.
   b. The scatter radiation is reduced.
   c. Contrast is reduced.
   d. Definition is increased.
14. The primary concern in radiation to the gonads is to prevent:
   a. Somatic effects.
   b. Chronic effects.
   c. Genetic effects.
   d. Erythema.

15. Sensitivity to radiation in humans is greatest:
    a. Immediately after birth.
    b. During the embryonic stage.
    c. During the teenage years.
    d. During the reproductive years.

BIBLIOGRAPHY

Barnett M, Morrison J: Reducing genetic risk from x-rays, *FDA Consumer Pub 77-8019*, Rockville, MD, 1980, HHS Publications.

Britian V: Radiation: benefit vs risk, *FDA Consumer Pub 75-8014*, Rockville, MD, 1980 HHS Publications.

Bushong SC: *Radiologic science for technologists: physics, biology, and protection*, ed. 8, St. Louis, 2004, Mosby.

Curry TS, Dowdy JE, Murry RC: *Christensen's introduction to physics of diagnostic radiology*, ed. 4, Philadelphia, 1990, Lippincott Williams & Wilkins.

Fodor III J, Malott JC: *The art and science of medical radiography*, ed. 7, St. Louis, 1993, Mosby.

Frankel R: *Radiation protection for radiologic technologists*, New York, 1976, McGraw-Hill.

Frigerio N: *Your body and radiation*, Washington, DC, 1969, US Atomic Energy Commission.

National Council on Radiation Protection and Measurements: Medical x-ray and gamma-ray protection for energies up to 10 MeV-equipment design and use, *NCRP Report No 34*, Washington, DC, 1973, NCRP Publications.

National Council on Radiation Protection and Measurements: Radiation protection for medical and allied health personnel, *NCRP Report No 48*, Washington, DC, 1979, NCRP Publications.

National Council on Radiation Protection and Measurements: Recommendations on limits for exposure to ionizing radiation, *NCRP Report No 91*, Washington, DC, 1987, NCRP Publications.

Price P: Equipment safety and risk management, *Radiol Technol* 17(3), Jan/Feb 2004.

Rados B: Primer on radiation, *FDA Consumer Pub 79-8099*, Rockville, MD, 1980, HHS Publications.

Renne RL: *Radiologic enhancement methodology*, Memphis 1976, UTCHS.

Selman J: *Fundamentals imaging physics and radiobiology*, ed. 9, Springfield, IL, 2000, Charles C Thomas.

Thompson MA, et al: *Principles of imaging science and protection*, 1994, WB Saunders.

Travis EL: *Primer of medical radiobiology*, ed. 2, Chicago, 1989, Year Book.

Allied Health Professions

LaVerne Tolley Gurley

OBJECTIVES

On completion of this chapter, you should be able to:

- Give a historical account of how the allied health professions developed.

- Describe the role of the nurse and the scope of the profession.

- Describe the role of the medical technologist and the scope of the profession.

- Describe the role of the dietitian and the scope of the profession.

- Describe the role of the physical therapist and the scope of the profession.

- Describe the role of the occupational therapist and the scope of the profession.

- Describe the role of the respiratory therapist and the scope of the profession.

- Describe the role of the emergency medical technician and the scope of the profession.

- Describe the role of the physician assistant and the scope of the profession.

- Describe the role of the histotechnologist and the scope of the profession.

- Describe the role of the cytotechnologist and the scope of the profession.

- Describe the role of the medical records administrator and the scope of the profession.

- Describe the role of the dental hygienist and the scope of the profession.

One of the most important changes that occurred during the evolution and progression of scientific medicine in this country was the tendency of

KEY TERMS

allied health
cytotechnologist
dietitian
emergency medical
    personnel
histologic technician
medical records
    personnel
medical technologist
nursing profession
occupational therapist
physical therapist
physician assistant
respiratory therapist
U.S. Department of
    Health and Human
    Services

CHAPTER OUTLINE

Nursing
Medical technology
Histotechnology
Cytotechnology
Medical records
    administration
Nutrition and dietetics
Physical therapy
Occupational therapy
Respiratory therapy
Physician assistant
Emergency medical
    technician/paramedic
Dental hygiene
The team approach to
    health care
Conclusion

health providers to specialize. **Allied health**, which is a group of specialized, complex, and highly technical professions, grew, developed, and proliferated out of this specialization, which brought with it the need to develop efficient working relationships among the numerous medical professionals as well as among the organizational components of health services. These relationships needed to extend beyond the health field into other areas, including science and industry. Specialization allowed health professionals to develop more complex skills and expertise in their fields.

As the population has increased and medical care has become more sophisticated, the role of allied health professions has greatly expanded. Many new professions have emerged as more duties and responsibilities once performed by physicians and dentists have shifted to allied health personnel. Allied health personnel can be trained more quickly and less expensively than physicians and dentists, who can now make better use of their time and skills.

Some of the allied health professions are well established and well known; others have just emerged and parallel the introduction of new technology. You should be aware of the tasks performed by allied health providers in your work environment and the role they play in the health care team. This chapter discusses some health professions you may encounter in your clinical experience, but it by no means covers all of them. The **U.S. Department of Health and Human Services**, a federal government department with the responsibility for providing services in health care, has identified more than 250 health-related occupations. The following descriptions introduce you to a few of these other health care team members.

NURSING

Nursing, although not considered an allied health profession, is listed here because of its health-related services. The **nursing profession** is the largest, oldest, and most readily identified of the health professions besides that of the physician. The nurse has around-the-clock contact with patients and must provide the physical and emotional support a patient needs because of illness or disability. The nurse often teaches patients and their families about illness and therapy, thereby alleviating many of their anxieties.

The registered nurse makes observations and assessments that are useful to other staff members, takes patient histories, gives physical examinations, and administers prescribed treatments.

The nursing student can consider three courses for becoming a registered nurse. The diploma program is administered in a hospital and is sometimes affiliated with a college or university; this program usually takes 3 years to complete. The associate degree program involves 2 years at a community college, technical institute, or university with course work in basic physical, biologic, and social sciences, humanities, and nursing. The baccalaureate program usually involves 4 to 5 academic years, and the graduate from this program most often receives a bachelor of science in nursing. Course work includes anatomy and physiology, biology, physical and social sciences, nursing, and humanities.

To become a registered nurse, the student must graduate from an approved nursing program, pass the state board examination, and meet individual state requirements for licensure.

Specialized areas of nursing include psychiatric nursing, community health nursing, and rehabilitation nursing. The individual nurse practitioner must have advanced nursing skills, which usually include a master of arts or master of science in nursing. The practitioner often establishes private practice and offers services in health teaching, assessment, and physical care; he or she often has close contact with a physician for patient referral and follow-up.

The nurse anesthetist must complete an advanced program to administer anesthesia to surgery and obstetrics patients. The nurse midwife must be certified or have a master of arts in midwifery. Critical care nursing has a core curriculum of advanced specialized study and a critical care registry examination.

Nursing, like radiologic technology, is experiencing the development of specialized functions that stimulate the growth of separate educational programs, professional organizations, and qualifying examinations and procedures.

MEDICAL TECHNOLOGY

The **medical technologist** functions within the clinical laboratory to provide diagnostic and therapeutic information to primary caregivers. This information is generated by the medical technologist through highly precise analysis of blood and body fluids to measure and identify the constituents (Fig. 19-1). There are several different disciplines or specialties within the profession of medical technology. Body fluid chemistry involves measurement of constituents such as glucose, cholesterol, blood acidity, and the various blood proteins. Hematologic analyses include counting red and white blood cells and using the microscope to identify abnormalities. Clotting abnormalities also can be identified by a variety of special tests. Medical technologists working in the blood banking discipline test donor and recipient blood to ensure compatibility of transfusion products. In the microbiology laboratory, medical technologists culture and analyze bacteria, fungi, parasites, and viruses to diagnose infectious diseases while also performing tests to determine the most effective therapeutic agents. Immunodiagnostic testing involves the detection of immune system products such as antibodies to determine infectious disease status as well as protective immunity. A newly emerging discipline in medical technology involves molecular testing such as analysis of DNA.

To perform these tasks, medical technologists must apply technical skills, while they also must understand the related chemical, physical, and biologic principles necessary to ensure accurate laboratory results. The

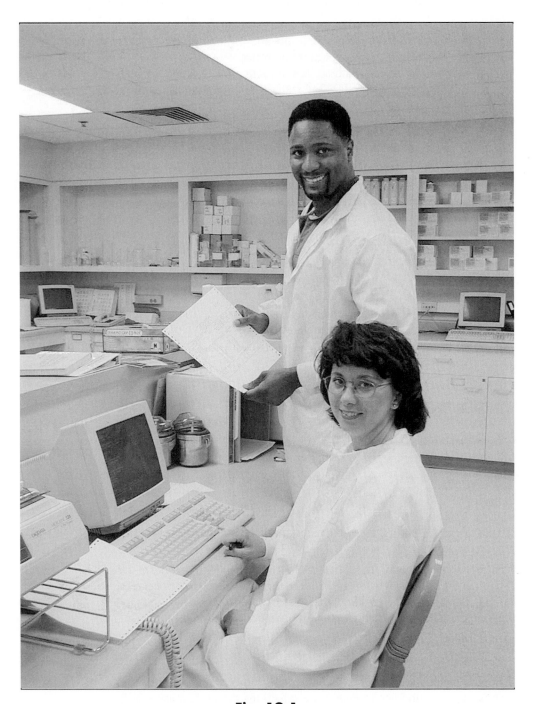

Fig. 19-1
Medical technologists.

educational requirements to become a medical technologist take approximately four years and involve completion of chemistry, biology, math, English, and elective prerequisites after which the student attends an accredited program of medical technology to focus on both classroom and practical experiences in all the disciplines to complete a baccalaureate degree. Once educational requirements are complete, the graduate is eligible to sit for one or more of the national certification exams in medical technology. The most recognized certification is offered by the American Society for Clinical Pathology, which results in the MT(ASCP) credential.

The traditional work settings for medical technologists are in the hospital clinical laboratory or in large independent laboratories. However, many medical technologists work in other settings such as research, education, or in the laboratory supply industry as technical representatives.

HISTOTECHNOLOGY

The field of histotechnology is fairly small; there are approximately 9,000 registered **histologic technicians** in the United States. The histologic technician processes tissue samples from surgical autopsies and research procedures. These technicians may work in university hospitals, research centers, or private laboratories. They must be skilled in processing tissue from surgical and autopsy procedures, embedding tissue into paraffin blocks, cutting ultra-thin, paraffin-embedded tissue samples, and identifying tissue by sight and stain.

The curriculum for the histologic technician requires instruction in medical terminology, medical ethics, chemistry, anatomy, histology, and histochemistry. The program also includes clinical education in instrumentation, microscopy, and processing techniques. Programs in histotechnology are accredited by the National Accrediting Agency for Clinical Laboratory Sciences.

The educational entrance requirements to an accredited program include a high school diploma or equivalent plus 1 year of supervised training in a qualified pathology laboratory or graduation from an accredited program of histologic technique. A college background in chemistry, biology, and mathematics may be helpful. Certification is through examination by the Board of Registry of Medical Technologists. Histologic technicians are given the designation HT(ASCP).

CYTOTECHNOLOGY

Cytotechnology is a growing field in the allied health sciences. It involves the microscopic study of cells that have been exfoliated or abraded from body tissues to reveal abnormalities that could implicate cancer. With the help of cytotechnology, the physician is often able to diagnose and treat cancer before symptoms occur or before it can be detected by other methods.

Cytotechnology originated as a method of detecting malignant and premalignant lesions in the female genital tract. This test, which is commonly known as the Pap smear, was named after Dr. George Papanicolaou, the test's developer. Today cytotechnology has expanded to include cancer detection in all body areas as well as the detection of other disease processes and genetic disorders.

Cytotechnologists work with pathologists in hospital laboratories, universities, and private laboratories and perform various specialized techniques used in the collection, preparation, and staining of cell samples; therefore, cytotechnology requires an extensive knowledge of anatomy, physiology, and the pathology of cells, tissues, and organ systems to interpret cell morphology.

Prerequisites for entering cytology programs are 2 years in an accredited college or university with an area of concentration in biologic sciences, certification as a registered medical technologist (ASCP), or a baccalaureate degree from an accredited college or university with an emphasis in biology. The clinical program is 1 year. Graduates of an accredited program are certified through the American Society of Clinical Pathologists and are recognized as CT (ASCP) cytotechnologists.

MEDICAL RECORDS ADMINISTRATION

The work of **medical records personnel** encompasses a wide variety of tasks including planning, organizing, and directing the activities of a medical records department; preparing, maintaining, and analyzing records and reports of patient illnesses; and assisting the medical staff in research studies and evaluation of the quality of medical care (Fig. 19-2). Medical records personnel also develop auxiliary records (such as physicians' indexes and statistics for medical staff and hospital administration) and summarize medical records for insurance or legal purposes. Medical records personnel bridge the gap between the increasing volume of medical data and the latest information-handling systems.

There are two levels of medical record personnel. The first is the registered records administrator, who must possess a baccalaureate degree with prerequisite courses in biology, business and office administration, English, psychology, and social science. Medical records administrators plan, design, develop, and manage systems of patient information, administrative and clinical statistical data, and patient medical records in all types of health care institutions.

The second level of medical record personnel is the medical record technician. This level may be completed through an approved 2-year program at a junior college or by completion of the American Medical Record Association's independent study program for medical record personnel.

The professional program includes anatomy and physiology, medical terminology, medical record administration, statistics, law, data processing, management, fundamentals of medical science, and organization

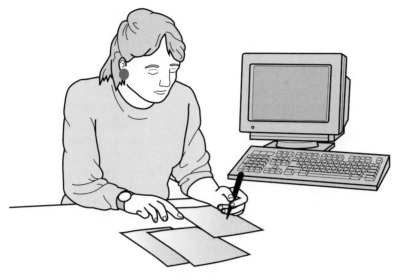

Fig. 19-2

One of the functions of a medical records worker is to organize patient reports.

and administration of health care facilities. These programs are accredited by the American Medical Record Association.

The registered record administrator is required to engage in continuing education and must earn 30 hours of continuing education credit every 2 years. A continuing education program is administered by the American Medical Record Association.

NUTRITION AND DIETETICS

A nutritionist or **dietitian** may work in a department of public health performing patient education and counseling or in a hospital operating food service, planning modified menus and therapeutic diets, and counseling patients. He or she may also work in a nursing home as a dietary consultant in both therapeutic and administrative functions or with a food-processing company aiding in the testing of food products.

A dietetics program includes a 4-year baccalaureate program with the addition of a dietetic internship. The internship may be completed concurrently with the undergraduate program, or a year's dietetic internship may be taken at an approved hospital, medical center, or commercial institution. The curriculum covers a broad range of topics including nutrition and disease, maternal and child nutrition, and nutrition and aging. Admission to the American Dietetic Association requires an advanced degree or a dietetic traineeship. Dietitians and nutritionists are accredited by the American Dietetic Association, which was founded in

1917. Continuing education is mandatory, and each member must complete 75 continuing education hours over a period of 5 years.

PHYSICAL THERAPY

The **physical therapist** performs therapeutic procedures that include exercise for increasing strength, endurance, coordination, and range of motion. Physical therapists also provide instruction in activities of daily living and the use of assistive devices. The physical therapist works with a team of personnel—as do other allied health care providers—including physicians, other health specialists, and members of the lay community. Physical therapists are mainly concerned with the restoration of function and the prevention of disability after disease, injury, or the loss of a body part; in some instances, this requires the physical therapist to spend a considerable amount of time with the patient.

A minimum of 2 years of college (or its equivalent) is required for admission to a program in physical therapy. The physical therapy program curriculum includes human anatomy and physiology, pathology, psychology, clinical medicine, tests and measurements, therapeutic exercise and assistive devices, physical agents, and clinical application of physical therapy theory. Graduates from an approved physical therapy program are eligible for a baccalaureate degree and may be licensed or registered in the state in which they wish to practice. Continuing education and professional growth is encouraged in the physical therapy profession, and the curriculum is designed so that students recognize their responsibilities to expand and improve their professional knowledge and skills and to foster continuing improvement in the delivery of health care.

OCCUPATIONAL THERAPY

Occupational therapy arose during World Wars I and II, when occupational therapists were sent to Europe out of a need for advanced rehabilitation of wounded servicemen. The profession has continued to become important to the promotion of health in physical, emotional, and social abilities. The **occupational therapist** evaluates the psychosocial and physical needs and capabilities of an individual, develops a treatment program, and determines the necessary therapeutic activities and procedures to make the treatment program effective. Through occupational therapy, the patient's motor functions are enhanced, and psychologic, social, and economic adjustments are promoted. Occupational therapists often work with patients who are regaining daily living skills with the use of artificial limbs and special equipment.

To become certified, the occupational therapy student must fulfill the baccalaureate requirements of an accredited program and the affiliated university or college. The program includes basic human sciences, human development processes, specific life tasks and activities, theory and application of occupational therapy, and at least 6 months of field experience. Some states require licensure through a state examination, although an American-Occupational-Therapy-Association (AOTA)–certified occupational therapist need not take the state examination.

RESPIRATORY THERAPY

The respiratory therapist has become an integral part of the health care team. The **respiratory therapist** administers therapy through such procedures as intermittent positive-pressure breathing (IPPB), aerosol therapy, postural drainage, airway management, and pulmonary function testing; he or she also handles respiratory emergencies and administers drugs that act in the cardiopulmonary tract.

The respiratory therapy student may attend either an 18-month community college program, which expands technician-level training, or a 4 year baccalaureate program. Studies include anatomy and physiology, pharmacology, pathology, chemistry, technical theory, and clinical practice. The RRT examination can be taken by graduates of an accredited therapist school, and some states also require licensure examinations.

PHYSICIAN ASSISTANT

The **physician assistant**, which is one of the newest allied health professionals, performs, under the direction and supervision of a physician, tasks that are usually conducted by the physician but that do not require such a level of expertise. These tasks include taking patient histories, physical examinations, follow-up care, patient teaching, counseling, and, in certain cases, diagnosis, therapy, and preventive medicine.

Prerequisites include high school graduation or its equivalent and 2 years of college course work or related health care experience. The program is usually 2 years and includes courses in anatomy, physiology, microbiology, pharmacology, medical ethics, and a clinical practicum. Certification is through the National Commission on Certification of Physician Assistants.

EMERGENCY MEDICAL TECHNICIAN/PARAMEDIC

Immediate care of the sick and injured is of paramount importance, and emergency medical technicians (EMT)/paramedics are often the first to tend to the patient's needs. **Emergency medical personnel** must have competence in the areas of prehospital care, patient transportation, patient and family counseling, providing medical care under the direction of an emergency physician, and maintaining emergency vehicles and biomedical equipment. The EMT is trained to administer basic life-support skills and definitive therapy via radio communication with a physician.

Prerequisites for an EMT program include high school or its equivalent. The program includes classroom and clinical work and a field internship. Students with military medical training may be exempt from some requirements. Certification is awarded after examination by the National Registry (or another designated agency) and 6 months of employment.

DENTAL HYGIENE

Dental hygiene is a preventive oral health profession whose practitioners support total health and are responsible for promoting optimal oral health for people of all ages. In doing so, dental hygienists facilitate the prevention and treatment of oral diseases such as dental caries (cavities) and periodontal (gum) disease. Dental hygienists, working with dentists, carefully monitor the oral health status of their patients and intervene as necessary with a variety of therapeutic services (Fig. 19-3). Specific professional activities of the dental hygienist may include:

- Initial screening examination and charting of a patient's teeth, soft tissue, and other oral structures
- Exposing and developing radiographs
- Developing individualized oral hygiene programs for control of dental biofilm
- Removing calculus and dental biofilm from above and below the gum line
- Applying caries-preventive agents such as fluoride and dental sealants

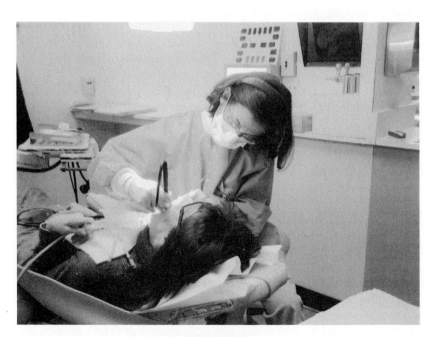

Fig. 19-3

Dental hygienist at work.

Educational requirements vary at different schools from associate degree to baccalaureate degree programs. Upon completion of an accredited dental hygiene program, graduates are eligible to take national, regional, and state licensing examinations in order to be licensed to practice. Personal qualifications needed for entry into this career include good general academic ability, a desire to be able to contribute to the health and well-being of people, and the ability to get along well with others. Good health, normal eyesight, and better than average finger and hand dexterity are important qualifications. In addition, patience, tact, emotional stability, and willingness to assume responsibility are necessary to practice dental hygiene successfully.

Employment opportunities are good for dental hygienists, and a shortage currently exists in many areas of the country, especially rural communities and the inner city. Most dental hygienists work in private dental offices and dental clinics. Other practice settings include:

- Public health departments
- Nursing homes
- Private industry
- Health maintenance organizations
- Hospitals
- School systems
- Correctional facilities
- Educational institutions and/or research

Opportunities exist for advanced training in specialized skills, as well as graduate study in dental hygiene. Master's program graduates are prepared to assume leadership roles in improving dental hygiene care and in advancing knowledge and practice of dental hygiene.

THE TEAM APPROACH TO HEALTH CARE

Of all of the organizations of the health care system, the hospital is perhaps the most complex. Hospitals provide for inpatient and outpatient services of treatment and diagnosis, and there are many subdivisions of medical care within these broad functions. Hospitals also must provide professional and technical in-service education to ensure that personnel are kept abreast of new developments within their fields. Research is another important aspect of hospital care, because the concentration of patients provides a database for investigation. Another function that hospitals are concerned with is the prevention of disease, and this concern is being given high priority in some areas for example, isolating patients with contagious diseases.

It is obvious that a hospital that is attempting to provide these services must have individuals with many diverse and highly technical skills. It is equally obvious that those individuals must work together if the goals of the health care facility are to heal the sick and to provide measures for preventive treatment. The above reasons are why the team approach to health care warrants special attention.

A team can be more than the sum of its parts, just as a clock is more than the sum of its parts. The clock's function is to indicate the time, and each of its parts is precisely tooled to work in concert with the other parts to achieve this objective; so, too, must the individuals that make up the health care team work together to achieve the mission or objectives of the hospital.

Three conditions are basic to the team's ability to work together successfully. First, there must be a clear understanding of the hospital mission by all members of the team. Second, there must be a defined purpose for each technical or professional role as it relates to the mission. Third, the care provided by the team needs to be of the highest possible quality. When these three conditions exist, the team's success is assured.

CONCLUSION

More people in America are engaged in health care than in any other occupation. Many factors have contributed to the establishment and rapid growth of new health occupations. Although the radiologic technologist will not deal with members of all of these occupations directly, it is essential to recognize the valuable contributions made by your colleagues on the health care team.

Specialization is a fact of life within the radiology department as much as it is in other segments of medicine. Chapter 22 provides a detailed exploration of some of the specializations available to radiologic technologists.

Review Questions

1. Allied health developed as a result of which of the following?
   a. Specialization
   b. Advancements in science and technology
   c. Medical economics
   d. All of the above
2. The nursing profession:
   a. Was the last of the health professions to require registration.
   b. Has the most members but the fewest registered.
   c. Has specialized in several areas.
   d. Was the last to accept specialization.
3. The medical technologist:
   a. Works independent of physicians.
   b. Analyzes and performs tests for diagnosis and treatment.
   c. Provides biomechanical and assistive devices for relieving pain.
   d. Evaluates the nature of medical emergencies.
4. Histotechnologists:
   a. Have round-the-clock patient contact.
   b. Perform diagnostic testing of the respiratory system.
   c. Administer temporary medical emergency help.
   d. Identify, mount, and stain human tissue.
5. The medical records administrator:
   a. Plans, designs, and manages patient records.
   b. Applies principles of nutrition.

c. Alters medical records for insurance agencies.

d. Alters medical records for hospital administration.

6. The dietitian:
   a. Performs tests for vitamin deficiency.
   b. Manages and administers institutional food service.
   c. Performs tests for nutritional status.
   d. Evaluates body fluids for dietary purposes.

7. The physical therapist:
   a. Performs chemical analysis to evaluate treatment plans.
   b. Is concerned mainly with restoring function.
   c. Tests muscle cells for bodily strength and range of motion.
   d. Tests bodily fluids for nutritional deficiency.

8. The occupational therapist:
   a. Matches skills and talents suited to the occupation.
   b. Counsels individuals to the most-needed occupations.
   c. Trains applicants for specific occupations.
   d. Develops and maintains a client's ability to perform daily living tasks.

9. The respiratory therapist:
   a. Must have a bachelor of science degree to become registered.
   b. Must have graduated from a school accredited by the American Medical Association.
   c. Administers therapeutic procedures for respiratory emergencies.
   d. None of the above.

10. The emergency medical technician/paramedic:
    a. Administers basic life support and definitive therapy.
    b. Provides long-term care for the functionally disabled.
    c. Provides rehabilitative and diagnostic testing.
    d. Performs restorative function procedures after an injury.

BIBLIOGRAPHY

American Medical Association: *American Medical Association Health Professions Career and Education Directory*, ed. 29, Chicago, 2001, The Association.

Carnegie Commission on Higher Education: *Higher education and the nation's health*, New York, 1970, McGraw-Hill.

Gerdin JA: *Health careers today*, ed. 2, St. Louis, 1997, Mosby.

Harris EL, et al: *The shadowmakers, a history of radiologic technology*, Albuquerque, NM, 1995, American Society of Radiologic Technologists.

Hepner JO, Hepner DM: *The health strategy game*, St. Louis, 1973, Mosby.

Horn, Marie L, MS, RDH: University of Tennessee Health Science Center, consultant 2005.

Rosen G: *From medical police to social medicine: essays on the history of health care*, New York, 1974, Science History Publications.

Wyatt, Diane, MS, MT (ASCP): University of Tennessee Health Sciences Center, consultant 2005.

III

Growing with the Profession

The American Registry of Radiologic Technologists

Neta B. McKnight

OBJECTIVES

On completion of this chapter, you should be able to:

- **Narrate the history of the American Registry of Radiologic Technologists.**
- **List the professions that the American Registry of Radiologic Technologists certifies.**
- **Describe the examination procedures.**
- **List the subject areas of the examination content.**
- **Explain how results are reported.**
- **Describe the rights and privileges of the registered technologist.**

Today, certification and registration with the **American Registry of Radiologic Technologists (ARRT)** is the internationally recognized standard of the profession. The ARRT is the only national certifying agency that is recognized by the **American Society of Radiologic Technologists (ASRT)**, the **American College of Radiology (ACR)**, and the American Medical Association (AMA). The symbol "(ARRT)" has been registered in Washington, DC, as the exclusive property of the ARRT, and it has become the passport to ethical employment in hospitals and clinics

KEY TERMS

American College of
  Radiology (ACR)
American Registry of
  Radiologic
  Technologists (ARRT)
American Society of
  Radiologic
  Technologists (ASRT)
certification
equated scores
Radiological Society of
  North America (RSNA)
registration
scaled scores

CHAPTER OUTLINE

The history of the ARRT
Organization
Examination procedures
  General qualifications
  Educational
    requirements
  Military
  Competency
    requirements
  Examination window
  Application forms
  Agreement of
    applicants
  Application Status
    Report
  Registry examinations
  Score report
Certification in radiologic
  technology
Conclusion

within English-speaking countries. Certification by the ARRT is accepted by all states with licensure laws for state licensing purposes.

THE HISTORY OF THE ARRT

In 1920, four members of the **Radiological Society of North America (RSNA)** presented a plan to their organization for the certification of operators of x-ray equipment. Working together with the American Roentgen Ray Society, these two organizations established operation of the ARRT in 1922. That year there were 89 certifications, the first of which was presented to Sister M. Beatrice Merrigan of St. Louis.

Also during this early period, the technicians themselves formed the American Association of Radiological Technicians (AART), which later became the American Society of X-ray Technicians (ASXT). In April of 1926, they voted to accept only registered technicians as members. The standard was set and has never been lowered. In 1936, a joint sponsorship between the RSNA and the ASXT was established, with the ARRT incorporated as a separate body. Sponsorship again changed in 1943, when the RSNA transferred its co-sponsorship to the American College of Radiology. The ASXT continued as the other sponsor of the ARRT. At about the same time, the Council on Medical Education and Hospitals of the AMA began to establish guidelines for x-ray courses; this helped to ensure quality education for students nationwide.

In 1960, work began on programs to educate and certify people in the specialties of radiation therapy and nuclear medicine technology. The first examinations for nuclear medicine were given in 1963, and the ones for radiation therapy were first given in 1964. Also in 1960, the ARRT moved to 2600 Wayzata Boulevard, Minneapolis, Minnesota. In August of 1989, the ARRT moved into its new headquarters in St. Paul.

As of publication, the preliminary end-of-the-year count of ARRT certificates in good standing is as follows:

Radiography: 233,965
Nuclear medicine technology: 10,906
Radiation therapy technology: 14,738
Cardiovascular-interventional technology (CV): 4,278
Cardiac-interventional technology: 47
Vascular-interventional technology: 133
Mammography: 46,114
Magnetic resonance imaging (MRI): 15,238
Computed tomography (CT): 23,360
Quality management: 1,331
Sonography: 42
Vascular sonography: 25
Bone densitometry: 592
Breast sonography: 20

This makes for a total of 350,789 certificates held by 245,795 certified professionals who are qualified to work in these fields.

Those who have served the ARRT can look back on a gratifying process of growth and acceptance: growth in professional competence and gradual acceptance by all medical, civil, and governmental organizations as the single authoritative source of qualified personnel in the disciplines that the ARRT serves. The ARRT has indeed come a long way from the first Board of Registry, in which the board members personally administered their 20-question certification examination, to the present ARRT. Today's ARRT includes government by a board of trustees; a full-time salaried staff; modern facilities with computerized records; criterion-referenced certification examinations in radiography, nuclear medicine technology, and radiation therapy; and advanced level examinations in cardiac interventional technology (CI), vascular interventional technology (VI), mammography, computed tomography (CT), quality management, sonography, magnetic resonance imaging (MRI), bone densitometry (BD), sonography (S), vascular sonography (VS), and breast sonography (BS).

ORGANIZATION

The ARRT is governed by a board of trustees that is composed of nine members. Five trustees are registered radiologic technologists appointed by the ASRT, and four are physicians appointed by the ACR. Trustees are appointed to serve 4-year terms. Each year, the board of directors of the ASRT and the board of chancellors of the ACR each appoint one new member to the board of trustees. Meetings of the board are held semiannually, although additional meetings can be held if circumstances require. Trustees serve without compensation, but meeting expenses are reimbursed. The board is served by a full-time salaried staff of 45 employees, who conduct the routine business of the board at the ARRT's office in St. Paul, Minnesota. The board is also served by consultants in radiography, nuclear medicine technology, radiation therapy, and physics (all disciplines to which the ARRT administers examinations) who serve without compensation but are reimbursed for expenses.

The *ARRT Certification Handbook* is furnished to all applicants for examination for registration, and the semiannual *ARRT Educator Update* is mailed to accredited educational programs and related organizations in radiologic technology. The *Directory of Registered Technologists* is available online at the ARRT's website (www.arrt.org). The *Annual Report to Registered Technologists* is mailed each spring to all radiologic technologists.

EXAMINATION PROCEDURES

General Qualifications

Candidates must be of good moral character. Generally, conviction for either (1) a felony or (2) any offense, misdemeanor, or felony indicates a lack of good moral character for ARRT purposes. Those who have been convicted of a crime may be eligible for **registration** (an official entry on a list of people who are certified as eligible by qualifications) if they have served their entire sentence, including parole, and have had their civil rights restored.

Educational Requirements

Candidates must have successfully completed a program of formal education that is accredited by a mechanism acceptable to the ARRT.

- Applicants for registration as radiographers must have completed an educational program in radiography.
- Applicants for registration as nuclear medicine technologists must have completed an educational program in nuclear medicine technology.
- Applicants for registration as radiation therapists must have completed an educational program in radiation therapy.
- Application for certification must be made within 5 years of program completion.

Accepted accreditation mechanisms in the United States are the Joint Review Committee on Education in Radiologic Technology (JRCERT), the Joint Review Committee on Education in Nuclear Medicine Technology (JRCNMT), and the branches of the six regional accrediting organizations that accredit degree-granting institutions. Outside the U.S., ARRT-accepted accreditation mechanisms include the Conjoint Secretariat of the Canadian Medical Association and the Australian Institute of Radiography.

Military

The U.S. Army and U.S. Air Force offer accredited educational programs in radiography. The U.S. Navy offers accredited educational programs in radiography and nuclear medicine technology. People who have completed all requirements of these programs may apply for ARRT examination under regular eligibility procedures. Those who did not satisfy all follow-up training requirements for one of these programs must enroll in and graduate from an educational program that is accredited by a mechanism that is acceptable to the ARRT. Individuals trained in the U.S. military should review Appendix E of this handbook for further information.

Competency Requirements

Applicants for ARRT primary certification (Radiography, Nuclear Medicine Technology, or Radiation Therapy) must demonstrate competency in didactic course work and an ARRT-specified list of clinical procedures. Details are available on the ARRT website (www.arrt.org) and in the *ARRT Certification Handbook*.

Examination Window

Applicants may schedule appointments to test at any time during a set examination window. Generally, examination windows begin on the Wednesday after the applications are processed and extend for 90 calendar days. For example, if an application is processed on April 15, 2005, the examination window begins on Wednesday, April 20, 2005, and ends on July 29, 2005.

If the educational program completion date as reported on the application form has not passed, the examination window will begin on the program completion date.

Applicants taking the examination for ARRT continuing education credit should be sure that their examination date occurs within the assigned continuing education biennium.

Application Forms

An application form is located at the back of the ARRT handbook. Requests for additional handbooks should be directed to ARRT Examination Services by phoning 651-687-0048, extension 560 or by writing to the ARRT at 1255 Northland Drive, St. Paul, Minnesota, 55120-1155.

The *ARRT Certification Handbook*, which includes the application form, is provided to each applicant. The purpose of the handbook is to help the applicant prepare for and understand the registration and examination procedures. The information in the handbook should be read very carefully.

Agreement of Applicants

Applicants for certification must, at the time of application and on subsequent occasions when the registration of the certificate is renewed, agree to abide by the agreement included in Article III, Section 3.02 of the *ARRT Rules and Regulations* (Box 20-1). A copy of the *ARRT Rules and Regulations* is included as an appendix of the *Certification Handbook*. Applicants should read the *ARRT Rules and Regulations* before signing and submitting an application for certification.

Application Status Report

The ARRT mails an Application Status Report to the candidate after the application is processed and certification eligibility has been determined. The Application Status Report contains candidate identification information, the six-digit ARRT ID number, and examination window dates.

Registry Examinations

The authority and responsibility for the construction of examinations for national registration in radiologic technology have resided with the

BOX 20-1—AGREEMENT OF CANDIDATES*

I hereby apply to ARRT for certification in the discipline of radiologic technology indicated elsewhere on this application and examination relative to that certification in accordance with and subject to the *Rules and Regulations* of ARRT. A full and complete copy of the *Standards of Ethics and Rules and Regulations* of ARRT is available to me upon request, and I understand that the *Rules and Regulations* are summarized in the current *Certification Handbook* issued by ARRT. By signing this document and filing it with ARRT, I understand and agree that I am in compliance with the *Standards of Ethics* of ARRT and that ARRT may confirm the information contained in the application and may also request information relating to my education, training, employment, and personal history. I further agree to be legally bound by and to abide by all the terms and conditions of this Application and Agreement and the *Rules and Regulations and Standards of Ethics* of ARRT. I agree that upon the issuance to me of a certificate, I shall become bound by the Bylaws of ARRT and shall remain bound by the *Rules and Regulations and Standards of Ethics* of ARRT, including, without limitation, provisions thereof pertaining to the denial or rejection of an application for renewal of registration of a certificate, the revocation or suspension of a certificate, and the censure of a registrant.

I hereby certify that the information given in this application is true, correct, and complete, that any photographs enclosed are recent photographs of me, and that I have read and accept the terms and conditions set forth in ARRT's *Rules and Regulations and Standards of Ethics*. I understand and agree that eligibility for ARRT's examinations is determined by, and that each examination will be supervised by persons who are responsible to, and are empowered by, ARRT to ensure that the examination is conducted ethically and in accordance with the *Rules and Regulations* of ARRT.

I understand and agree that (i) any misrepresentation in this application or in any other document or other information I submit to ARRT (including the verification of my identity when I submit this application and when I take the examination), or (ii) any offer of financial benefit to a trustee, officer, employee, proctor, or other agent or representative of ARRT in order to obtain a right, privilege or benefit not usually granted by ARRT to similarly situated candidates, or (iii) any irregular behavior during the examination, such as copying or recording questions or answers, sharing information, using notes, or otherwise giving or obtaining any unauthorized information or aid, evidenced by observation, statistical analysis of answer sheets, or otherwise, on any portion of the examination will be reported to ARRT and will constitute grounds for ARRT to bar me permanently from all future examinations, to terminate my participation in the examinations, to invalidate the results of my examinations and any prior examinations, to withhold my scores or certificate, to revoke or suspend my certificate, to deny or reject my application for renewal of registration of a certificate or otherwise to refuse to renew the registration of a certificate, to censure me, and/or to take any other appropriate action, and that ARRT's decision on any such matter is final.

I also understand and agree that ARRT may withhold my scores and may require me to retake one or more portions of an examination if ARRT is presented with evidence demonstrating to ARRT, in its sole discretion, that the security of those portions of the examination have been compromised, notwithstanding the absence of any evidence of my personal involvement in the com-

Continued

promising activities. I recognize that the examination booklets and related materials utilized in ARRT's examinations are copyrighted as the sole property of ARRT and must not be removed from the test area or reproduced in any way and that reproduction of copyrighted material, in whole or in part, is a federal offense and may subject me to the sanctions listed above. I understand and agree that the decision as to whether my grades and other performances on ARRT's examinations qualify me for a certification rests solely and exclusively in ARRT, and that its decision is final.

I understand that if I am certified and registered by ARRT and/or if the registration is renewed by ARRT, ARRT may issue to me one or more forms of printed certificate or card to evidence such certification and/or registration. I understand and agree that each such form of printed certificate or card remains the property of ARRT and shall be returned to ARRT upon its request. I understand and agree that I may indicate my certification and/or registration by ARRT by (a) displaying any such certificate or card in my place of practice as a Radiologic Technologist, and (b) a factual statement on stationery, in advertisements, and in resumes, biographical sketches and the like, using the name of ARRT or a recognizable abbreviation of the name. I further understand and agree that the name of ARRT and the logo of ARRT shall not be used by me on any other certificate or material displayed, prepared, or distributed by or for me, or on any other sign or display used by or for me, without ARRT's prior written permission.

I hereby waive and release, and shall indemnify and hold harmless, ARRT and persons in their capacities as ARRT's trustees, members, officers, committee members, employees, and agents from, against, and with respect to any and all claims, losses, costs, expenses, damages, and judgments (including reasonable attorney fees) that arise or are alleged to have arisen, from, out of, with respect to, or in connection with any action which they, or any of them, take or fail to take as a result of or in connection with this application, any examination conducted by ARRT which I apply to take or take, the grade or grades given me on the examination, and, if applicable, the failure of ARRT to issue to me a certificate or to renew the registration of a certificate previously issued to me, ARRT's revocation of any certificate previously issued to me, or ARRT's notification of legitimately interested persons of such actions taken by ARRT. I understand and agree that in the event of my breach of or default in any provision of this Application and Agreement in any respect whatsoever, ARRT shall have the absolute right, in its absolute discretion, to revoke or suspend any certificate issued to me, refuse to issue to me any certificate or renewal of the registration thereof, censure me, and/or cancel my registration with ARRT and to provide information regarding such circumstances to all legitimately interested persons without restriction.

I hereby authorize the Registry to release the results of my examination to appropriate state agencies for credentialing purposes. I also authorize the Registry to identify me and to report the fact of my certification or non-certification to prospective employers, universities, colleges, schools, federal, state and local agencies, hospitals, health departments and similar organizations and agencies."

*Excerpt, with permission granted, has been taken from the *ARRT Certification Handbook*, St. Paul, MN. The American Registry of Radiologic Technologists.

ARRT board of trustees since 1922. In the early days, the trustees set up the test specifications, wrote all test items, and administered the examinations entirely without outside help. However, as the ARRT grew in number and complexity, it became necessary to use nontrustee help to get the job done. The position of executive secretary was established on a part-time basis to assist the board. Eventually, that position evolved into a full-time executive office to which the board could delegate portions of its examination construction work.

The construction of present-day ARRT examinations is actually a combined effort of the board, its staff, and carefully selected examination committee members and item writers. The board approves the specifications for each test, including the format and item writing style. The staff assembles the first draft of each test form according to the specifications from a library of several thousand test items. At the semiannual meeting of each of the examination committees, the first draft of the new test form is reviewed and revised where necessary. Revisions are incorporated into a second draft, which the committee then reviews. Revisions are made, and a third draft is produced. The committee then approves the final draft.

The examinations consist of multiple-choice questions designed to measure the examinee's abilities to apply current knowledge in radiologic technology. There are 200 scored questions on the radiography, nuclear medicine technology, and radiation therapy examinations. The numbers of scored questions on the advanced level exams are noted on ARRT's website (www.arrt.org). In addition to the scored questions, there may be up to 20% more pilot questions included that do not count towards the examinee's scores. The examinations are objective tests that cover knowledge, understanding, and application of radiologic technology practices and principles. Table 20-1 presents a breakdown of the content categories and provides the number of questions in each area.

The copyright for the examinations in radiologic technology is owned by the ARRT, and any attempt to reproduce all or parts of the examination is prohibited by law unless written permission is obtained from the ARRT.

All examinations are administered by computer at test centers designated by the ARRT.

Score Report

Approximately 3 to 4 weeks after the test date, the ARRT mails score reports to all examinees. Examination results are not given over the telephone.

In reporting scores on the examinations in radiologic technology, two statistical procedures are used.

The first one is **equated scores**, which takes into account the difficulty level of each version of the examination and the ability level of each group tested. Although the difficulty level of the examination and the ability level of the group tested may vary, examinees are always statistically compared with the same reference group, and their scores are reported in relation to that group. The equating procedure is used because questions in each content area of the examinations in radiologic technology are different for

TABLE 20-1

CONTENT SPECIFICATIONS FOR THE EXAMINATION IN RADIOGRAPHY, NUCLEAR MEDICINE TECHNOLOGY, AND RADIATION THERAPY

Content Category	Weight	Number of Questions
Examination in Radiography		
A. Radiation protection	20%	40
B. Equipment operation and quality control	12%	24
C. Image production and evaluation	25%	50
D. Radiographic procedures	30%	60
E. Patient care and evaluation	13%	26
Total	100%	200
Examination in Nuclear Medicine Technology		
A. Radiation protection	10%	20
B. Radionuclides and Radiopharmaceuticals	12%	24
C. Instrumentation and quality control	18%	36
D. Diagnostic and therapeutic procedures	50%	100
E. Patient care and education	10%	20
Total	100%	200
Examination in Radiation Therapy		
A. Radiation protection and quality assurance	17.5%	35
B. Clinical concepts in radiation oncology	27.5%	55
C. Treatment planning	27.5%	55
D. Treatment delivery	12.5%	25
E. Patient care and education	15%	30
Total	100%	200

© 2004 The American Registry of Radiologic Technologists.

each form of a test, and multiple test forms are in use at any given time. These differences may affect the difficulty level of the test form. Specifically, the statistical equating process is designed to identify examinees of comparable ability, regardless of the group with which the examinee is tested or the difficulty level of the test form used.

The second statistical procedure deals with **scaled scores**. Scaling is the process by which examinees of comparable ability who are taking different versions of the examination can be given the same reported score. Passing or failing is determined by the examinee's total score, but the total score is reported as a scaled score. The scaled score does not equal the number of questions answered correctly or the percent of the questions answered correctly. Total scores for all examinees are converted to a score scale ranging from 1 to 99, with a scaled score of 75 defined as passing. The number of correct answers necessary to achieve a scaled score of 75 is based on the ARRT's judgment regarding what level of performance constitutes a minimal passing score and the examination of the actual scores and historical data available.

Although section scores are reported, they are not used in determining whether an examinee passes or fails but rather to provide data to the examinee that may be useful for self-evaluation purposes. The section scores are reported on a scale that ranges from 0 to 10. It should be reiterated that these scores are advisory only.

A passing score does not constitute certification unless all other requirements are also satisfied.

CERTIFICATION IN RADIOLOGIC TECHNOLOGY

Applicants for certification shall agree to abide by the ARRT rules and regulations and the ARRT standards of ethics.

To those who have passed the examination and are otherwise eligible, **certification** is issued to confer on the applicant the right to use the title *registered technologist* and its abbreviation, RT(ARRT), in connection with her or his name so long as the registration of the certificate is in effect. Technologists certified by the ARRT are advised to designate by the initial (R), (N), or (T) their specialty of certification following the RT and to use the symbol "(ARRT)" in connection with RT to avoid confusion with certification from any other source. Individuals who have successfully passed advanced level examinations should use the appropriate credentials pertaining to the specific examination, such as CV, M, CT, MR, QM, S, BD, VS, CI, VI, and BS.

The formal certification of successful candidates is made effective as of the date of the examination. Pocket credentials and a certificate of registration are included when the ARRT mails the score report to the successful candidates. The certificate at time of issue is valid through the individual's next birth month. The certificate can be renewed from year to year on application and payment of the renewal fee as fixed by the board of trustees as long as the applicant remains qualified and meets continuing education requirements. Registrants are sent renewal applications according to their month of birth.

CONCLUSION

The ARRT is one of the oldest—as well as the second largest—certifying agency in the health professions, second only to nursing. The purposes of the ARRT include encouraging the study and elevating the standards of radiologic technologists, examining and certifying eligible candidates, and periodically publishing a listing of registrants. The mission of the ARRT is to promote high standards of patient care by recognizing individuals who are qualified in medical imaging, interventional procedures, and therapeutic treatment. To ensure that registrants would remain qualified, continuing education became a requirement in 1997. The modalities of interest include (but are not necessarily limited to) radiography, nuclear medicine technology, radiation therapy, mammography, cardiovascular-interventional technology, computed tomography, magnetic resonance imaging, quality management, sonography, vascular sonography, breast sonography, bone densitometry, cardiac interventional technology, and vascular interventional technology.*

Review Questions

1. The ARRT is the national organization for:
   a. The continuing education of radiologic technologists.
   b. The certifying of qualified technologists.
   c. Monitoring technologists' ethical conduct.
   d. All of the above.
2. Eligibility to sit for the ARRT examination in radiography requires:
   a. Completion of an ARRT-recognized accredited program in radiography.
   b. A baccalaureate degree in radiation physics.
   c. A master's degree in radiation biology.
   d. All the above.
3. The ARRT offered its first certificate in:
   a. 1895.
   b. 1906.
   c. 1920.
   d. 1922.
4. The ARRT:
   a. Registers technologists in radiation therapy, radiography, and nuclear medicine.
   b. Examines technologists for advanced-level specialties.
   c. Awards certificates in basic and advanced-level technology.
   d. All of the above.
5. The ARRT:
   a. Approves the curriculum for radiologic education.
   b. Surveys programs in radiologic education for accreditation.
   c. Sets standards for educators in radiologic technology.
   d. Develops tests and examines applicants in radiologic technology.

*All information pertaining to the ARRT is presented with the permission of the ARRT and is accurate as of publication. However, all ARRT policies and procedures are subject to periodic evaluation and revision. For more information, contact The American Registry of Radiologic Technologists, 1255 Northland Drive, St. Paul, Minnesota 55120-1155; 651-687-0048.
NOTE: The ARRT does not review, evaluate, or endorse publications. Permission to reproduce ARRT copyrighted materials within this publication should not be construed as an endorsement of the publication by the ARRT.

6. The ARRT examination consists of a:
   a. 200-question computerized test plus pilot questions.
   b. 200-question paper-and-pencil test and a practicum.
   c. 200-question paper-and-pencil test and a sample radiograph.
   d. 200-question paper-and-pencil test and a physician's statement of competence.

7. A score is defined as passing provided that:
   a. A score of 75 is made on all sections of the test.
   b. A score of 75 is made in radiation protection.
   c. A composite score of 75 is made.
   d. A score of 75 is made on at least two sections of the test.

8. In 1997, which of the following became a requirement for recertification?
   a. Passing an updated examination
   b. Showing evidence of continuing education
   c. Documenting evidence of ethical conduct
   d. Presenting evidence of continued employment

9. The ARRT is one of the oldest certifying agencies in the health professions and is also:
   a. The largest.
   b. The second largest.
   c. The third largest.
   d. The most regulated.

10. The purpose of the ARRT is to:
    a. Encourage education.
    b. Elevate standards of radiologic technologists.
    c. Examine and certify eligible candidates.
    d. All of the above.

BIBLIOGRAPHY

American Registry of Radiologic Technologists: *ARRT certification handbook*, St. Paul, MN, 2004, The Registry.

Harris EL: *The shadowmakers, a history of radiologic technology*, Albuquerque, NM, 1995, American Society of Radiologic Technologists.

The Joint Review Committee on Education in Radiologic Technology

Joanne S. Greathouse

OBJECTIVES

On completion of this chapter, you should be able to:

- Define accreditation and describe its characteristics.

- State the two primary types of educational accreditation, and describe the difference.

- State the purpose of program accreditation.

- Discuss the evolution of radiologic sciences education and accreditation.

- List the three groups of individuals who collaborate in the operation of the Joint Review Committee on Education in Radiologic Technology, and describe the responsibilities of each group.

- List and briefly discuss the components of the accreditation process.

- Discuss the process of programmatic self-study and its role in the accreditation process.

- Discuss the purpose of a site visit, and list the individuals involved and their roles.

- List the benefits of programmatic accreditation to various groups of individuals.

Continued

KEY TERMS

accreditation
compliance
peer review
self-study
site visit
STANDARDS

CHAPTER OUTLINE

Introduction
History of the JRCERT, radiologic sciences education, and accreditation
JRCERT mission statement
Types of programs
Organization
 Board of Directors
 Staff
 Site visitors
Standards
The accreditation process
 Definition
 Self-study
 Site visit
 Exit interview
 Report of findings
 Board's consideration
 Categories of accreditation awards
 Maintenance of accreditation
 Allegations
The value of JRCERT accreditation
Services of the JRCERT
Conclusion

OBJECTIVES — CONT'D

- **Describe the process for submitting complaints to the Joint Review Committee on Education in Radiologic Technology, and explain how complaints are handled.**

INTRODUCTION

Accreditation is a process of external quality control. Through a process of peer review, a nongovernmental agency attests to the adequacy of an institution or program in meeting established standards. Students enrolled in a program of study in the radiologic sciences will likely encounter accreditation in several ways: the educational program in which they are enrolled will be accredited; the educational and/or hospital institution that sponsors the educational program will be accredited; and the clinical settings in which they receive clinical education and experience will be housed in accredited institutions.

There are two forms of educational accreditation: institutional and specialized. Institutional accreditation seeks to assess the overall quality and integrity of an institution. Most postsecondary educational institutions that sponsor radiologic sciences programs are accredited by one of several regional (institutional) accrediting agencies. Specialized accreditation, on the other hand, seeks to address educational endeavors at the program level. These agencies, of which the Joint Review Committee on Education in Radiologic Technology (JRCERT) is an example, evaluate the quality and integrity of individual programs. Although the specific process is somewhat different for each type of accreditation, the general principles are the same.

In the broadest sense, accreditation exists to safeguard the public. For example, when a health care organization voluntarily meets the standards established by an accrediting organization, the public can be assured that the quality of the services it provides meets certain minimum levels. Educational accreditation also has a role in safeguarding the public by assuring the adequacy of the preparation of practitioners. An educational institution that meets accreditation standards of regional accrediting agencies is able to assure prospective and enrolled students and others that it meets, at the least, the minimum standards developed by educational communities of interest. At the program level, particularly in the health fields, the adequacy of education is of significant concern to the general public. The accreditation of programs in radiologic sciences that voluntarily meet standards establishes that these programs adhere to nationally developed professional education standards in their preparation of these health care professionals. It assures the public, the profession, and the students that graduates are adequately prepared for professional practice as determined by the profession.

HISTORY OF THE JRCERT, RADIOLOGIC SCIENCES EDUCATION, AND ACCREDITATION

From the earliest days following Roentgen's discovery of the x-ray in 1895, the need for proper training in the use of this powerful force was recognized. The first physicians who experimented with the use of the Roentgen ray in the diagnosis of disease informally trained x-ray technicians on an as-needed basis; this training followed the apprentice model. The individual observed procedures and then performed them with progressively less supervision; there were no organized classroom activities.

The onset of more formal training programs began with radiologists and technicians working together to establish instructional programs in a few hospitals. The American Medical Association (AMA) was recognized as the official accrediting agency, but it delegated the responsibility for the inspection and evaluation of educational programs to the American College of Radiology (ACR). In 1944, x-ray technology (the predecessor of radiologic technology) became the fifth health occupation (after occupational therapy, clinical laboratory sciences, physical therapy, and medical records administration) to establish standards of education and qualifications for program accreditation. The first criteria published in "Essentials of an Acceptable School for X-ray Technicians" on June 12, 1944, in the Journal of the American Medical Association were the product of negotiations between the American Society of X-ray Technicians (now the American Society of Radiologic Technologists [ASRT]) and the Council on Medical Education and Hospitals of the American Medical Association. A limited didactic curriculum was required, but the emphasis was on clinical learning and proficiency through repetitive practice and skills development. By 1950, approximately 125 schools offered training in x-ray technology.

The Commission on Technologist Affairs of the ACR carried out program evaluation from 1944 to 1969. The review of programs was a joint effort that involved both radiologists and radiologic technologists. During the latter part of this period, "education" replaced "training" as the curricula evolved to include significant didactic components in support of clinical experience. The idea of progression from classroom to clinical learning began to take hold, and radiologic technologists rather than radiologists increasingly assumed primary responsibility for the educational programs.

In 1964, radiation therapy was recognized as a distinct discipline separate from radiography, and the first "Essentials" recognized for the support of radiation therapy programs were implemented in 1968. Nuclear medicine became recognized as a distinct discipline in 1969. Educational programs in nuclear medicine technology are accredited by the Joint Review Committee on Educational Programs in Nuclear Medicine Technology. As the radiologic sciences have continued to advance, additional disciplines have evolved. The first standards for magnetic resonance programs were adopted by the JRCERT in 2003, and standards for educational programs in medical dosimetry were adopted in 2004.

The number of educational programs grew dramatically, and the evaluation of their **compliance** (the agreement with published educational standards) became more complex. In 1969, the ASRT and the ACR established the JRCERT. It became incorporated in 1971, and it assumed the responsibilities for evaluating educational programs in radiography and radiation therapy. At that time, the JRCERT operated as part of the AMA Council on Medical Education. In 1976, the AMA Council on Medical Education delegated responsibility for allied health accreditation to a newly formed Committee on Allied Health Education and Accreditation (CAHEA). The JRCERT worked with this agency until 1992, when the dissolution of CAHEA was announced.

In the early 1970s, more than 1,300 radiography and radiation therapy programs were accredited by the American Medical Association. Today, the JRCERT accredits approximately 600 radiography and 75 radiation therapy programs. In the past 30 years, many of the program closures have been the result of hospitals withdrawing from program sponsorship. Many of these institutions, however, have not removed themselves completely from education; instead, they now affiliate with academic institutions and serve as recognized clinical education settings for the academic programs. The JRCERT currently recognizes more than 3,300 clinical education settings as affiliates for radiography programs and nearly 400 for radiation therapy programs.

During this same period, radiologic sciences education continued to evolve. Educational programs became more structured, the curriculum was significantly expanded, and competency became a defining principle. Instead of prescribing the experiences that students must have and the number of hours of instruction students must complete, the emphasis shifted to the outcome of the process (i.e., whether graduates are capable of performing as entry-level radiologic technologists or radiation therapists). Programs were structured to guide students from basic theoretic knowledge and laboratory experience to limited clinical experience. As students progressed through educational programs, the level of clinical involvement increased as the level of supervision decreased.

The JRCERT became an independent agency and petitioned the United States Department of Education (USDE) for recognition; this recognition was granted in 1992. The JRCERT is the only agency recognized by the United States Department of Education to accredit educational programs in radiography and radiation therapy. Just as programs must submit applications and self-study reports to be accredited by the JRCERT, the JRCERT must periodically submit a petition and documentation of its compliance with federal regulations to the USDE to maintain recognition.

JRCERT MISSION STATEMENT

The Joint Review Committee on Education in Radiologic Technology promotes excellence in education and enhances the quality and safety of patient care through the accreditation of educational programs in the radiologic sciences.

Types of programs

The JRCERT may accredit programs that are sponsored by health care facilities; colleges or universities; or proprietary, government, military, or other institutions if the program and the sponsoring institution meet the JRCERT's educational standards. Program length ranges from 1 to 4 years depending on the completion award, which may be a certificate, an associate degree, or a baccalaureate degree. Regardless of the type of program sponsorship, each program's competency-based curriculum must include didactic instruction (classroom sessions) and clinical education that are consistent with a nationally recognized professional curriculum.

Organization

The effective operation of the JRCERT requires the efforts and collaboration of three distinct groups of people.

Board of Directors

The JRCERT is incorporated in the state of Illinois as a not-for-profit corporation. Although the corporate directors are volunteers who serve without compensation, they have a legal duty and responsibility to protect the interests of the JRCERT as an organization. These directors establish policy and have professional responsibilities specific to the accreditation process. In support of the concept of peer review (a review process conducted by a qualified site-visit team and accrediting agencies), the Board of Directors is made up of representative radiologic technologists (from education, administration, and clinical practice), radiologists, and radiation oncologists. At least one member of the general public is also a member of the Board of Directors.

Staff

The professional staff of the JRCERT consists of certified radiologic technologists with experience in education and accreditation. These individuals are responsible for the administration of the accreditation process and the implementation of JRCERT policy as established by the Board of Directors. Professional staff work closely with institutional and program officials in the achievement and maintenance of educational program accreditation.

Site Visitors

Consistent with the concept of peer review, individuals who are assigned to visit programs are radiologic technologists, radiation therapists, radiologists, and radiation oncologists who are involved in the educational process at their home institution. They volunteer their time as site visitors and provide an important service to both the profession and to the programs accredited by the JRCERT; they are an integral component of the JRCERT structure. Without these individuals, who serve without compensation, the process of peer review would not be possible.

Most site-visit teams are comprised of two members. The site-visit team evaluates a program by reviewing the application and self-study materials submitted by the program and by visiting the sponsoring institution and its clinical affiliates.

STANDARDS

The standards that an educational program are required to meet to achieve and maintain accreditation are developed over time, through consensus building, and with input from professional organizations, educators, practitioners, students, and other communities of interest. Because accreditation is a peer-review process, it is important to have agreement among major communities of interest about the standards that must be met. Through consensus-building with a variety of constituencies, the JRCERT has developed the following accreditation standards: Standards for an Accredited Educational Program in the Radiologic Sciences (**STANDARDS**-RS; as revised in 2002, for radiography and radiation therapy); Standards for an Accredited Educational Program in Magnetic Resonance (STANDARDS-MR; adopted in 2003); the Standards for an Accredited Educational Program in Medical Dosimetry (STANDARDS-MD; adopted in 2004). These standards define requirements in the areas of mission and goals, integrity, program organization and administration, curriculum and academic practices, resources, students, radiation and/or general safety, and program effectiveness and satisfaction.

Students should be aware of the accreditation standards that their programs are required to meet. Many educational programs provide a copy of the accreditation standards in their student handbooks or post them on a bulletin board that is accessible to the student body. Students can also access this information by visiting the JRCERT website or by contacting the JRCERT office.

To maintain accreditation standards that are responsive to what is going on in the educational community, the JRCERT adheres to a cycle of evaluation that results in new standards at least every 10 years. When revisions to the accreditation standards are considered, feedback from a wide variety of interested groups and individuals is sought; student comments are always welcome.

THE ACCREDITATION PROCESS

Definition

Accreditation is the process of voluntary, external peer review in which a nongovernmental agency grants public recognition to an institution or specialized program of study that meets established qualifications and complies with educational standards as determined through initial and subsequent periodic evaluations. In the radiologic sciences, the JRCERT, which is a nongovernmental agency, evaluates educational programs in radiography, radiation therapy, magnetic resonance, and medical dosimetry to determine their level of compliance with standards that have been established nationally by radiologic science professionals. Programs that are found to be in substantial compliance with the standards—either initially or later according to predetermined schedules—are recognized by the JRCERT as accredited programs.

Because accreditation is a voluntary process, evaluation of a radiologic sciences educational program is undertaken only after the program has submitted an application for initial or continuing accreditation. For initial accreditation, the sponsoring institution initiates the process by submitting an application for accreditation. For accredited programs, the JRCERT initiates the process for review approximately 1 year before the date for renewal of accreditation.

Self-Study

Whether for initial or continuing accreditation, each program submits an application for accreditation and a self-study report. The process of self-study is integral to the accreditation process (see Fig. 21-1). During the period of **self-study**, the program reviews all aspects of its operation and its outcomes to determine both its assessment of its degree of compliance with the relevant accreditation standards and how well it has adhered to its unique mission and goals. The results of the self-study are written in a format prescribed by the JRCERT and submitted with the application for accreditation.

The self-study process usually involves several people. Most programs include representatives from the academic and clinical components of the program and from hospital and/or college administration. Some programs include representatives of their advisory committees and/or students.

Site Visit

After submission and JRCERT staff review of the self-study report, a **site visit** to the program is scheduled. The site-visit team is charged with verifying that the self-study report is an accurate portrayal of the program's operation and with evaluating the program's compliance with the established educational standards. The on-site evaluation usually takes 2 days. Site visitors review the program's master plan of education; program and student records; and the program's physical resources, including classrooms, laboratories, libraries, and clinical education settings. They interview institutional and program administrators and faculty, clinical personnel, and students. In addition to assessing the program's compliance with the relevant accreditation standards, site visitors may also provide suggestions to the sponsoring institution and to the program for improving the educational process.

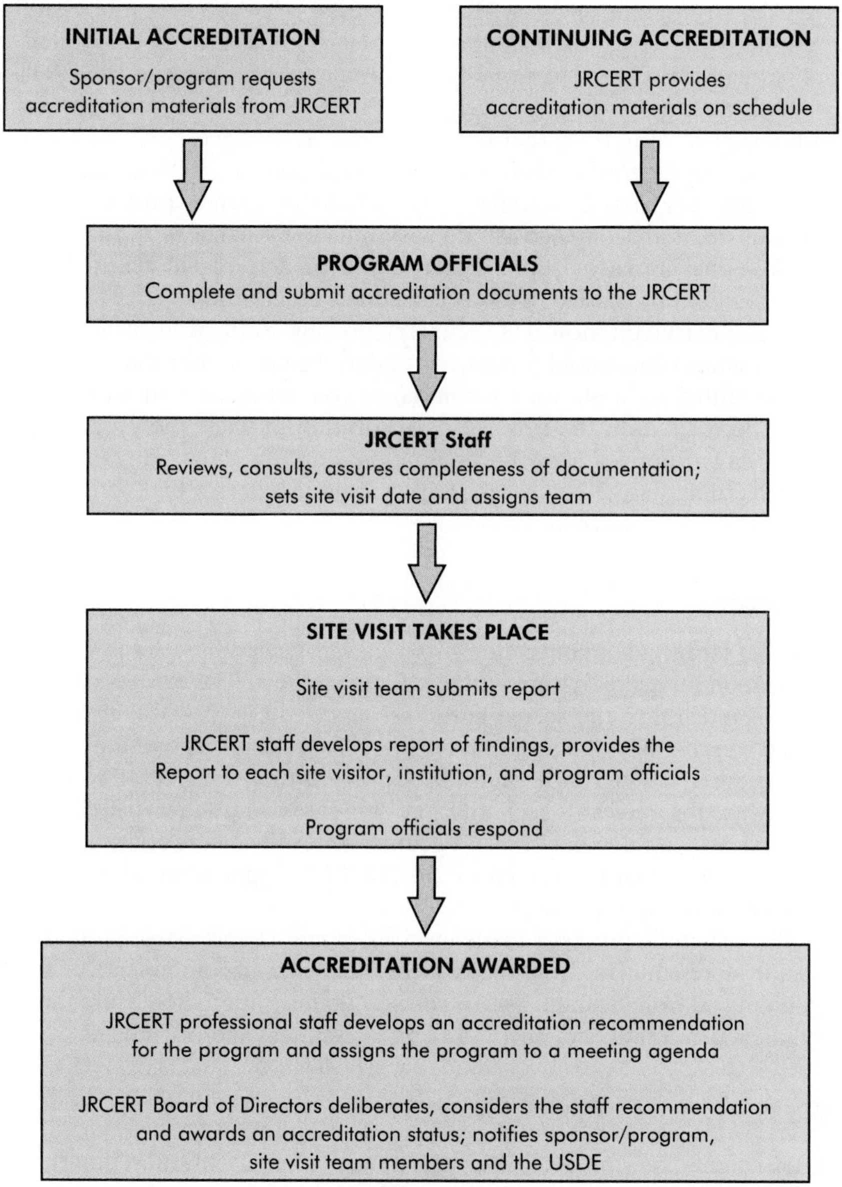

INITIAL ACCREDITATION	CONTINUING ACCREDITATION
Sponsor/program requests accreditation materials from JRCERT	JRCERT provides accreditation materials on schedule

PROGRAM OFFICIALS
Complete and submit accreditation documents to the JRCERT

JRCERT Staff
Reviews, consults, assures completeness of documentation; sets site visit date and assigns team

SITE VISIT TAKES PLACE

Site visit team submits report

JRCERT staff develops report of findings, provides the Report to each site visitor, institution, and program officials

Program officials respond

ACCREDITATION AWARDED

JRCERT professional staff develops an accreditation recommendation for the program and assigns the program to a meeting agenda

JRCERT Board of Directors deliberates, considers the staff recommendation and awards an accreditation status; notifies sponsor/program, site visit team members and the USDE

Fig. 21-1

The accreditation process.

Exit Interview

At the conclusion of the site visit, the site-visit team provides an oral report of its findings in an exit interview. This exit summation is typically attended by institutional administrators and program faculty. Some programs also invite clinical personnel and/or students to attend. During the exit summation, the site visitors cite program strengths and any findings that indicate possible noncompliance with educational standards. The site-visit team does not make an accreditation recommendation or decision but rather sends a written report of its findings to the JRCERT office.

Report of Findings

A member of the JRCERT professional staff considers the program's self-study report, the report of the site-visit team, and any other relevant information and develops an official report of findings. The report cites program strengths and identifies any standards with which the program is determined to not be in substantial compliance. The report may also provide suggestions to the program; these suggestions do not address areas of noncompliance with accreditation standards but rather indicate ways that the program might improve beyond just meeting the minimum standards.

The program is required to respond to the report of findings before the Board of Directors will consider an accreditation action for the program. In the response, the program may provide additional information about the program and demonstrate how it has already addressed issues identified by the site visitors. The program's response is part of the material considered by the Directors in determining a program's accreditation award.

Board's Consideration

At regularly scheduled meetings, the Board of Directors considers programs for accreditation action. For each program on the agenda, the Directors review the current report of findings, the program's response to the report of findings, the JRCERT staff evaluation, and, where applicable, the program's previous report of findings.

After consideration, the Board awards initial or continuing accreditation or decides to withhold or withdraw accreditation. The maximum period of accreditation is 8 years, but a program may receive less than the maximum period. A program that is not in substantial compliance with one or more of the standards may be awarded probationary accreditation. A program is generally limited to 1 year of probationary accreditation; at the end of the year, the program must qualify for accreditation, or accreditation will be withdrawn.

Categories of Accreditation Awards

The JRCERT may award any one of a variety of accreditation categories to a program:

Initial Accreditation: Initial accreditation is awarded to a program that has not been previously accredited or to a program that has had an interruption in its accreditation history.

Continuing Accreditation: This is awarded to programs that are already accredited when the accreditation review process confirms that the program continues to operate in substantial compliance with the educational standards.

The JRCERT may award less than the maximum 8 years' duration of accreditation to a program with some deficiencies; it may require a progress report by a specific date to discuss how the program is addressing those deficiencies. On the basis of this report, the original duration of the accreditation period may be maintained, lengthened, or reduced without another full review process.

Probationary Accreditation: Probationary accreditation is awarded when a program is not in substantial compliance with one or more educational standards and the deficiencies threaten the capability of the program to provide acceptable education. Probationary accreditation is usually limited to 1 year; however, probationary accreditation is an accreditation category, so the program remains accredited. A new application and self-study report must be submitted, usually within 1 year; a site visit will follow. Failure to come into substantial compliance with the educational standards will result in the withdrawal of accreditation.

Administrative Probationary Accreditation: This may result when a program does not comply with one or more of the administrative requirements for maintaining accreditation such as submitting reports, notifying the JRCERT of changes, agreeing to a site-visit date, and paying accreditation fees within a period determined by the JRCERT.

Withholding of Accreditation: Accreditation may be withheld from a program that is seeking initial accreditation if the program is not in substantial compliance with the educational standards.

Withdrawal of Accreditation: Accreditation may be withdrawn from a program with a status of probationary accreditation or administrative probationary accreditation if, at the conclusion of the specified period, the accreditation review process confirms that the program is not in substantial compliance with the educational standards or with the administrative requirements for maintaining accreditation.

Voluntary Withdrawal of Accreditation: An institution that is sponsoring a program may voluntarily withdraw from the JRCERT accreditation system at any time by informing the JRCERT, in writing, of the effective date. Students who complete a program after an institution's withdrawal from accreditation are not considered graduates of a JRCERT-accredited program.

Maintenance of Accreditation

Accredited programs must comply with requirements for maintaining accreditation. Failure to comply with established requirements will result in the program being placed on probation. Some of the requirements for maintaining accreditation include appropriate notification to the JRCERT of program official changes, significant changes in the operation or content of a program, and the submission of annual reports.

Allegations

The JRCERT is required by the USDE to be responsive to allegations that an accredited program is not in compliance with educational standards. Allegations against an accredited program must be submitted in writing to the JRCERT; they must be signed, and they must relate to the accreditation standards relevant to the particular program. Efforts to resolve the allegations within the program and/or institution should always precede any action to involve the accrediting agency. Allegations can be submitted by any individual or group of individuals, including students, faculty, graduates, clinical staff, or the public.

Upon receipt of signed allegations, the JRCERT acknowledges the complaint and presents the allegations to the institution and program, without revealing the identity of the complainant. The program is given a deadline by which it must respond to the allegations. A summary of the allegations and the program's response is presented to the Board of Directors for consideration and action. After deliberation, the Board may decide that the allegations are without merit; that the allegations are true but that the program has taken appropriate action; or that the program is in noncompliance with one or more of the educational standards.

The program may be required to submit one or more progress reports to demonstrate that changes have been made to achieve compliance with the educational standards in question. The program may have its accreditation status reduced to a shorter period of time, or the JCERT may accelerate the continuing accreditation process of the program. After the conclusion of the investigation and deliberation, the sponsoring institution, the program, and the complainant are notified of the JRCERT's disposition of the allegations.

THE VALUE OF JRCERT ACCREDITATION

The impact of accreditation is diverse, as it affects students, institutions, and society in general. Perhaps the most significant benefit of JRCERT accreditation is assurance to the public that graduates have met the minimum level of competency as defined nationally by the profession.

In its broadest sense, accreditation ensures acceptable educational quality. The process of accreditation, including an external peer assessment of program quality, contributes to the continuing improvement of an educational program. The process of peer review based on national educational standards established by radiologic science professionals assures prospective students that their educational programs will provide them, as graduates, with the requisite knowledge, skills, and values to competently perform the expected range of professional responsibilities.

Some state licensing boards require graduation from a JRCERT-accredited program in addition to certification by the national credentialing agency. Some employers, as well, require graduation from a JRCERT-accredited program. Thus, graduation from a JRCERT-accredited program makes students more marketable and assists in ensuring mobility of practice because the graduates have met national standards. By hiring graduates of an accredited program, employers are also assured that their personnel have met national standards.

SERVICES OF THE JRCERT

The principal purpose of the JRCERT is to guarantee the delivery of quality education in the radiologic sciences. In recognition of these responsibilities, the directors and staff of the JRCERT are committed to providing services to the communities of interest: students, educational programs, institutional sponsors, and the public. The professional staff of the JRCERT, with years of experience in education and accreditation, are available by telephone to accredited programs and to those that seek accreditation to assist the programs in achieving and maintaining compliance with established educational standards; they are also available to students and others with an interest in accreditation issues. Professional staff and the Board of Directors also attend a variety of professional meetings and continuing education functions to discuss education and accreditation issues.

The JRCERT maintains a web site that contains information of interest to its various constituencies. Some of the items that can be found there include a directory of accredited programs, accreditation standards, policies and procedures, a listing of Directors and staff, and an allegations reporting form. Students are encouraged to visit the site at www.jrcert.org to review information of interest to them.

CONCLUSION

Radiologic sciences education has evolved from an apprentice model to today's academic model, in which classroom instruction and laboratory competency precede clinical competency. Accreditation is the process of voluntary, external peer review in which a nongovernmental agency grants public recognition to an institution or a specialized program of study that meets established qualifications and complies with educational standards. Compliance is determined through initial and subsequent periodic evaluations.

The JRCERT is the organization whose primary function is to document the compliance of educational programs in the radiologic sciences with the standards that have been established by the radiologic sciences profession. The process for programmatic accreditation is rigorous but well defined and organized and serves to assure the public and the profession that accredited programs meet the profession's minimum standards for quality.

Contact Information:
Joint Review Committee on Education in Radiologic Technology
20 North Wacker Drive, Suite 2850

Chicago, IL 60606-3182
312-704-5300
www.jrcert.org

Review Questions

1. What governmental agency is responsible for the oversight of institutional and programmatic accreditation?
    a. American College of Radiology (ACR)
    b. Committee on Allied Health Education and Accreditation (CAHEA)
    c. Council on Medical Education
    d. United States Department of Education (USDE)
2. In what way does JRCERT accreditation benefit students?
    a. By lowering tuition costs
    b. By making it easier to gain entry into a program
    c. By mandating that all programs have identical courses
    d. By ensuring that a program meets nationally established professional standards
3. Site visitors' responsibilities include which of the following?
    a. Evaluating a program through an on-site visit of the sponsoring institution and clinical practice settings
    b. Recommending an accreditation status to a program during an on-site visit
    c. Developing a report of findings from the on-site evaluation of a program
    d. Both a and c
4. Which of the following is likely when a program's deficiencies threaten the capability of a program to provide acceptable education?
    a. Accreditation is withheld by the JRCERT.
    b. Accreditation is immediately withdrawn by the JRCERT.
    c. The program is awarded administrative probationary accreditation.
    d. The program is awarded probationary accreditation.
5. Educational standards address which of the following?
    a. Program effectiveness
    b. Curriculum
    c. Radiation safety
    d. All of the above
6. The JRCERT is:
    a. An accreditor of educational institutions.
    b. An accreditor of educational programs.
    c. A not-for-profit corporation.
    d. Both b and c.
7. The JRCERT Board of Directors includes:
    a. Radiologic technologists, physicians, and site visitors.
    b. Radiologic technologists, physicians, and a representative of the public.

   c. Radiologic technologists, physicians, students, and a representative of the public.

   d. Radiologic technologists, physicians, and JRCERT staff.

8. The JRCERT investigates complaints that:
   a. Relate to a program's compliance with the educational standards.
   b. Relate to student grades.
   c. Relate to graduate job opportunities.
   d. All of the above.

9. Which of the following is a responsibility of the JRCERT?
   a. Development of professional curricula
   b. Credentialing of radiologic science professionals
   c. Evaluation of educational programs
   d. Provision of job placement services for professionals

10. The accreditation process includes:
    a. Submitting documents, a peer site visit, and JRCERT action.
    b. Submitting documents, a site visit by the JRCERT Board of Directors, and JRCERT action.
    c. A peer site visit, JRCERT action, and USDE approval.
    d. Submitting documents, a peer site visit, and USDE approval.

11. JRCERT-accredited programs may exist in which of the following settings?
    a. Health care facilities
    b. Colleges
    c. Proprietary schools
    d. All of the above

12. What is the maximum length of an accreditation award from the JRCERT?
    a. 1 year
    b. 3 years
    c. 5 years
    d. 8 years

13. Responsibilities of JRCERT directors include which of the following?
    a. Accreditation, corporate, policy development
    b. Accreditation, corporate, policy implementation
    c. Accreditation, corporate, site visits
    d. Accreditation, corporate, development of reports of findings

14. Services offered by the JRCERT include which of the following?
    a. Identification of accredited programs for prospective students
    b. Administration of national credentialing examinations
    c. Maintenance of a placement service for educators
    d. Both a and b

15. Which of the following is true of accreditation?
    a. It is a voluntary process.
    b. It is generally conducted by a nongovernmental agency.
    c. It is a peer-review process.
    d. All of the above.

16. Which of the following is true of a program's self-study report?
    a. It is an evaluation of the program by the JRCERT.
    b. It is an evaluation of the program by program personnel.
    c. It includes information about the program's outcomes in relation to its mission and goals.
    d. Both b and c
17. Which of the following individuals may serve as site visitors?
    a. Radiologic technology educators
    b. Radiologists/radiation oncologists
    c. Students
    d. Both a and b
18. Radiologic sciences education has evolved from the _____ to the _____ model.
    a. Apprentice, academic
    b. Academic, apprentice
    c. Formal, informal
    d. Apprentice, repetitive practice

BIBLIOGRAPHY

Council on Medical Education and Hospitals of the American Medical Association: Essentials of an acceptable school for x-ray technicians, JAMA, June 12, 1944.

Files of the Joint Review Committee on Education in Radiologic Technology, Chicago, 2005, The Committee.

Harris EL, et al: *The shadowmakers, a history of radiologic technology*, Albuquerque, NM, 1995, American Society of Radiologic Technologists.

Millard RM: Whither accreditation in the health professions, *Educ Rev* 65(4): 31-35, 1984.

Stull GA: Commentary, *J Allied Health* 18(5): 425-435, 1989.

Weithaus B: New directions for allied health accreditation, *J Allied Health* 22(3); 239-247, 1993.

Professional Associations

William J. Callaway

OBJECTIVES

On completion of this chapter, you should be able to:

- Explain the primary mission of the American Society of Radiologic Technologists (ASRT).

- Describe the ASRT's involvement in testing and program review.

- List the goals of the American Healthcare Radiology Administrators (AHRA).

- Explain the purpose of the Association of Collegiate Educators in Radiologic Technology (ACERT)and the Association of Educators in Radiological Sciences (AERS).

- List other organizations to which technologists may belong.

- Explain how membership in a professional organization will benefit your personal practice of radiologic technology.

- List the member organizations of the Summit on Radiologic Sciences and Sonography.

- List the organizations to which your instructors belong.

- List the many activities provided by the organizations described in this chapter by visiting each of their websites.

KEY TERMS

American Healthcare
  Radiology
  Administrators (AHRA)
American Society of
  Radiologic
  Technologists (ASRT)
Association of Collegiate
  Educators in Radiologic
  Technology (ACERT)
Association of Educators
  in Radiological
  Sciences (AERS)
Summit on Radiologic
  Sciences and
  Sonography

CHAPTER OUTLINE

An association for all
  radiologic science
  professionals
Practice standards for
  medical imaging and
  radiation therapy
Socioeconomics
Legislation
State and local affiliates
Educators
Radiology managers and
  supervisors
Other technologist
  organizations
Radiologist and physicist
  organizations
The Summit on Radiologic
  Sciences and
  Sonography
Conclusion

As the field of radiologic technology has grown from its beginnings at the turn of the twentieth century, organizations have been formed to carry out the business of the profession. Primary responsibilities include testing, certification, representation, and education (Fig. 22-1). Chapter 20 explained the role of the American Registry of Radiologic Technologists

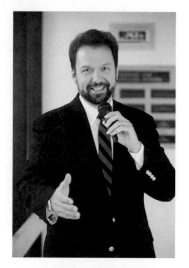

Fig. 22-1

Several professional organizations have formed to benefit the growth of the radiography profession. These organizations give members the opportunity to meet other radiologic technologists, to conduct business, and to give educational presentations.

in testing and certification. This chapter highlights some of the associations to which many technologists belong.

THE AMERICAN SOCIETY OF RADIOLOGIC TECHNOLOGISTS: AN ASSOCIATION FOR ALL RADIOLOGIC SCIENCE PROFESSIONALS

The **American Society of Radiologic Technologists (ASRT**; www.asrt.org) was founded in 1920 by a small, dedicated group of technologists who felt the need to meet and share their knowledge with each other. It has grown from a charter membership of 46 technologists to over 112,000 members. The ASRT is the only nationally recognized professional society that represents all radiologic technologists in the United States today.

The organization, purposes, and functions of the ASRT are directed through the bylaws of the society. These bylaws state, "The purposes of this Society shall be to advance the professions of radiation and imaging disciplines and specialties; maintain high standards of education; and, to enhance the quality of patient care; and, to further the welfare and socioeconomics of radiologic technologists."

To accomplish these aims, there must be a well-defined organization. The house of delegates is the governing and legislative body of the society; the board of directors must carry out the policies and procedures that are established by the house. The members of the board of directors, the president, the vice president, the president-elect, the secretary-treasurer, and the immediate past president are elected by the membership at large. All members of the board of directors must be actively employed in the field of radiologic technology.

The ASRT supports an executive office staff that carries out the wishes of the board as it serves the members. The ASRT has the following staff: executive director, vice president of communications, director of continuing education, director of customer service (who handles thousands of contacts per month), vice president of education and research, executive vice president of operations, chief financial officer, director of government relations, director of information services, director of marketing, director of public relations, executive vice president of professional development, and director of shipping and receiving.

The board of directors holds formal meetings immediately before the annual conference, immediately after the annual conference, and at least once between annual conferences to conduct the business of the ASRT. There is also a great deal of work carried on by this board via email and conventional mail. Serving on this board is truly a commitment of time and energy.

One of the primary reasons that the ASRT was organized was to present education and educational opportunities to the radiologic technologists of the United States. This is still a primary purpose, and the involvement is on many different levels of education.

The ASRT has been instrumental in formulating accreditation standards for the various modalities within radiologic technology. These documents are the sources for the organization and correct operation of the educational programs in the various disciplines. The ASRT has played a key role in the approval process for accreditation documents that affect educational programs in the following areas: radiography, radiation therapy, nuclear medicine, and sonography. Such documents are revised every 5 years, and the ASRT always contributes to their revision.

All educational programs in the field of radiologic technology rely heavily on the curriculum guides that the ASRT has developed for the various disciplines. These guides are written with a behavioral objective format and assist the program directors of the various programs in knowing what should be taught within the curriculum of their programs.

The ASRT believes that a great amount of education can take place among radiologic technologists when they are provided with a forum in which to meet and share their knowledge. The ASRT annual conference is one such event that is provided for technologists to accomplish this goal. There is an extensive educational program presented, and there are also commercial exhibits. The ASRT also provides an educational program formulated for radiation therapy technologists that is presented at the meeting of the American Society for Therapeutic Radiology and Oncology (ASTRO).

Another valuable source of education for technologists is the ASRT scientific journal, *Radiologic Technology*, which is published six times each year. This journal provides radiologic technologists with the latest developments within the profession.

The ASRT has always been committed to continuing education as well as to basic education for all radiologic technologists. A reconfirmation of this commitment was the establishment of the ASRT Educational Foundation in 1984. The foundation is a separate corporation that has responsibility for all educational activities of the ASRT; it has a separate budget and depends on grants and gifts. In addition to radiologic science professionals and affiliate societies, many companies that do radiology-related business and that are interested in the education of radiologic technologists have contributed to the foundation. The foundation awards research grants and scholarships and sponsors self-study materials that technologists can use within their own employment setting or home to further their education. These include a supply of slide/tape sets, videocassette programs on various subjects, and self-study booklets.

More evidence of the commitment of the ASRT to education for radiologic technologists in the United States is the appointment of radiologic technologist trustees to the American Registry of Radiologic Technologists (ARRT), of committee members to the Joint Review Committee on Education in Radiologic Technology (JRCERT), of committee members to the Joint Review Committee on Education in Nuclear Medicine Technology

(JRCENMT), and of one committee member to the Joint Review Committee on Education in Diagnostic Medical Sonography (JRCEDMS). All of the ASRT appointees to these boards of directors represent radiologic technology.

The ASRT has been involved for many years with helping the radiologic technologist attain professional status; however, it takes more than recognition to be considered a professional. Important documents have been developed that define the fundamental role of the radiologic technologist. These documents are identified as the Practice Standards for Medical Imaging and Radiation Therapy, and details are included in Chapter 23. These standards are of extreme importance to the profession of radiologic technology and are especially pertinent to you as you define your role within the profession.

The radiologic technologist is qualified by education and the achievement of technical skills to provide patient care in diagnostic or therapeutic radiologic modalities under the direction of radiologists. In the performance of their duties, the application of proper radiologic techniques and radiation protection measures involves both initiative and independent professional judgment by the radiologic technologist. Inasmuch as it is both desirable and necessary for all disciplines of radiologic technology to be recognized as professionals by government and other agencies, the American College of Radiology supports this position and recognizes the radiologic technologist as a professional member of the health care team (ACR, 1980). This statement was adopted by the American College of Radiology in support of recognizing the professional status of radiologic technologists.

PRACTICE STANDARDS FOR MEDICAL IMAGING AND RADIATION THERAPY

Practice standards have been published for each of the following specialties:
Radiography
Radiation therapy
Nuclear medicine
Diagnostic medical sonography
Magnetic resonance imaging (MRI)
Mammography
Computed tomography
Cardiovascular-interventional technology (CIT)

If professional status is to be maintained, the radiologic technologist has to do more than just be recognized as a professional; he or she must also perform in a professional manner. The measure of a professional is a very complex matter; it is the result of a combination of how we see ourselves and how our patients, our peers, and other health professionals see us. The ASRT has done very thorough research in this area to help the radiologic technologist clarify just what a professional radiologic technologist does and what constitutes professional behavior. Professionalism is a very dynamic process that must be continually practiced. Technologists must continually assess their own performance as professionals, and hold themselves accountable to the patients and their peers.

SOCIOECONOMICS

The ASRT bylaws state that one of the goals of the organization is to "improve the welfare and socioeconomics of radiologic technologists." The accomplishment of this goal demands a many-faceted approach. *Scanner*, which is a monthly newsletter published by the ASRT, keeps its members abreast of current happenings within the profession. This vehicle for communication with radiologic technologist members of the ASRT has an ever-changing format to meet the needs of the time.

The ASRT is constantly gathering data relative to staffing and compensation of radiologic technologists within the United States. The results of this data are published periodically for members to refer to when negotiating for new positions or upgrading their present positions. The best source for this information is the ASRT's website at www.asrt.org.

LEGISLATION

Legislation that mandates the licensing of radiologic technologists by the states in which they work has been a goal of the ASRT for decades. The members believe that it is important that the public be protected from unnecessary exposure to radiation that is administered by people who are not adequately educated in the operation of radiation-emitting equipment. The only way to do this is to make it mandatory that operators of radiation-emitting equipment be tested to ensure that they have a fundamental knowledge of radiation, its uses, and its effects.

To attain this goal, the ASRT is very active in working for the passage of national legislation that would serve to protect the public from unnecessary medical radiation exposure. Such legislation would provide for standards to be passed by the states for the education and credentialing of people who administer radiologic procedures. After the legislation is passed, the ASRT will continue to play a key role in seeing that the public is protected by the law. Radiologic technologists can monitor the progress of such legisltation on the ASRT website.

STATE AND LOCAL AFFILIATES

Radiologic science professionals can maintain their professional involvement locally through state societies. Each state society is considered an affiliate of the ASRT and conducts its business according to ASRT standards. Most state societies conduct an annual educational conference, and many sponsor more than one such session each year.

Mandatory continuing education in many states has prompted the need for additional educational activities throughout the year. These sessions are generally conducted locally through districts within each state society. In addition, the members of these districts elect officials to conduct the business of the district society (e.g., publicity, fund-raising, political action). Thus, the goals and values of the ASRT are shared and propagated from the national to the local level.

As already mentioned, the ASRT maintains an active liaison with the Radiological Society of North America (RSNA) and the American Society for Therapeutic Radiology and Oncology (ASTRO) through joint educational and political efforts. Active communication is also maintained with the American College of Radiology (ACR), the **American Healthcare Radiology Administrators (AHRA)**, the **Association of Collegiate Educators in Radiologic Technology (ACERT)**, and the **Association of Educators in Radiological Sciences (AERS)** to promote the common goal of safe radiology. The ASRT also has active membership in the International Society of Radiographers and Radiologic Technicians (ISRRT).

The ASRT is a multifaceted organization of, by, and for radiologic science professionals. It is the obligation of every radiologic technologist and radiation therapist—as professionals—to join the organization that represents them and therefore contribute to the advancement of the profession. Browse the many pages of www.asrt.org to see how your professional association functions and what it offers to you.

Educators

A specialty in radiologic technology is education. Being an educator in the field today means keeping up with the latest developments in rapidly changing technology as well as educational theory and methodology. This is one of the fastest growing specialties within radiologic technology and represents a dynamic career choice for those interested in teaching the next generation of radiologic technologists.

Both the Association of Collegiate Educators in Radiologic Technology (ACERT; www.acert.org) and the Association of Educators in Radiologic Sciences (AERS; www.aers.org) exist to provide forums for educators to share ideas, strategies, and solutions in their quest for excellence in radiologic science education. Although these are separate and distinct organizations, their primary goals are quite similar. These organizations represent several hundred program directors, clinical coordinators, and clinical instructors of radiologic technology education, and they are incorporated and governed by bylaws. The officers include a president, a president elect, a secretary, and a treasurer.

Members may become involved by serving on one of the many committees, running for office, or presenting a paper or project at the annual conference.

Specializing in radiologic technology education is an important career decision. It requires individuals with strong communication skills, competency in the field itself, and a desire to work hard. It is highly rewarding both professionally and personally.

RADIOLOGY MANAGERS AND SUPERVISORS

As the delivery of radiology services has become more detailed and involved, the role of the radiology administrator has also expanded. To meet their needs as radiology managers, seven administrators founded the American Healthcare Radiology Administrators (AHRA; www.ahra.com) in 1973. Now a nationally recognized organization with several thousand members, the AHRA addresses the issues and concerns of this very important subspecialty of radiology.

The stated goals of the AHRA include the education and training of radiology administrators, the maintenance of high ethical standards, and communication among members. The primary focus of these goals is on the skills needed for leading people and for dealing with the changing health care environment.

The AHRA sponsors national, regional, and local meetings, and it also awards continuing education units (CEUs). Written communication takes place through several publications. An annual directory provides members with names, addresses, and telephone numbers to facilitate the exchange of information among colleagues. A journal, *Radiology Management*, is published quarterly; it covers topics that are pertinent to radiology administration such as management skills, equipment purchasing, and fiscal matters.

The AHRA Link is a monthly newsletter that is distributed to keep members current (particularly with regard to meetings and job openings) between issues of the journal. Because of the proliferation of information about the field, each year the AHRA publishes the *Bibliography for the Radiology Administrator*.

Surveys are conducted by the AHRA, and the data are made available to members. Topics of such surveys have been salaries, productivity, equipment, and position descriptions, among others. By combining the knowledge of many, members have at their disposal publications that would be difficult to produce individually. AHRA provides, for a fee, several manuals containing invaluable information and guidance to the radiology administator.

Membership in the AHRA is open to individuals who practice radiology administration at the level of executive or department head. Associate members include supervisors and educators with some management responsibilities. Other membership categories cover those who wish to contribute to the goals of the organization but who are not eligible to be active or associate members.

It is never too early to begin considering supervision as a career in radiologic technology. Just as in patient care, people of high quality and expertise will always be necessary for leadership positions within radiology departments.

OTHER TECHNOLOGIST ORGANIZATIONS

Each specialty within radiologic technology has its own topics, concerns, and issues; therefore, each has formed its own professional association. An in-depth look at each is not possible here. However, each has as its primary goal the welfare of its patients, its members, and the profession itself.

Technologists who specialize in any aspect of radiologic technology would be wise to maintain membership in the ASRT and in whichever organizations pertain to their chosen specialty. The following professional societies currently serve more than a quarter million radiologic technologists in the United States:

American Association of Medical Dosimetrists
American Healthcare Radiology Administrators
American Registry of Diagnostic Medical Sonographers
American Registry of Radiologic Technologists
American Society of Radiologic Technologists
Association of Collegiate Educators in Radiologic Technology
Association of Educators in Radiological Sciences
Magnetic Resonance Managers Society
Radiology Business Management Association
Society of Computed Body Tomography
Society of Diagnostic Medical Sonographers
Society of Nuclear Medicine, Technologist Section
Society for Magnetic Resonance Imaging
Society for Magnetic Resonance Technologists
Society for Radiation Oncology Administrators

As the field continues to grow, radiologic technologists will band together to form new associations. This networking strengthens the entire profession; it adds to the ranks of dedicated professionals who are willing to put forth the time and effort to learn, to grow, and to promote their respective specialties.

RADIOLOGIST AND PHYSICIST ORGANIZATIONS

To satisfy the needs and demands of radiologists and physicists in diagnostic imaging and therapy, several organizations have been formed over the past 100 years:

American Academy of Health Physics
American Academy of Oral and Maxillofacial Radiology
American Association of Academic Chief Residents in Radiology
American Association of Physicists in Medicine
American Association of Women Radiologists
American College of Medical Physics
American College of Nuclear Physicians
American College of Radiology
American Institute of Ultrasound in Medicine

American Nuclear Society
American Osteopathic College of Radiology
American Radium Society
American Roentgen Ray Society
American Society of Clinic Radiologists
American Society of Emergency Radiology
American Society of Head and Neck Radiology
American Society of Neuroradiology
American Society for Therapeutic Radiology and Oncology
Association of University Radiologists
Health Physics Society
Radiation Research Society
Radiological Society of North America
Society of Breast Imaging
Society of Cardiovascular and Interventional Radiology
Society of Chairmen of Academic Radiation Oncology Programs
Society of Chairmen of Academic Radiology Departments
Society of Gastrointestinal Radiology
Society for Magnetic Resonance in Medicine
Society of Nuclear Medicine
Society for Pediatric Radiology
Society of Radiologists in Ultrasound
Society of Thoracic Radiology
Society of Uroradiology

In addition, The American Radiological Nurses Association exists to serve those nurses who work in radiology departments.

THE SUMMIT ON RADIOLOGIC SCIENCES AND SONOGRAPHY

The **Summit on Radiologic Sciences and Sonography** is a coalition of organizations that represent more than 350,000 health care professionals. These organizations communicate about and plan for issues that affect diagnostic imaging and therapy:

American College of Medical Physics
American College of Radiology
American Healthcare Radiology Administrators
American Hospital Association
American Osteopathic College of Radiology
American Registry of Diagnostic Medical Sonographers
American Registry of Radiologic Technologists
American Society of Radiologic Technologists
American Society of Therapeutic Radiology and Oncology
Association of Educators in Radiological Sciences
Joint Review Committee on Education in Diagnostic Medical Sonography
Joint Review Committee on Education in Radiologic Technology
Joint Review Committee on Educational Programs in Nuclear Medicine
  Technology

Nuclear Medicine Technology Certification Board
Radiology Business Management Association
Society of Diagnostic Medical Sonographers
Society of Nuclear Medicine
Society of Nuclear Medicine, Technologist Section
Society for Radiation Oncology Administrators

CONCLUSION

Never before have there been so many different associations within the profession; never before have true professionals been this willing to work together. As a student radiologic technologist, it is not too early to become involved at the local and state level and to join your national organization. Radiologic technology is not weaker because of specialization in imaging and therapeutic modalities, education, and administration; rather, it is stronger through diversity, because each group represents a pillar of strength that supports all for which we stand.

Review Questions

1. A national organization for radiologic technology educators is the:
   a. AHRA.
   b. ASRT.
   c. RSNA.
   d. ACERT.
2. A national organization for radiologic technology managers is the:
   a. AHRA.
   b. ASRT.
   c. RSNA.
   d. AERS.
3. A national organization for all radiologic technologists is the:
   a. AHRA.
   b. ASRT.
   c. RSNA.
   d. ACERT.
4. Which of the following was the primary reason that the ASRT was formed?
   a. Education
   b. Representation
   c. Unionization
   d. Testing and certification
5. Today, the ASRT serves its members with which of the following?
   a. Continuing education and scholarly publications
   b. Professional representation
   c. Education program curricula
   d. All of the above

6. A group that represents over 350,000 health care professionals, including all radiologic science practitioners, is the:
   a. AHRA.
   b. Summit on Radiologic Sciences and Sonography.
   c. Radiological Society of North America.
   d. AAPM.
7. The professional journal published by the ASRT is called:
   a. *X-Ray Today*.
   b. *Radiology Management*.
   c. *Radiographic Technology*.
   d. *Radiologic Technology*.
8. The ASRT currently represents how many radiologic technologists?
   a. Fewer than 25,000
   b. 10% of those registered
   c. More than 100,000
   d. More than 300,000
9. Other professionals who work in diagnostic imaging and therapy include:
   a. Radiologists.
   b. Physicists.
   c. Nurses.
   d. All of the above
10. The ASRT was founded in:
    a. 1895.
    b. 1960.
    c. 1945.
    d. 1920.

BIBLIOGRAPHY

American Healthcare Radiology Administrators: www.ahra.com, Sudbury, MA, 2005, The Association.

American Society of Radiologic Technologists: *Articles of incorporation and bylaws*, Albuquerque, NM, 2005, The Society.

American Society of Radiologic Technologists: *Practice standards for medical imaging and radiation therapy*, Albuquerque, NM, 2005, The Society.

Association of Collegiate Educators in Radiologic Technology: www.acert.org, Ogden, UT, 2005, The Association.

Association of Educators in Radiological Sciences: www.aers.org, Albuquerque, NM, 2005, The Association.

Specialization in Radiologic Technology

Peggy D. Franklin

OBJECTIVES

On completion of this chapter, you should be able to:

- Discuss the history of the several areas of specialization in radiologic technology.

- Describe the scope and practice of the specialized areas.

- List the requirements for entry into the specialty programs and qualifications for certification.

- Describe special equipment required for ultrasound, nuclear medicine, computed tomography, and magnetic resonance imaging.

- Describe the curriculum content specific to the areas of specialization.

- Compare images produced with ultrasound, computed tomography, and magnetic resonance imaging to images produced with radiation from the perspective of diagnostic quality.

Diagnostic radiology has progressed significantly since its beginning in 1895. It began as a means of determining a patient's illness by recording radiographic images on photographic film, identifying fractures, and examining internal organs for tumors or other physiologic disturbances. Today, however, diagnostic radiology encompasses much more than the simple procedures begun at the end of the last century (Box 23-1).

KEY TERMS

bone densitometry
computed tomography
  (CT)
interventional
  radiology
magnetic resonance
  imaging (MRI)
mammography
nuclear medicine
radiation therapy
radiologist assistant (RA)
sonography
special procedures
  radiography

CHAPTER OUTLINE

Radiation therapy
  History
  Responsibilities of the
    radiation therapist
  Education and
    certification
  Employment
    opportunities
Nuclear medicine
  History
  Responsibilities of the
    nuclear medicine
    technologist
  Equipment and
    procedures
  Education and
    certification
  Employment
    opportunities

Continued

Sonography
  History
  Responsibilities of the
    sonographer
  Education and
    certification
  Employment
    opportunities
Special procedures
  radiography
  History
  Responsibilities of the
    special procedures
    technologist
  Equipment and
    procedures
  Education and
    certification
  Employment
    opportunities
Mammography
Computed tomography
  History
  Responsibilities of the
    CT technologist
  Equipment and
    procedures
  Education
  Employment
    opportunities
Magnetic resonance
  imaging
  History
  Responsibilities of the
    MRI technologist
  Equipment and
    procedures
  Education
  Employment
    opportunities
Bone densitometry
Radiologist assistant
Conclusion

BOX 23-1 — RADIOLOGIC TECHNOLOGIST OR DIAGNOSTIC MEDICAL RADIOLOGIC TECHNOLOGIST

Scope of Practice

Radiography—Practice Comprehensive

Position Summary

Provides health care services by applying x-ray energy to assist in diagnosis or treatment. Performs radiographic procedures and related techniques to produce images for the interpretation by or at the request of a licensed practitioner. Exercises professional judgment in the performance of services and maintains a demeanor complementary to medical ethics. Provides appropriate patient care and recognizes patient conditions essential for successful completion of the procedure.

Duties and Responsibilities

- Performs diagnostic radiographic procedures
- —Corroborates patient's clinical history with procedure; ensures that information is documented and available for use by a licensed practitioner
- —Prepares patient for procedures; provides instructions to obtain desired results, gain cooperation, and minimize anxiety
- —Selects and operates radiography equipment, imaging, and/or associated accessories to successfully perform procedures
- —Positions patient to best demonstrate anatomic area of interest while respecting patient ability and comfort
- —Immobilizes patients as required for appropriate examination
- —Determines radiographic technique exposure factors
- —Applies principles of radiation protection to minimize exposure to patient, self, and others
- —Evaluates radiographs or images for technical quality; ensures that proper identification is recorded
- —Assumes responsibility for the provision of physical and psychologic services to patients during procedures
- —Practices aseptic techniques as necessary
- —Understands methods for and is capable of performing venipunctures
- —In agreement with state statute(s) and/or where institutional policy permits, prepares, identifies, and/or administers contrast media and/or medications as prescribed by a licensed practitioner
- —Verifies informed consent for and assists licensed practitioner with interventional procedures
- —Assists licensed practitioner with fluoroscopic and specialized interventional radiography procedures
- —Performs noninterpretive fluoroscopic procedures as appropriate and consistent with applicable state statutes (where applicable)
- —Initiates basic life support when necessary

Continued

- Provides patient education
- Assists in maintaining records, thereby respecting confidentiality and established policy
- Assumes responsibility for assigned area; reports equipment malfunction
- Provides input for equipment purchase and supply decisions
- Provides practical instruction for students and/or other health care professionals
- Participates in the department's quality assessment and improvement plan; may be responsible for specific quality control duties in assigned area
- May be responsible for control of inventory and purchase of supplies for assigned area
- Maintains knowledge of and observes universal precautions
- Understands and applies patient-relation skills
- Pursues appropriate continuing education

Qualifications

- Graduate of JRCERT accredited program or a USDE institutional accreditation
- Certification by the ARRT in radiography, or equivalent
- Possesses valid state credential, if applicable

The American Society of Radiologic Technologists (ASRT) *Job Description and Scope of Practice* reflects the expanded role of today's radiologic technologist.

The role of the radiologic technologist has increased in complexity and responsibility since its rather simple early beginnings. In addition to development within diagnostic radiography, specialized areas have evolved for the diagnosis and treatment of disease. These areas, which provide many opportunities for today's radiologic technologists, include special procedures radiography, mammography, computed tomography, magnetic resonance imaging, nuclear medicine, radiation therapy, and sonography.

RADIATION THERAPY

History

Radiation therapy, which is often referred to as radiation oncology, began approximately a year after x-rays were discovered in 1895. A medical student, Emil H. Grubbe, together with a physician friend, treated an advanced case of breast cancer with x-rays in 1896. Grubbe continued his research for many years but eventually contracted skin cancer and lost his left hand. Neither radiation nor its potential dangers were yet understood.

Rather, radiation was thought to be a cure-all. After discovering that radiation produced epilation (loss of hair), it was suggested that shaving would no longer be necessary. Radiation was also used to cure blindness, epilepsy, acne, and warts, as well as various bacterial and viral infections. Almost every form of malignant and benign disease was treated. Because so little was known about the effects of radiation, the results were disappointing. The damaging effects of radiation were realized as the number of injuries was brought to public attention. Some people even demanded that the use of radiation be abandoned altogether, but techniques and equipment improved, with a moderate number of good results.

In 1904, Bergonie and Tribondeau announced their landmark findings about tissue response to radiation. They discovered that, at certain times, living cells are more sensitive to the effects of radiation.

Unlike the other specializations in radiology, radiation therapy is not used to diagnose disease. Therapy involves treating a patient who is already known to have a disease. Radiation therapy is practiced by exposing a diseased area to various types of radiation while also trying to protect the unaffected parts of the patient's body from radiation exposure. Most of the diseases treated with radiation today are cancerous; there was a time when nonmalignant diseases were successfully treated with radiation, but today other forms of therapy are preferable for most noncancerous conditions.

Responsibilities of the Radiation Therapist

The radiation therapist applies ionizing radiation to the patient in accordance with the prescription and instructions of the radiation oncologist. The radiation therapist checks the physician's prescription for mathematic errors. Accurate technical details of treatment administered must be recorded at the time of treatment. The patient must be properly positioned, and the area of interest must be correctly marked. In addition, the radiation therapist assists in the calibration of equipment and must be able to detect malfunctions and maintain control if a radiation accident occurs. The radiation therapist may be required to prepare molds and casts of various body parts, and he or she must understand the use of wedge and compensating filters for treatment.

An understanding of minor surgical procedures and aseptic technique may also be required. Finally, the radiation therapist must render care and comfort to the patient. Unlike diagnostic radiography, where the radiologic technologist has brief contact with patients, radiation therapy patients are seen on a regular basis. Because of the traumatic emotional aspects that may be associated with a patient who is undergoing treatment for a malignancy, the radiation therapist must be empathetic to patients' needs and refer them, when necessary, to social services.

Education and Certification

An individual who wishes to become a certified radiation therapist must attend a radiation therapy program approved by the Joint Review

Committee on Education in Radiologic Technology or its equivalent. Therapy programs are generally 1 year in length or 1 to 2 years in conjunction with a baccalaureate degree and may be established in community colleges, universities, hospitals, or clinics. Applicants may have prior qualifications from a clinically related allied health profession with a minimum of 2 years of education from an accredited educational program. The therapy curriculum generally includes courses in medical ethics and law, patient care, human structure and function, oncologic pathology, radiobiology, radiation physics and protection, clinical dosimetry, and computer applications. In addition to classes, the student spends time in the clinical environment learning a suitable variety and quantity of patient treatments.

At the successful completion of the educational program, a student is eligible to take the certification examination offered by the American Registry of Radiologic Technologists (ARRT). Upon successful completion of the examination, a certified radiation therapist is qualified to work in any major cancer treatment center or in large hospitals that have both diagnostic equipment and high-energy radiation therapy units. Individual state licensure may also be required.

A certified technologist may also wish to pursue additional training in medical dosimetry. A dosimetrist plans patient treatments and analyzes the radiation distribution and dose for accuracy and safety. Additional training can be up to 2 years of academics and 1 year of supervised work experience under a certified medical dosimetrist or certified medical physicist before examination by the Medical Dosimetrist Certification Board (MDCB).

Employment Opportunities

Opportunities for employment are available throughout the country. Positions are generally found in larger clinics or medical centers. Salaries vary according to location, employer, education, and work experience.

The ASRT *Job Description and Scope of Practice* for radiation therapists differs distinctly from that for the radiologic technologist. The description clearly indicates the difference in the body of knowledge required to develop the necessary skills for therapeutic techniques (Box 23-2).

NUCLEAR MEDICINE

History

Radioactivity, which was co-discovered by Marie Curie, Pierre Curie, and Henri Becquerel in 1898, is a phenomenon in which the nucleus of an atom contains excess energy and is considered excited or unstable; the nucleus spontaneously emits this energy in the form of radiation to reach a more stable state. The three types of rays emitted are alpha, beta, and

BOX 23-2—RADIATION THERAPIST RT (T)(ARRT)

Scope of Practice

The curriculum base for a Radiation Therapist is outlined in the ASRT Professional Curriculum for Radiation Therapy Technology. Education program standards are those defined in the Essentials and Guidelines of an Accredited Educational Program for the Radiation Therapy Technologist. Radiation therapy technology professional educational programs prepare the radiation therapist to, but are not limited to, the following:

- Provide radiation therapy services by contributing as an essential member of the radiation oncology treatment team through the provision of total quality care of each patient undergoing a prescribed course of treatment
- Assess treatment delivery components
- Provide radiation therapy treatment delivery services to cure or improve the quality of life of patients by accurately delivering a prescribed course of treatment
- Evaluate and assess daily the physiologic and psychologic responsiveness of each patient to treatment delivery
- Maintain values congruent with the profession's code of ethics and scope of practice and adhere to national, institutional, and/or departmental standards, policies, and procedures regarding treatment delivery and patient care

Domains of Practice: Organizational and Work Role Competencies

- Coordinates and meets multiple patient needs and requests; sets priorities
- Participates effectively in a therapeutic team approach to provide optimum therapy
- Adapts to contingency planning in response to variables that influence workload or schedule
- Maintains a flexible stance toward patients, visitors, and staff, technology, and bureaucracy
- Coordinates daily activities in an effort to devote complete attention to all necessary tasks involved in treatment delivery

Administering and Monitoring Radiation Therapy Treatments

- Implements a planned course of treatment
- Administers treatment accurately and safely; reports untoward effects, reactions, therapeutic responses, and incompatibilities
- Withholds treatment when conditions warrant, and consults with a radiation oncologist before proceeding
- Participates in total quality management system to ensure safe and accurate patient care
- Detects equipment malfunctions and takes appropriate action
- Accurately documents details of treatment procedures, and maintains daily treatment records
- Always applies principles of radiation protection

Continued

- Takes appropriate action with regard to real or potential radiation hazards
- Understands the function of equipment, accessories, treatment methods, and protocols, and applies such knowledge appropriately
- Simulates and plans a course of treatment by defining and identifying tumor volume, target volume, and treatment volume as directed and prescribed by the radiation oncologist
- Constructs and/or prepares immobilization devices, beam directional devices, and the like, which facilitate treatment delivery
- Performs daily and periodic quality assurance checks and related tasks as appropriate
- Performs dosimetric calculations and treatment planning procedures
- Monitors doses to normal tissues within the irradiated volume to assure that tolerance levels are not exceeded
- Prepares and/or assists in the preparation and use of brachytherapy sources

Caregiving

- Creates climate for and establishes commitment to healing or improving quality of life
- Provides comfort measures and facilitates the preservation of patient self-image and dignity
- Is a source of support and encouragement for each patient and his or her family
- Provides patient education to maximize patient compliance with his or her plan of care, and provides family education as needed
- Monitors and interprets side effects and/or complications to create a management strategy that fosters prevention, healing, and comfort
- Monitors the patient's physical and psychologic response to treatment, and refers patient for appropriate management, when indicated
- Detects, documents, and reports significant changes in patients' conditions

gamma. Alpha and beta particles are small pieces of the nucleus that have been ejected. Gamma rays are identical to x-rays except that they originate from the nucleus of an unstable atom, whereas x-rays are generated in a radiographic tube.

Radioactive elements can be naturally occurring or artificially produced in cyclotrons and nuclear reactors. All of the radioactive compounds used in nuclear medicine, often called *radionuclides* or *radiopharmaceuticals*, are artificially produced.

Radiopharmaceuticals are used as tracers in nuclear medicine studies. A tracer is a substance that emits radiation and that can be identified when placed in the human body. By detecting the tracer, information about the structure, function, secretion, excretion, and volume of a particular organ can be obtained.

Responsibilities of the Nuclear Medicine Technologist

Nuclear medicine (NM) involves the use of radioactive materials for diagnostic and therapeutic studies both inside (in vivo) and outside (in vitro) the body. Under the direction of a qualified physician, the nuclear medicine technologist prepares and administers radiopharmaceuticals to patients by intravenous, intramuscular, subcutaneous, and oral methods; the nuclear medicine technologist also manages the quality control of the substances. The radiologic technologist must understand and use radiation detection devices and other laboratory equipment that measures the quantity and distribution of radionuclides deposited in a patient or in a patient's specimen. In addition, in vivo and in vitro procedures must be performed safely, with the radiologic technologist applying the principles of radiation protection to limit the amount of radiation exposure to the patient, the public, and other employees. The radiologic technologist must also be able to develop film and make the calculations of a biologic specimen analysis for the physician's interpretation.

Equipment and Procedures

NM procedures provide physicians with essential molecular level information about both the structure and function of organs and body systems. Utilizing small amounts of radioactive materials administered to the patient by oral, IV, subcutaneous, and/or direct introduction, NM imaging and analysis provides essential information to a broad range of medical specialties including cardiology, oncology, psychiatry, and pediatrics. The use of NM procedures often permits earlier identification of pathology, thus permitting more timely diagnosis and effective treatment. New and developing NM diagnostic and therapeutic procedures are revolutionizing the understanding of a wide host of disease and conditions.

NM imaging equipment works with computers, producing images and data used to detect and analyze the biodistribution of radionuclides and radiopharmaceuticals in the body. Both 2-D planar and 3-D tomographic (SPECT and PET) images are utilized in NM. Other detecting equipment utilized by the NMT includes Geiger counters, dose calibrators, well counters, and single-/multi-channel analyzers.

In diagnostic imaging, the NMT administers the radioactive material to the patient and operates the imaging/detecting equipment. The NMT is also responsible for performing the majority of the imaging equipment's daily quality control and management procedures.

Education and Certification

There are several different paths to becoming a NMT. Educational programs approved by the Joint Review Committee on Education Programs in Nuclear Medicine Technology (www.jrcnmt.org) range from 1 to 4 years dependant on the individual's past education and prerequisites of the specific school. Interested parties can visit www.nmtcb.org, www.arrt.org, and www.snm.org for more detailed information.

In general the nuclear medicine curriculum includes clinical experience and didactic instruction in radiation safety and protection, patient management, medical ethics, radiopharmacy, NM imaging and non-imaging procedures, physics, math, and instrumentation.

Upon completion of the NMT education program, a student is eligible to sit boards given by two nationally recognized certifying agencies: *American Registry of Radiologic Technologists* (www.arrt.org) and/or *Nuclear Medicine Technology Certification Board* (www.nmtcb.org).

Employment Opportunities

The field of nuclear medicine technology has developed rapidly, and there is a growing demand for well-trained personnel. Opportunities for employment are varied and include hospitals, clinics, nuclear pharmacies, research facilities, mobile imaging services, and relief agencies. Because of the growing number of training programs, there is also a need for instructors in nuclear medicine technology.

Salaries may vary according to location, employer, work experience, and level of education.

The ASRT *Job Description and Scope of Practice* for the nuclear medicine technologist differs markedly from those for the radiologic technologist and the radiation therapy disciplines. It is obvious that this area developed as a separate discipline (Box 23-3).

SONOGRAPHY

History

Sonography, which is often referred to as *ultrasound*, uses high-frequency sound waves to form an image. A sound beam is like an x-ray beam in that it is composed of waves that transfer energy from one point to another. However, radiation passes through a vacuum, whereas sound waves can only pass through matter. Sound waves are simply vibrations that pass through a material. If no material exists, there is nothing to vibrate, and sound cannot exist.

Sonography was first successfully used during World War I to detect submarines, but not until after World War II did testing begin on human tissue for diagnostic purposes. In the late 1940s and early 1950s, three physicians—working independently—discovered that if ultrasound waves were sent through the body, echoes reflected from the different tissues would return and could form an image of the anatomic structures, and a permanent photograph could be made of the image.

BOX 23-3 — NUCLEAR MEDICINE TECHNOLOGIST RT (N)(ARRT)

Scope of Practice

Nuclear Medicine—Practice Comprehensive

Position Summary

Provides health care services using radionuclides to assist in diagnosis or treatment. Performs nuclear medicine procedures and related techniques to produce images for the interpretation by and at the request of a licensed practitioner. Exercises professional judgment in the performance of services and maintains a demeanor complementary to medical ethics. Provides appropriate patient care and recognizes patient conditions essential for successful completion of the procedure.

Duties and Responsibilities

- Performs diagnostic and therapeutic procedures
  —Corroborates patient's clinical history with procedure; ensures that information is documented and available for use by a licensed practitioner
  —Prepares patient for procedures; provides instructions to obtain desired results, gain cooperation, and minimize anxiety.
  —In agreement with state statute(s) and/or where institutional policy permits, prepares, calculates, identifies, and/or administers radiopharmaceuticals and/or medications as prescribed by a licensed practitioner.
  —Selects and operates radiation detection, imaging, and/or associated equipment to successfully perform procedures
  —Positions patient and equipment to best demonstrate the anatomic area of interest while respecting patient ability and comfort
  —Immobilizes patients as required for appropriate examination
  —Applies principles of radiation protection to minimize exposure to patient, self, and others
  —Evaluates images and data for technical quality; ensures that proper identification is recorded
  —Verifies informed consent for and assists a licensed practitioner with interventional procedures
  —Practices aseptic technique
  —Assumes responsibility for provision of physical and psychologic services to patients during procedures
  —Understands methods for and is capable of performing venipunctures
  —Initiates basic life support action when necessary
- Provides patient education
- Assists in maintaining records, thereby respecting confidentiality and established policy
- Assumes responsibility for assigned area, and reports equipment malfunction
- Provides input for equipment purchase and supply decisions

Continued

- Provides practical instruction for students and other health care professionals
- Participates in the department's quality assessment and improvement plan; may be responsible for specific quality control duties in assigned area
- May be responsible for control of inventory and purchase of supplies for assigned area
- Maintains knowledge of and observes universal precautions
- Understands and applies patient-relation skills
- Pursues appropriate continuing education

Qualifications

- Graduate of Committee-of-Allied-Health-Education-and-Accreditation (CAHEA)-accredited nuclear medicine program, or equivalent
- Certification by the American Registry of Radiologic Technologists in nuclear medicine, the Nuclear Medicine Technology Certification Board, the American Society of Clinical Pathologists, or equivalent
- Possesses valid state credential, if applicable

The components necessary to produce an ultrasonic image are a transducer, an ultrasound beam, and an image display on a cathode ray tube or television monitor. The transducer serves two purposes: it transmits sound in pulses or bursts (approximately 2,000-15,000/second), and it senses the echoes that are returning from the previous pulse. The radiologic technologist positions the transducer on the patient and moves it around the area of interest to produce echoes while adjusting the television controls to achieve the optimum image. The electronic image is made one bit at a time from each returning echo and is displayed much like a TV image. The radiologic technologist must have a thorough knowledge of anatomy and pathology to be able to interpret the images as they appear on the monitor.

X-rays are produced when electrons are accelerated to a very high speed and then decelerated or suddenly stopped. Sound waves are produced in the transducer by a vibrating crystal. When the transducer is placed in contact with the body, the vibrating crystal causes the particles in the body to vibrate; the vibrations are then passed from one layer of tissue to another. Reflections of the ultrasound pulses are created at the borders between two different body structures. With both ultrasound and radiographic images, adjacent structures to be visualized must differ in physical characteristics, such as atomic number or thickness. One significant difference between sonography and radiography is that the ultrasound pulse continually loses energy as it passes through the body, whereas an x-ray photon loses its energy all at once.

The first sonograms were incomplete; they were not two-dimensional images. Immersing the patient in a tank of water improved the image, but the biggest improvement came with the development of compound scanning, in which the transducer is moved simultaneously in two different patterns over the area of interest. A lubricating gel is placed on the patient's skin, thereby minimizing friction and air gaps between the skin surface and the transducer and enhancing the image.

Responsibilities of the Sonographer

The sonographer plays an important role on the medical team as technical assistant to the radiologist. A certified sonographer performs various ultrasound examinations for the diagnosis of tumors, the malfunction of organs, and evaluation during pregnancy. Ultrasound is also used as a therapeutic tool. Muscle treatment, removal of plaque from teeth, and the dissolution of cataracts are a few examples of the therapeutic uses of ultrasound.

Any soft tissue area of the body may be examined with the use of ultrasound—from abdominal organs to the evaluation of blood flow (Fig. 23-1). Transducers have even been developed to evaluate the skull; this type of examination was usually referred to computed tomography.

In addition, the radiologic technologist is responsible for the maintenance of existing equipment and for recommending replacement and modification. Other duties include developing film, maintaining statistical records, ordering and storing supplies, and maintaining services in accordance with the standards established by the radiologist.

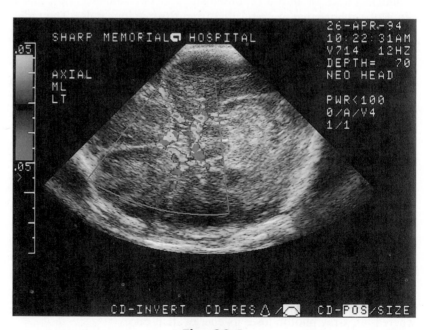

Fig. 23-1

With ultrasound, a sonographer can examine any soft tissue of the body, from abdominal organs to the evaluation of blood flow.

Education and Certification

There are several options for education in sonography. A person may enroll in an ultrasound program or a 2-year accredited allied health occupational program that is patient-care related in addition to a minimum of 12-month, full-time clinical ultrasound/vascular experience. An individual may also study on a full-time basis in a clinical setting (such as a private practice) under the supervision of a physician and a registered sonographer. Regardless of the type of education, most applicants to the American Registry of Diagnostic Medical Sonographers (ARDMS) for certification must have 12 to 24 months of clinical ultrasound training experience. The curriculum in an accredited school may include courses such as physics, equipment instrumentation, anatomy and physiology, patient care, positioning, and scanning procedures.

Upon graduation, a candidate may apply to the ARDMS for one of four credentials: certification in abdomen, obstetrics, gynecology, and neurosonology (RDMS); certification in pediatric or adult echocardiography (RDCS); certification in vascular technology (RVT); or certification in ophthalmology.

Employment Opportunities

A certified diagnostic medical sonographer is qualified to work in a hospital, clinic, or private practice. Salaries vary according to location, employer, and work experience.

The ASRT *Job Description and Scope of Practice* for sonography is limited to specific anatomic regions by credentialing standards (Box 23-4).

SPECIAL PROCEDURES RADIOGRAPHY

History

Special procedures radiography began soon after Roentgen's discovery of x-radiation. One of the most successful early investigators was Walter Bradford Cannon, who began his work in 1896 when he was still a medical student. Cannon placed animals that had ingested radiopaque buttons and balls in front of an x-ray tube and followed the movement of the digestive tract. Eventually he used barium sulfate suspension, which is still used today, to study the digestive system.

By 1920, investigators began to develop agents that produced radiocontrast in specific organs. As more complicated procedures were developed, these examinations quickly became the routine daily diagnostic contrast procedures used in radiology departments.

Special procedures radiography involves giving a patient a substance to produce radiographic contrast in certain anatomic structures that lack natural contrast with surrounding tissues and organs; this allows the

BOX 23-4 — DIAGNOSTIC MEDICAL SONOGRAPHER RDMS (ARDMS)

A diagnostic medical sonographer is a practitioner who is responsible for the administration of high-frequency sonic energy to humans or animals for diagnostic or research purposes.

RDMS (ARDMS) indicates the following:

1. Completion of an accredited 2-year American Medical Association or equivalent allied health training program that is patient-care related in addition to a minimum of 12 months of full-time clinical ultrasound/vascular experience

OR

2. Completion of didactic education and clinical experience acceptable to the American Registry of Diagnostic Medical Sonographers

AND

Certification by the American Registry of Diagnostic Medical Sonographers

The art and science of diagnostic medical sonography requires that the sonographer achieve a specific level of knowledge and skill in each subspecialty performed. These subspecialties include abdomen, obstetrics-gynecology, echocardiography, ophthalmology, vascular technology, Doppler, and neurosonology. For each subspecialty, the sonographer must possess and demonstrate knowledge of and competency in, but not limited to, the following areas:

Computer literacy and applications: An understanding of generic terminology, keyboard operations, menu selection strategies, and logistics of program flow

Human structure and function: General anatomy, anatomic relationships, sectional anatomy, and organ and system functions to perform accurate procedures for the defined discipline and to accurately identify the area of interest on resulting images

Instrumentation: An understanding of the operation of devices; transducer selection (A-mode, B-mode, T-M-mode, real-time, and Doppler); hard copy image recorders; and other processing techniques

Medical ethics: Legal considerations that affect the scope of practice and a respect for an established code of ethics and risk management

Medical terminology: An understanding of disease descriptions, abbreviations, symbols, terms, or phrases necessary to successfully communicate with other health care professionals

Pathology: Knowledge of disease and abnormalities that influence performance or outcome of an ultrasound procedure; ultrasonic characteristics of pathophysiology and abnormal tissues

Patient care: Attention and concern for the physical and psychologic needs of the patient; recognition of a life-threatening condition and ability to implement basic life-sustaining actions

Positioning: Accurate placement of the body with respect for the patient's comfort, ability, and safety to achieve prescribed results and best demonstrate the anatomic area of interest; use of techniques to physically manipulate and apply appropriate transducers and equipment to produce a desired image

Physical science: Knowledge of propagation properties, transducer parameters, beam profile, Doppler effect, interaction properties with human tissue, and possible biologic effect

Continued

Quality control: Preventive maintenance and knowledge of equipment capabilities; calibration of and care for equipment with respect to operating standards, sensitometry characteristics, and monitoring of image processing systems for accuracy and consistency

Scanning procedures: Ability to select appropriate equipment and scanning techniques to optimally visualize areas of interest

The practice of diagnostic medical sonography is stated as the performance of service including, but not limited to, the following:

- Ultrasonic examinations of all body parts for diagnostic interpretation
- Optimal patient care using established and accepted protocols
- Supervision of other peers and students, where applicable
- Evaluation of responsibilities and recommendations for improvements

The practice of diagnostic medical sonography includes both initiative and independent judgment by performance, in appropriate settings, of service as identified above.

radiologic technologist to make a good radiograph of the structure. Examinations that involve the vascular and nervous system are usually designated as special radiographic procedures.

Interventional radiology, which is a rapidly growing subspecialty of special procedures, consists of examinations that may improve a patient's condition and perhaps even negate the need for surgery. Examples of interventional procedures include removal of bile duct or renal stones, postoperative abscess drainage, and selective cancer therapy.

Special and interventional radiology procedures require not only specialized equipment but also a highly trained team to successfully perform the techniques required to obtain optimal diagnostic information. The radiologic technologist is an important part of this team and is responsible for operating the equipment, making preparations for the procedures, and assisting the physician during the examination.

Responsibilities of the Special Procedures Technologist

A special procedures technologist performs radiographic procedures of a highly technical nature without supervision of technical detail. This position requires thorough knowledge of the application of sterile technique and the use of sophisticated equipment.

A special procedures technologist prepares all equipment for use, chooses technical factors for producing optimal radiographs, positions the patient for proper anatomic visualization, and assists the physician in sterile application of the procedure.

The radiologic technologist prepares the patient for the examination and observes the patient for any unusual reactions. In addition, the radiologic technologist maintains inventory and accessory supplies.

Equipment and Procedures

Many examinations may be included under special procedures radiography; however, studies of the circulatory system are generally considered the most common.

Angiography refers to the study of the circulatory structures by opacifying the blood vessels with a positive contrast medium (Fig. 23-2). Many different angiographic studies are performed in a radiology department; the examination is identified by the particular vascular structure demonstrated and the method of injection of contrast media.

Arteriography is the study of arterial vessels, which may be broken down further into peripheral studies of the extremities and visceral

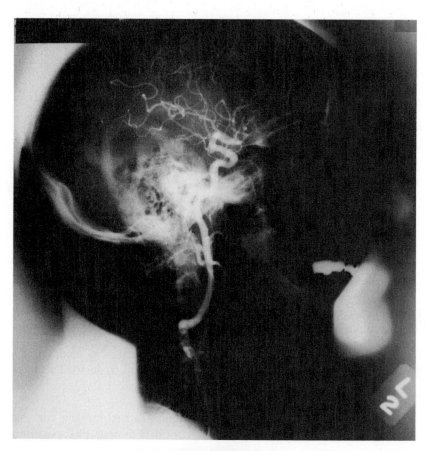

Fig. 23-2

Cerebral angiographic study.

studies of various organs in the chest or abdomen. Venography is the study of the venous system; cerebral angiography is the examination of the vessels in the brain; angiocardiography is the opacification of the heart and great vessels; aortography is the study of the thoracic or abdominal aorta; and lymphography is the study of the lymph vessels and nodes.

Injection of contrast media can be made directly into the vessel of interest or indirectly through another vessel through a catheter.

Angiographic studies are performed to demonstrate any vascular abnormalities or pathology in the surrounding tissue and organs, such as tumors. Examinations are also performed to demonstrate organ function, as in a study of the heart valves or kidneys.

Simple angiographic studies, such as peripheral venography, are performed with regular radiographic equipment. More complex examinations involving motion studies, such as angiocardiography, require the use of rapid film changers, which can take several images a second, or movie cameras.

A cine or movie camera is used for motion picture radiography when dynamic function is of interest. The camera's shutter is synchronized with the pulses of x-ray, and this allows multiple picture frames to be taken each second. Some cameras have capabilities of 120 frames per second. The film is then viewed in the same manner as a movie film.

Image intensification equipment is essential for performing complex angiographic studies. The examinations are viewed on a television monitor or a videotape system.

Contrast media can be injected by hand, or frequently an electromechanical or compressed air device, called a *pressure injector*, is used.

Accessory equipment other than radiographic equipment is needed for special procedures radiography. Monitoring devices that record electric impulses of the heart and pressure within the heart and great vessels are often used. Anesthesia equipment might be necessary, and so might an emergency apparatus such as a crash cart that contains drugs, defibrillators, suction machines, and other resuscitation devices.

Education and Certification

A few schools offer education in special procedures radiography, but this specialized training is usually in conjunction with a baccalaureate degree. Registered radiologic technologists may apply to sit for the ARRT examination. Upon passing the examination, they receive a certificate in cardiovascular intervention technology and can use the designation "RT (R)(CV)(ARRT)."

Employment Opportunities

Employment opportunities vary. There is not as large a demand for special procedures technologists as there is for general diagnostic radiologic technologists. Most special procedures are performed in large hospitals and medical clinics. Salaries vary, but special procedures technologists usually earn a higher salary than radiologic technologists do.

MAMMOGRAPHY

Breast cancer has been recognized as a major condition that affects our population; it has received a great deal of attention in recent years. Increased chances for a cure depend on early detection. Radiographic examinations of the breast are used to screen large segments of the population (Fig. 23-3). **Mammography**, which is the radiographic examination of the breast with the use of specialized equipment, has become a

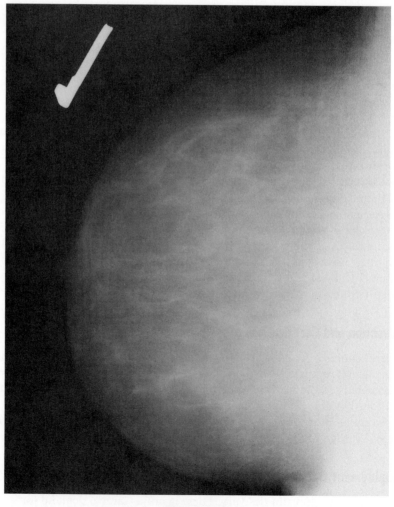

Fig. 23-3

Mammogram (radiographic examination of the breast).

specialized discipline, because the nature of breast tissue requires unique technical procedures. A dedicated radiographic unit and equipment are required for optimal diagnostic results. In October 1991, the first examination was given to certify radiologic technologists in this discipline. Those who have passed the examination receive the certificate of advanced qualifications in mammography, and they use the designation "RT(R)(M)(ARRT)."

Closely associated but not limited to the field of mammography is quality management (QM). QM technologists use standardized data collection tools and methods to monitor radiologic quality while identifying and solving problems associated with medical images and processes. Because QM is part of the basic radiologic technology curriculum, there is no separate examination for certification, although the ARRT offers an advanced certificate in mammography and QM. After the examination has been passed, the designation "RT(R)(QM)(ARRT)" may be used.

COMPUTED TOMOGRAPHY

History

Computed tomography (CT), which is the gathering of anatomic information from a cross-sectional plane of the body and presenting it as a three-dimensional image, was introduced in 1972 at the annual congress of the British Institute of Radiology by G.N. Hounsfield, a senior research scientist at EMI Limited in Middlesex, England. A CT image is formed by scanning a thin cross-section of the body with a narrow x-ray beam and measuring the transmitted radiation with a detector similar to the ones used in nuclear medicine. The detector does not form the image; rather, it adds all of the energy from the transmitted rays. The information is numeric in form and must be processed by a computer to construct an image.

Responsibilities of the CT Technologist

A CT technologist must be able to perform computed tomographic procedures without constant supervision of technical detail. As in ultrasonography, it is very important that the technologist have a thorough knowledge of anatomy. Judgments about the formation of the image may have to be made without the direct guidance of a radiologist. Other responsibilities include maintaining inventory and stock level of contrast media, film, magnetic tapes, and other required materials. Equipment must be maintained and kept orderly, and any mechanical difficulties must be reported for service. The technologist must maintain visual and audible contact with the patient during the examination and observe for unusual emergency situations. A knowledge of sterile technique in administering contrast media is essential for the radiologic technologist, and all emergency equipment must be maintained in case of a reaction to contrast media. In addition, examinations must be scheduled with physicians' offices, and complete history and diagnosis records of each patient must be kept.

Equipment and Procedures

Most CT units have three functional components involved in the production of an image: the scanning unit, the computer, and the viewing unit. The scanning unit uses a very small beam (1 mm in thickness). After the beam has passed through the body, it is picked up by a detector that produces an electric signal in proportion to the intensity of the x-ray beam. A profile of the body section is obtained by moving the x-ray beam over the body or by simultaneously using several beams (Fig. 23-4). Within the CT system is a digital computer that forms the image from the multiple x-ray beams; this process is mathematic, and the image created is numeric. For viewing, the numeric image is usually converted into a video-type signal that is displayed on a TV screen; the video signal is represented by varying shades of gray. Very dense structures are demonstrated as white areas; less dense structures are dark gray (Fig. 23-5).

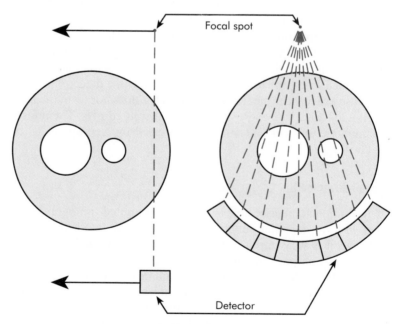

Fig. 23-4

Two methods for obtaining a penetration profile of a body section are illustrated. **Left**, A single-beam translate system. **Right**, A fan-beam system.

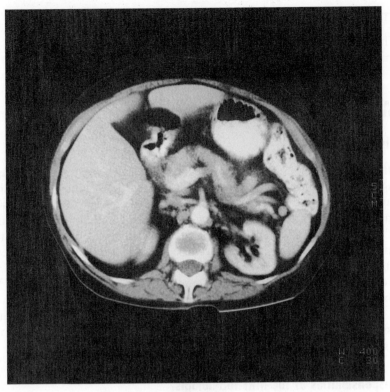

Fig. 23-5

In the CT scan image, very dense structures are demonstrated as white areas, and less dense structures are dark gray.

The field of computed tomography is perhaps the most rapidly changing field in radiology. Numerous CT units have been constructed, and the related computer programs change often.

Although the first scanners were designed for evaluating the brain, now any part of the body can be scanned by most CT systems. In addition, contrast media can be administered to highlight any low-contrast areas.

CT has made possible the diagnosis of disease processes of organs such as the liver and pancreas that, before this time, could not be demonstrated by normal radiographic methods.

Education

At this time no specialized schools offer education in CT, and there is no separate examination for certification. However, the ARRT offers an advanced certification in CT. Most CT technologists are certified radiologic technologists who have been trained by a radiologist, a neurologist, or another CT technologist in a clinical setting.

Employment Opportunities

There are many opportunities for radiologic technologists interested in this type of imaging, usually in a hospital or large clinic.

MAGNETIC RESONANCE IMAGING

History

One of the newest of the imaging devices is the **magnetic resonance imaging (MRI)** scanner. This imaging technique was first introduced in the early 1980s. Originally it was introduced as the nuclear magnetic resonance scanner (NMR). The word *nuclear* caused some confusion because of the association with radioactive nuclear medicine used in diagnostic imaging, and so it was dropped, because no nuclear radiation is involved. The imaging technique is new, but nuclear magnetic resonance has been around for quite some time; it was employed in chemistry and physics to obtain information about complex molecules and molecular motion.

MRI provides cross-sectional, three-dimensional images without using x-rays or radioactive materials; it produces images with the use of a strong magnetic field and radio waves.

Responsibilities of the MRI Technologist

The MRI technologists must be able to perform MRI procedures without constant supervision of technical detail. As in other imaging modalities, it is important that the radiologic technologists have a thorough knowledge of anatomy. Judgments about the MRI pulsing sequence, gradient magnetic fields, and anatomic slice orientation must be made.

Knowledge about the characteristics of magnetic fields, electromagnets, and atomic structure is useful in this type of imaging. A computer is used in magnetic imaging just as one is in CT, and thus a basic knowledge of how a computer constructs the image is helpful. Patient care responsibilities apply in MRI very much the same as in other types of diagnostic imaging. Knowledge of sterile technique in the administration of contrast media is needed, and all emergency equipment must be maintained in case of a patient reaction. In addition, there are other tasks that must be accomplished, such as maintaining records and scheduling.

Equipment and Procedures

The equipment used for imaging consists basically of large electromagnetic coils that surround a second electromagnetic coil that is capable of delivering pulses of radio waves. The patient lies inside the hollow, cylindrically arranged magnetic coils and is subjected to a magnetic field that is thousands of times more powerful than the earth's magnetic field. When the magnetic field acts on the patient's body, the nuclei of the body's atoms—

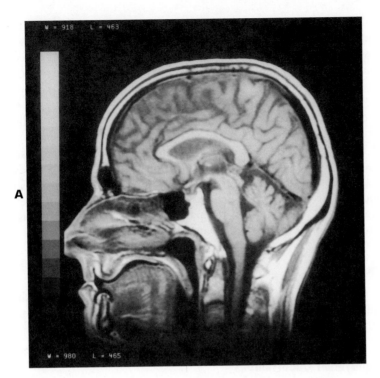

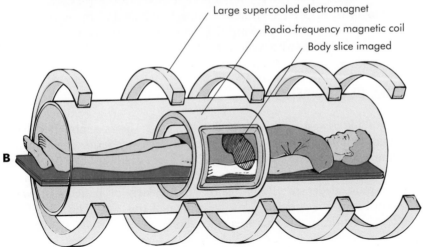

Large supercooled electromagnet

Radio-frequency magnetic coil

Body slice imaged

Fig. 23-6

A and **B**, Since its inception in the 1980s, MRI has become a significant diagnostic technique.

particularly of the hydrogen atoms—arrange themselves parallel to each other like rows of tiny magnets. Normally the spinning atoms' nuclei point randomly in different directions. When the patient is in the magnetic field, some of the spinning hydrogen nuclei line up in the same direction as the polarity of the magnetic waves. At this instant, a pulse of radio waves is emitted by the second inside electromagnetic coil; this causes the spinning nuclei within the tissue to change their angle of rotation because of the absorbed energy of the radiofrequency pulse. The wobbles produced by the changing angles of rotation produce signals that are analyzed to produce an image that shows varying densities of hydrogen in the body part.

The MRI produces images of body parts that are surrounded by bone in clear, unobstructed detail; this characteristic makes it especially useful for studying the brain and spinal cord (Fig. 23-6). MRI can show the detail of nerve damage by such diseases as multiple sclerosis; it can also detect brain tumors that may be obscured by bone in other imaging procedures.

There is an obvious disadvantage in the MRI scanning. Because the body is placed in a strong magnetic field, metallic objects on the patient (e.g., jewelry) as well as in the patient (e.g., hip joint prosthesis plates, screws in bones, surgical clips) are also affected by the magnet.

Education

In the same class as CT procedures, MRI imaging is part of the basic radiography curriculum. Therefore, there is no separate examination, although the ARRT offers an advanced MRI certification.

Employment Opportunities

Employment in MRI is found in large hospitals and many outpatient clinics. It is a rapidly growing field, and many opportunities exist for those technologists who wish to work with this modality.

BONE DENSITOMETRY

One of the newest fields is **bone densitometry**. This is a modality that is gaining in importance because of the public's concern for detecting and treating osteoporosis. Special equipment is required for bone densitometry; it makes use of x-ray energy, but it is specially designed to measure bone mineral density. Bone health—particularly of patients in whom osteoporosis is suspected—can be evaluated this way. The ARRT has offered certification in this area since January 2001.

Radiologist Assistant

The **radiologist assistant (RA)** is an advanced level radiologic technologist who works under the supervision of a radiologist to assist in the diagnostic imaging clinical environment.

The radiologist assistant is an ARRT certified radiographer who has successfully completed an advanced academic program. The programs, although limited in number at this time, offer a nationally recognized PA curriculum and a radiologist-directed clinical preceptorship.

The programs offered vary in length and prerequisites. By the year 2006 it is expected that there will be 10 programs available.

The focus of the radiologist assistant is to perform selected radiology procedures including, but not limited to, fluoroscopy and patient assessment and management, along with patient education. Radiologist assistants will participate in the systematic analysis of the quality of patient care delivered within the radiology environment. The radiologist assistant will also make initial observations of diagnostic images, with official interpretations and written reports being supervised by the radiologist (as defined by the American College of Radiology (ACR) standards for communication in diagnostic radiology).

Additional information about the radiologist assistant programs nationwide can be found on the ASRT website (www.asrt.org).

CONCLUSION

Several areas for specialization exist in the profession of radiologic technology. The three areas for certification by the ARRT are radiography, nuclear medicine, and radiation therapy. In addition, advanced levels of certification may be obtained in several areas of specialization. Entrance into these areas is usually a matter of the technologist's preference, but other factors may also be included in the decision, such as employment opportunities, educational requirements, and access to educational programs.

Review Questions

1. Which specialty is specific to the imaging of breast tissue?
   a. Special procedures
   b. Radiation therapy
   c. CT
   d. Mammography
2. Which procedure is not an x-ray examination?
   a. CT
   b. MRI
   c. Mammogram
   d. Bone densitometry
3. The distinguishing difference between CT and MRI is:
   a. Cross-sectional images.
   b. Digital imaging.
   c. Magnetic field versus radiation.
   d. Use of contrast.
4. Which imaging modality is most useful in studying the brain and spinal cord through visualization of soft tissue detail?
   a. CT
   b. MRI
   c. Special procedures
   d. Ultrasound

5. The formulation of radiopharmaceuticals and the localization of each within the body are unique to what discipline?
   a. Sonography
   b. Radiation therapy
   c. Nuclear medicine
   d. Special procedures
6. The specialty that allows the most patient contact is:
   a. Special procedures.
   b. Ultrasound.
   c. MRI.
   d. Radiation therapy.
7. Which subject in the curriculum is not common to all disciplines discussed in this chapter?
   a. Knowledge of anatomy
   b. Medical ethics
   c. Patient care
   d. Treatment planning
8. Which specialty is involved in the treatment of disease rather than its diagnosis?
   a. CT
   b. MRI
   c. Radiation therapy
   d. Both a and b
9. In which specialty may national certification be obtained through an organization other than the ARRT?
   a. Special procedures
   b. MRI
   c. Ultrasound
   d. Radiation therapy
10. An advantage of ultrasound over other imaging modalities is that:
    a. It can be used to monitor fetal development.
    b. No radiation is used.
    c. It includes the use of radiopharmaceuticals.
    d. Both a and b.

BIBLIOGRAPHY

American Medical Association: *Health professions career and education directory*, ed. 29, Chicago, 2001, The Association.

Ballinger PW: *Merrill's atlas of radiographic positions and radiologic procedures*, ed. 10, St. Louis, 2004, Mosby.

Bergonie J, Tribondeau D: *Acad Sci* 143:983, 1906.

Bushong SC: *Radiologic science for technologists: physics, biology, and protection*, ed. 7, St. Louis, 2001, Mosby.

Christensen ET, Curry TS, Dowdy J: *An introduction to the physics of diagnostic radiology*, ed. 4, Philadelphia, 1990, Lippincott Williams & Wilkins.

Clifton, Nancy, RT, CNMT, Program Director, School of nuclear medicine technology, Methodist University Hospital, 2/15/2005, consultation.

Harris EL, et al: *The shadowmakers, a history of radiologic technology,* Albuquerque, NM, 1995, American Society of Radiologic Technologists.

Holmes J: *Diagnostic ultrasound during the early years of* AIUM Journal of Clinical Ultrasound, New York, 1980, Wiley & Sons.

Selman J: *The fundamentals of imaging physics and radiobiology,* ed. 9, Springfield, IL, 2000, Charles C Thomas.

Sprawls P: *The physical principles of medical imaging,* Baltimore, 1993, University Park.

Professional Development and Career Advancement

Wanda E. Wesolowski

OBJECTIVES

On completion of this chapter, you should be able to:

- Discuss upward-mobility career routes for radiologic technologists.
- Describe the requirements and functions of the radiologist assistant (RA).
- Describe the requirements for radiology administrators.
- Describe the requirements for radiology educators.
- Discuss the impact of computers in radiology.
- List the skills required for in-service educators, and describe their role in radiology.
- Describe the upward-mobility route for radiography educators.
- List the duties of a radiology program director.

Professionals continually investigate opportunities for career mobility. Student radiologic technologists should begin looking at the opportunities in their chosen profession. A **radiologic technologist** is a health care professional who is skilled in the theory and practice of the technical

KEY TERMS

accreditation
angiographer
career mobility
carte blanche credits
formative evaluations
nuclear medicine
    technologist
quality assurance
    technologist
radiation therapy
    technologist
radiologic technologist
radiologist
radiologist assistant (RA)
sonography
summative evaluations

CHAPTER OUTLINE

Short-term postgraduate
    education
Long-term educational
    commitment
Radiologist assistant (RA)
Administrative radiology
The radiologic
    technologist-educator
Computer science
The quality assurance
    technologist
Radiation safety
    officer/health physicist
Continued

The equipment specialist
Commercial
   representatives
Conclusion

aspects of the use of x-rays in the diagnosis and treatment of disease. In the past, the radiologic technologist was faced with minimal opportunities for mobility. After the completion of their training, radiologic technologists usually began their careers as staff radiologic technologists. Promotions were based on seniority and the amount of responsibility an individual assumed. Such promotions were usually to a senior radiologic technologist, who was responsible for supervising a particular area in the department of radiology, then to assistant chief radiologic technologist, and finally to chief radiologic technologist. Promotions were not necessarily based on formal educational background and preparation; instead, they were based on a process of self-education that often was the result of many years of employment and experience.

Over the years, significant changes have occurred in the field of radiology, and with these changes have come opportunities for greater career mobility for the radiologic technologist. Mobility today, however, is based primarily on the formal educational background of an individual, and it is the individual who decides the direction of advancement and how much education is needed.

Student radiologic technologists who are interested in career mobility must examine their career priorities, assess their individual capabilities and interests, and then begin investigating opportunities. The need for additional education depends on an individual's area of interest. Student radiologic technologists who are seeking upward mobility must consider the amount of time they want to invest in additional education, their financial status, and the opportunities this career decision and additional education will offer them. In radiography, a short-term commitment to education usually involves an additional year of postgraduate work. A long-term commitment can include undergraduate, graduate, and even doctoral studies. Students should carefully read course descriptions and compare them to their own career goals; then they can direct the course of their careers. It is important, however, to stress that in choosing a career path, an individual must determine goals, explore opportunities, and then make a final commitment.

In addition to the multitude of postgraduate educational opportunities, there are also several nontraditional educational programs available to radiologic technologists.

College and universities offer nontraditional off-campus courses; most offer online courses, as well. Although most students in nontraditional courses are past the usual college age, this is rapidly changing. Younger students are now taking advantage of this option, and some earn entire degrees at home; they can spend time with family or continue to work while studying toward the degree with little disruption in their lives.

Continuing education programs are offered by the American Society of Radiologic Technologists and by state and local societies throughout the country. Such informal educational programs offer the radiologic technologist an opportunity to improve expertise without a long-term collegiate commitment and without extensive financial output. Programs

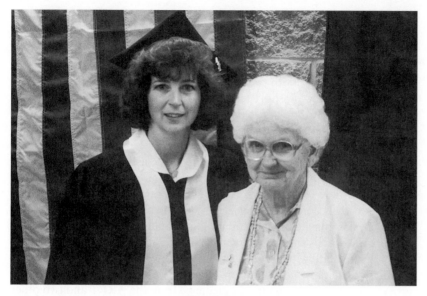

Fig. 24-1

In choosing a career path, the radiologic technologist must consider post-graduate educational commitments.

sponsored by national, state, and local societies assist radiologic technologists in keeping abreast of the newest innovations in the field of radiologic technology, provide them with the opportunity to improve skills, and show that individuals in this field are not stagnating but are endeavoring to improve in their chosen profession (Fig. 24-1).

Short-Term Postgraduate Education

As mentioned earlier, postgraduate education can take one of two routes. The first is short-term postgraduate education, which requires approximately 1 year of formal education following the 24-month program of a radiologic technologist. One of four separate areas may be pursued in this short-term educational program: radiation therapy, nuclear medicine, sonography, or interventional radiographic procedures.

The **radiation therapy technologist** assists the radiation oncologist in radiation therapy treatments by exposing specific areas of the patient's body to prescribed doses of ionizing radiation. In this field, the radiation therapy technologist operates therapeutic equipment such as high-energy linear accelerators, particle generators, cobalt-60 units, and superficial therapy equipment. The curriculum as recommended by the American Society of Radiologic Technologists (ASRT) includes courses such as radiation and radionuclide physics, mathematics, pathology, radiation therapy, radiation safety, oncology, brachytherapy, treatment planning, and records and statistics. After postgraduate training, the candidate is eligible to take the certifying examination of the American Registry of Radiologic Technologists (ARRT) in therapy. Many radiologic technologists are certified in both radiography and radiation therapy.

The second area of short-term educational commitment is that of a nuclear medicine technologist. Frequently during training in radiography, students rotate through the nuclear medicine area on an elective basis; they can then decide whether nuclear medicine might be an area of interest they wish to pursue. A **nuclear medicine technologist** attends to patients, abstracts data from patient records, assists the physician in the operation of scanning devices, and makes dose calculations for in vivo studies. Curricula usually consist of nuclear physics, instrumentation and statistics, health physics, biochemistry, immunology, radionuclide chemistry, radiopharmacy, administration, radiation biology, clinical nuclear medicine, radionuclide therapy, and computer applications. In nuclear medicine, as in radiation therapy, graduates of accredited programs are qualified for certifying examinations in nuclear medicine from the ARRT and two other certifying bodies. Nuclear medicine offers many job opportunities for qualified individuals in hospitals throughout the country.

Sonography, which is the radiologic technique in which deep structures of the body are visualized by recording the reflections of ultrasonic waves directed into the tissues, offers a short-term commitment in education, or it can be included in a long-term commitment. Throughout the country, there are several 1-year programs available in which the candidate majors in sonography techniques; there are also several 4-year programs that lead to a bachelor of science degree in radiologic technology that include sonography courses in the curriculum. Whichever commitment an individual chooses, the courses in sonography usually include sonography techniques, acoustic physics, ultrasound for gynecology and obstetrics, medical sonography for abdominal and pelvic scanning, and diagnostic sonography for cardiopulmonary and neurologic specialties. In addition, the individual is involved in clinical practice using modern sonography equipment, and he or she has the opportunity to practice in various clinical areas (Fig. 24-2).

Recently, interventional radiographic procedures have offered another avenue of **career mobility**. For those interested in this specialty, two types of education can be pursued. The first is on-the-job training in a particular department of radiology under the supervision of an **angiographer**, who is a physician engaged in radiography of the blood vessels. In an informal manner, the radiologic technologist learns about the techniques of interventional radiography, the equipment used, and the procedures themselves. There are also programs available in which an individual can pursue a formal education in interventional radiography. Courses in special procedures should include image processing, medical radiographic equipment, computer applications, management communications, emergency patient care procedures, medical-surgical diseases, imaging procedures in neurovascular and cardiovascular interventional

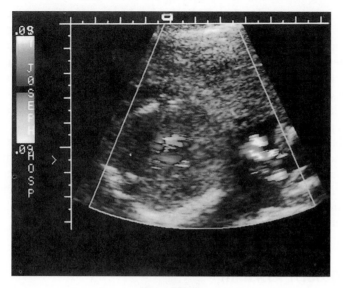

Fig. 24-2

A sonographic scan allows the sonographer to visualize deep structures of the pregnant abdomen. This Doppler image demonstrates a fetal heart and umbilical cord. (From Hedrick WR: *Ultrasound physics and instrumentation,* ed. 3, St. Louis, 1995, Mosby.)

radiography, computed tomography (CT) with special emphasis on transsectional anatomy, clinical practice, and digital subtraction angiography (DSA).

LONG-TERM EDUCATIONAL COMMITMENT

The decision to pursue a long-term educational program is not made on the spur of the moment; the radiologic technologist must first look at the present and future needs of the profession, which may influence a decision. He or she must also make an assessment of personal abilities, career needs, and desired challenges. It is then important to examine the areas in radiology that can be entered, such as radiologist assistant, management, education, or computer science. Having made a decision about the area of interest, an individual should inquire into various programs offered by undergraduate schools. The radiologic technologist has several choices: some institutions offer **carte blanche credits**, which are discretionary credits awarded by an institution of higher learning for radiologic technology training, or the credits may be earned through challenge examinations.

In essence, the radiologic technologist begins undergraduate school either at the end of the second year of college or in the third year of college. When such a program is not available, the radiologic technologist should inquire into local undergraduate schools that offer courses in the area of interest and obtain college catalogs to review available programs and course descriptions. An individual who is interested in pursuing this long-term educational commitment should speak to other radiologic technologists who are currently in the same field and discuss the needs of the course of study. The individual must also look at the additional financial burden of long-term education and decide whether an educational pursuit should be achieved as a full-time student or on a part-time basis. A long-term educational commitment can range from 2 ½ years to 8 or more years of work. After the decision and commitment have been made, every effort should be made toward completion of the program. The long-term rewards of education, such as self-esteem, professional satisfaction, challenges, and financial benefits, must also be examined.

RADIOLOGIST ASSISTANT

In the 1990s, a shortage of practicing radiologists became evident, and predictions for an increased shortage in the 21st century were ominous.

The predictions of a shortage became a reality in the 21st century, and in the summer of 2002, the American College of Radiology (ACR) decided to move forward in developing, with the American Society of Radiologic Technologists (ASRT), the **radiologist assistant (RA)** program. The first class of RAs began at Loma Linda University in California in fall of 2004 with anticipated graduation in 2006. Applicants must be certified in good standing by the American Registry of Radiologic Technologists (ARRT), with additional prerequisites established by each sponsoring education institution, resulting in a baccalaureate (BS) degree. The American Society of Radiologic Technologists (ASRT) has identified 13 educational RA programs, the names of which can be obtained from the ASRT.

The ASRT has been mandated to develop a standardized curriculum to include patient assessment, management and education, pharmacology, radiation safety, radiobiology, health physics, pathophysiology, and clinical preceptorship. A certification examination is to be administered through the American Registry of Radiologic Technologists (ARRT).

It is to be stressed that the RA does not interpret images or make diagnosis. The RA is supervised by a radiologist, and is intended to be a supplement, not a substitute, for the radiologist. The exact responsibilities of the RA are established by each employing clinical site and can include:

- Patient assessment and management
- Obtaining consent for and injecting agents that facilitate or enable diagnostic imaging
- Obtaining clinical history from patient or medical record
- Performing preprocedure and postprocedure evaluation of patients undergoing invasive procedures

- Assisting radiologist with invasive procedures
- Performing fluoroscopy for noninvasive procedures with the radiologist providing direct supervision of the service
- Monitoring and tailoring selected exams under direct supervision (e.g., IVU, CT urogram, GI studies, voiding cystourography (VCUG), and retrograde urethrograms)
- Communicating the reports of the radiologist's findings to the referring physician or an appropriate representative with appropriate documentation
- Providing nasoenteric and oroenteric feeding tube placement in the uncomplicated patients
- Performing selected peripheral venous diagnostic procedures

ADMINISTRATIVE RADIOLOGY

In the past, the department of radiology was a small, contained unit within the hospital that could easily be managed by a chief radiologic technologist whose expertise was primarily in the technical area. However, the department of radiology has now become a large department that employs numerous professional and nonprofessional staff and that requires an expanded budget. In addition, the regulations specified by federal and state authorities of radiation control must be met, and detailed planning for future departmental expansion is always on the drawing board. Because the chief radiologic technologist cannot have expertise in all of these areas, the demand has grown for individuals with business and management backgrounds to administer the department of radiology.

The ideal radiology administrator has a combined technical and management background, thereby possessing both radiologic expertise and management training or experience. In the past, this combination of skills has been difficult to find; however, today's radiologic technologist realizes that an administrative position requires business and management acumen as well as technical abilities. The radiology administrator is involved in purchasing, personnel management, union negotiations, budget preparation, regulatory specifications, decision making, and planning (Fig. 24-3).

A radiologic technologist who is interested in radiology management can consider two specific areas. He or she should initially investigate colleges that have a program in health care administration; many colleges offer degree programs in this area. Courses in health care administration might include principles of management, an introduction to data processing, statistics, industrial relations or personnel management, financial accounting, health care administration, health planning, and legal aspects of health services administration. Some institutions require a clinical management practicum. Such courses lead to a baccalaureate degree in health care management. After the completion of such a degree program, some institutions offer a master's degree in health administration or a master's of business administration in health administration.

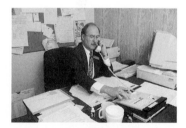

Fig. 24-3

The radiology administrator is ultimately responsible for all aspects of the operation of a department of imaging, which is one of the largest departments in any health care institution.

If local institutions do not offer a degree in health administration, an undergraduate degree in business administration should be considered. A radiology administrator needs courses in accounting, economics, finance, law, management, marketing, personnel management, and labor relations. Such an undergraduate program could be followed by an MBA program.

The role of the radiology administrator must grow simultaneously with the entire field of radiology, and such growth requires administrators with a variety of management skills. An individual who combines management abilities with technologic expertise is a valuable asset to the radiologist, the radiology department, and the hospital. There is a need for such individuals, and opportunity awaits the radiologic technologist who plans to fill this need. Careful planning in choice of undergraduate schools and programs will help ensure a stable future of great opportunities.

THE RADIOLOGIC TECHNOLOGIST-EDUCATOR

Roentgen's discovery of x-rays in 1895 established the need for specialists such as the **radiologist** (a physician who specializes in the medical science of x-rays and other radiation energy forms to diagnose and treat disease) and the radiologic technologist or, in the terminology of that time, the technician. Educators for the radiologists and technicians were needed so that enough people could be trained to enter the field. The need for the educator in Europe was established in France during World War I. During this bloody conflict, the Polish scientist Marie Sklodowska Curie (1867-1934) realized that radiologic units were needed to x-ray the wounded. She designed several "x-ray cars," which were mobile x-ray units available for surgeons and physicians at the front. From 1916 to 1918, Curie trained 150 technicians—the first formally trained x-ray technicians in Europe—to operate these mobile units.

During this same period, the formal training of x-ray technicians began in the United States. Eddy Clarence Jerman (1865-1936) was employed by the Victor X-ray Corporation, and in 1917 he was assigned to develop an educational program for x-ray technicians; this was the beginning of a formal educational program for operators of x-ray equipment. In 1920, 13 of these technicians met with Jerman at the Victor X-ray Corporation in Chicago to organize a professional society, which today is known as the ASRT.

With the beginning of formal training in x-ray technology, it became apparent that a means and method were necessary for the examination and certification of individuals trained in the profession. In 1922, the American Registry of X-ray Technicians was established. In 1933, formal training of x-ray technicians was recognized, and the ARRT began its list of accredited training schools. Over the years, hundreds of thousands of individuals trained in the art and science of radiography have become registered and certified by the ARRT.

The educator in radiologic technology has always been held in esteem, because it is the educator who trains the future professional radiologic technologist. With the dynamic growth of radiology and radiologic technology, the need for radiologic technologist-educators is greater today than ever before. Hospital certificate programs and collegiate degree programs in radiologic technology require the services of educators who are experts in radiologic technology and who are able to communicate this knowledge to the student radiologic technologist. The title "radiologic technologist-educator" indicates precisely the expertise an individual must bring to the classroom; this expertise includes not only radiography but should also include education itself. Today, when educators are held accountable not only by the profession but also by their students, it is the responsibility of the radiologic technologist-educator to enter the classroom with knowledge and experience in both radiologic technology and education.

Collegiate programs throughout the country offer a baccalaureate degree in radiologic technology, with core courses in education; on completion of such a program, the individual has a background in both radiologic technology and education. There are, however, individuals who choose to follow the traditional 24-consecutive-month radiologic technology program either in a hospital-based or collegiate program, and they then enter the profession as radiologic technologists. However, this does not exclude them from the area of education, because they may continue earning their undergraduate degrees. Graduates of collegiate associate degree programs who have strong backgrounds in radiologic technology can pursue continuing education toward a baccalaureate degree by majoring in education. Graduates of certificate hospital-based programs should inquire about collegiate programs that offer carte blanche credits for their technologic training or credits by examination to enable them to pursue educational core courses.

The radiologic technologist-educator must demonstrate competency in curriculum design and program planning. The individual should be able to design a model program, with particular attention given to course outlines, lesson plans, and use of textbooks and course materials.

The radiologic technologist-educator should also take courses in the historic foundations of education and the philosophic and psychologic foundations of education. Student counseling is very important, and it often occupies a great amount of time. A radiologic technologist who is pursuing a degree in education should complete several undergraduate courses in educational psychology and counseling. Instructional skills can be developed in numerous ways, and many educational programs require that candidates prepare microcourses and present them to their peers. Preparing such microcourses is an excellent opportunity for the education major candidate to write objectives for the course, prepare course outlines and lesson plans, and prepare audiovisual aids for the presentation of a microcourse. Many undergraduate programs offer candidates courses in audiovisual preparation in which the individual has the opportunity to learn the techniques of the preparation and use of various A-V modalities, as well as computer-assisted presentations.

Evaluating and testing are also important to the educator, because **formative evaluations** (in-depth, individualized assessments of knowledge) and **summative evaluations** (in-depth appraisals of knowledge that result in final grades or a certifying examination) are valuable tools for gauging the progress of class presentations and for determining final grades. Educational programs throughout the country offer courses in interpreting educational research and in methods of item writing that will be important throughout an individual's career.

Building on sound undergraduate educations, many radiologic technologist-educators are continuing toward doctoral degrees. Throughout the country, education centers are providing advanced programs geared toward allied health education.

The science of radiography is becoming more sophisticated and requires top-quality educators. It is the radiologic technologist-educator's responsibility to present a background that is indicative of the profession and the educational knowledge and skills to transmit this information to future generations of radiologic technologists.

The qualifications for a full-time program director, didactic program faculty, full-time clinical coordinator, and clinical instructor are addressed in Standard Six as published by the Joint Review Committee on Education in Radiologic Technology (JRCERT) in the *Standards for an Accredited Educational Program in Radiologic Sciences*, effective January 1, 2002.

Requirements for a full-time program director include:

- Minimum of a master's degree
- Proficient in curriculum design, program administration, evaluation, instruction, and counseling
- Equivalent 3 years full-time experience in professional discipline
- Two years experience as an instructor in a JRCERT accredited program
- Holds *American Registry of Radiologic Technologists (ARRT)* certification or equivalent in pertinent discipline

Requirements for a didactic program faculty include:

- Qualified to teach subject
- Knowledgeable of course development, instruction, evaluation, and academic counseling
- Holds appropriate professional credentials, if applicable

Requirements for a full-time clinical coordinator include:

- Minimum baccalaureate degree
- Proficient in curriculum development, supervision, instruction, evaluation, and counseling
- Two years full-time experience in the professional discipline
- One year experience as an instructor in a JRCERT accredited program
- Holds *American Registry of Radiologic Technologists (ARRT)* certification or equivalent in pertinent discipline

Requirements for a clinical instructor include:

- Proficient in supervision, instruction, and evaluation
- Two years full-time experience in the professional discipline

- Holds *American Registry of Radiologic Technologists (ARRT)* certification or equivalent in pertinent discipline

COMPUTER SCIENCE

In the field of radiology, computers are used in radiation therapy dosimetry, imaging, reporting, accounting, and billing. When computed tomography (CT) was introduced in the 1970s, the radiologic technologist became part of computerized radiology. Unfortunately, the radiologic technologist was unprepared at that time for the world of computer science. However, in today's world, computerized imaging is a daily occurrence. Unless radiologic technologists prepare themselves with the proper educational background, computer operations will be relegated to computer technicians. Programs in radiologic technology now require students to take courses in computer science.

Radiologic technologists who are interested in computer science should investigate several undergraduate programs before making a final decision. Programs may not be geared exclusively to the medical use of computers but rather to general computer science that is applicable to medical use. Courses in computer science should include an introduction to computer science (which should include basic concepts, language, programming, and flowcharting), computer mathematics and logic, programming applications, systems analysis, and computer operations. A background in radiography matched with a background in computer science is a necessity for radiologic technologists. Careful planning in educational endeavors will help ensure a professional future in this dynamic area of radiology.

THE QUALITY ASSURANCE TECHNOLOGIST

The health care industry today is very aware of its accountability and commitment to the patient. Awareness of this responsibility has caused many hospitals to voluntarily submit to **accreditation**, which is a process that a health care institution, provider, or program undergoes to demonstrate compliance with the standards developed by an official agency (in this case, the Joint Commission on Accreditation of Healthcare Organizations [JCAHO]). Such accreditation demands that each and every department within the hospital meet certain specific standards (see Chapter 21). The imaging department is required to meet very stringent standards in light of the fact that personnel use ionizing radiation on the patient. Such standards require that the radiology department have a quality assurance program and a quality control program to maintain film excellence on a day-to-day basis. The quality assurance radiologic technologist has the responsibility to oversee the equipment in the department and to guarantee that such equipment meets the standards set not only by the JCAHO but also by many federal, state, and local agencies. The **quality assurance technologist** is often a radiologic technologist with a baccalaureate degree or a radiologic technologist who holds a master of science degree with specialization in physics, radiation health physics, medical physics, or occupational safety.

The one most pressing responsibility of the quality assurance technologist is to oversee daily processor quality assurance/quality control. All too often the quality assurance technologist is called on to initiate minor in-house repairs on the processor, and the quality assurance technologist who is mechanically inclined is an asset to the department of radiology, primarily for the preventive maintenance of the processor. When service is required on the processor, however, the quality assurance technologist must interact with the service company. Having a good rapport with service personnel may mean that the processor can be repaired expeditiously with as little downtime as possible. Chemistry checks of all processors within the department are done routinely throughout the day to guarantee that quality assurance is maintained. In addition, the quality assurance technologist is called on to check radiographs for problems of a nontechnical nature that may occur as a result of processor problems.

Equipment quality assurance/quality control is another important aspect of the quality assurance technologist's responsibilities. Every month, each fluoroscope must be checked for image quality, resolution, and leakage radiation. Problems that may arise with the equipment must be checked out immediately by the quality assurance technologist, and such problems must be rectified by a service company; it must also be assured that there will be minimal downtime of the equipment. The quality assurance technologist is also responsible for acceptance testing and shielding surveys on all new installations of radiographic and fluoroscopic equipment. The fact that the department of radiology functions on a daily basis to produce radiographs of reproducible quality is dependent on the quality assurance technologist.

RADIATION SAFETY OFFICER/HEALTH PHYSICIST

To draw a fine line between the radiation safety officer and the health physicist is very difficult. The ideal situation is to have a physicist for the radiation therapy department whose primary duties include dosimetry and therapy treatment planning, a second physicist for nuclear medicine, and a third physicist for diagnostic radiology. Such an ideal situation rarely exists, and therefore the physicist involved in radiation therapy is also the radiation safety officer for all of radiology. Although hospital administration is ultimately responsible for employee radiation safety, the radiation safety officer ensures that radioactive materials and radiation-producing machinery are properly handled so that personnel and patient exposure does not exceed normally accepted levels.

The radiation safety officer holds a master's of science degree in radiation physics and is certified by the American Board of Health Physicists and the American Board of Radiology. The duties of the radiation safety officer are numerous: overseeing the safe use of all ionizing radiation, monitoring radiation exposure of all personnel, maintaining radiation monitoring reports, and providing surveillance of laboratories that use radioactive materials. The radiation safety officer oversees the proper handling and disposal of radioactive materials and supervises areas that may have been contaminated by radioactive materials.

All diagnostic radiographic and fluoroscopic equipment must be routinely checked by the radiation safety officer to guarantee that such equipment operates within the specified guidelines. Tabletop dose rate must be recorded, filtration must be checked, and collimators must be monitored, all to guarantee that the best image is produced with the least exposure to the patient. An important aspect of the surveillance of all radiographic and fluoroscopic equipment is the calculation of the fetal dose that may occur during the radiography of a pregnant patient. Lead aprons used in fluoroscopy and all protective garments are routinely checked by the radiation safety officer. Safelight testing in the processing areas also falls within the realm of the duties of the radiation safety officer. The radiation safety officer also instructs staff and students about new techniques in personnel and patient exposure limits and reviews concepts in the field of radiation protection and imaging.

THE EQUIPMENT SPECIALIST

In many large teaching hospitals, the department of imaging has an equipment specialist on staff whose sole purpose is the maintenance of all equipment in the imaging department. The equipment specialist must have a very strong electronics background, a high mechanical aptitude (60% to 70% of equipment problems are mechanical), and a working knowledge of computers and their application in radiology. The equipment specialist in the radiology department does not install the equipment, but he or she is involved on a day-to-day basis with the maintenance of the equipment. At the time of installation, the equipment specialist spends a great deal of time with the service engineers who are installing the equipment to learn the proper operation of the equipment and the methods of preventive maintenance to keep the equipment at its peak performance.

In such large teaching institutions, the equipment specialist is part of the equipment selection committee, and he or she interacts with service engineers, sales representatives, and applications specialists before and during the purchase and installation of equipment for the department. In today's busy department, the equipment specialist is an important asset for solving frequently occurring minor problems. Preventive maintenance guarantees that equipment downtime is kept to a minimum. The practicing radiologic technologist is well advised to befriend equipment specialists and to pick their brains, so to speak, for in most instances they are more familiar with the new equipment at the time of its installation than even the sales representatives and applications specialists.

COMMERCIAL REPRESENTATIVES

Commercial representatives of various film and equipment companies are frequent visitors to the radiology department. The category of commercial representative could probably be best divided into two groups: applications specialists and sales representatives. A technical background is important for applications specialists, because they will be dealing with the radiologist regarding new equipment and the applications of that equipment to a particular area of radiology. Their background will allow them to knowledgeably discuss the technical use of the equipment in the production of a quality image. Sales representatives, however, should possess a baccalaureate degree and a business background. Their interactions are primarily with the radiologist and other hospital administrators on a high finance level. Commercial representatives should possess a high degree of maturity and be confident, able to communicate, likable, good listeners, and hesitant to back down; they should believe in the product that they are selling or representing.

When dealing with the radiologist, commercial representatives must keep in mind that they are dealing with an individual whose time is very valuable. Commercial representatives have often described a "caste system" of radiologist/radiologic technologist that is particularly evident when the commercial representative has come from the ranks of radiologic technologists; this caste system must be overcome if commercial dealings are to be culminated. Many companies provide a training program for those individuals who are coming into the commercial field without a previous sales or applications background; this provides support during a very crucial transition period.

Commercial representatives may be required to travel a great deal with their job, because they often cover extensive territories. In addition, they must be flexible enough to relocate at any given time should they be reassigned to an area where their abilities are needed. Many of the commercial representatives are salaried employees for various companies; others are commissioned employees who are required to meet quotas set by the employer.

CONCLUSION

The growth of radiography since Eddy Jerman and Marie Curie trained x-ray technicians has been indicative of a science that is continually striving to serve and protect life. The radiologic technologist cannot stand still while the profession moves forward; it is the responsibility of the radiologic technologist to pursue the education necessary to keep abreast of professional development.

Radiologic technologists interested in career mobility have several options for investigation. Regardless of the option that they choose, advanced education holds the key to upward and lateral mobility.

Review Questions

1. In today's radiology department, upward and lateral mobility depends primarily on which of the following?
   a. Seniority
   b. Education
   c. Responsibility assumed
   d. Age
2. Short-term postgraduate education for the radiologic technologist would be in which of the following areas?
   1. Sonography
   2. Education
   3. Radiation therapy
   4. Vascular interventional angiography
      a. 1, 2, and 3 only
      b. 1, 3, and 4 only
      c. 2, 3, and 4 only
      d. 1, 2, 3, and 4
3. Which of the following is included in the responsibilities of the RA?
   1. Performing fluoroscopy of noninvasive procedures with radiologist direct supervision
   2. Performing invasive procedures with radiologist direct supervision
   3. Interpreting images and making diagnosis
   4. Performing pre- and postprocedure evaluation of patients undergoing invasive studies
      a. 1 and 2 only
      b. 1 and 3 only
      c. 1 and 4 only
      d. 1, 2, 3, and 4
4. Personnel management, budget preparation, union negotiations, and purchasing are a few of the areas of involvement of the:
   a. Equipment specialist.
   b. Department administrator.
   c. Quality assurance technologist.
   d. Staff radiologic technologist.
5. The formal training of x-ray technicians in the United States began in:
   a. 1895.
   b. 1917.
   c. 1933.
   d. 1970.
6. Formal training of x-ray technicians in Europe was first undertaken by:
   a. Wilhelm C. Roentgen.
   b. Eddy C. Jerman.

c. Marie Curie.
d. None of the above
7. The ASRT was established in:
   a. 1895.
   b. 1916.
   c. 1920.
   d. 1970.
8. Qualifications for radiologic science program director, faculty, clinical coordinator, and clinical instructor are addressed by the:
   a. ARRT
   b. ASRT
   c. JRCERT
   d. JCAHO
9. The JCAHO requires that radiology departments establish a(n):
   a. Educational program for radiologic technologists.
   b. Preventive maintenance procedure.
   c. Computer-enhanced imaging system.
   d. Quality assurance/quality control program.
10. Which of the following is of utmost importance in a quality assurance/quality control program?
   a. Acceptance testing
   b. Radiation badge monitoring
   c. Processor monitoring
   d. Radiographic equipment monitoring
11. The monitoring of personnel radiation exposure is the responsibility of the:
   a. Administrator.
   b. Educator.
   c. Quality control technologist.
   d. Radiation safety officer.
12. Minor radiographic and fluoroscopic equipment problems are often serviced by the:
   a. Commercial representative.
   b. Applications specialist.
   c. Equipment specialist.
   d. Administrator.

BIBLIOGRAPHY

American College of Radiology, www.acr.org
American Medical Association: *Health Professions Career and Education Directory*, ed. 29, Chicago, 2001, The Association.
American Registry of Radiologic Technologists, www.arrt.org
American Society of Radiologic Technologists, www.asrt.org
Curie E: *Madame Curie: a biography*, Garden City, NY, 1937, Garden City Publishing.
Easterling C (RTR, FASRT, Duke University): Personal communication, 1991.
Grigg ERN: *Train of the invisible light*, Springfield, IL, 1965, Charles C Thomas.

Kelly, T (Hospital of the University of Pennsylvania, Department of Radiology, Philadelphia): Personal communication, 1991.

Loma Linda University, www.llu.edu

Nunno M (MS, Albert Einstein Medical Center, Northern Division, Department of Radiology, Philadelphia): Personal communication, 1991.

Price T (RTR, MS, Pennsylvania Hospital, Department of Radiology, Philadelphia): Personal communication, 1991.

Rensch S (RTR, BA, Community College of Philadelphia, Philadelphia): Personal communication, 1991.

Sterling S (RTR, FASRT, Eastman Kodak Company): Personal communication, 1991.

Weber State University, www.weber.edu

Continuing Education for the Radiologic Technologist

Barbara A. Burnham-Rupp

OBJECTIVES

On completion of this chapter, you should be able to:

- **Understand the required number of credits needed to renew registration with the American Registry of Radiologic Technology (ARRT).**

- **Document proof of participation in obtaining continuing education credits.**

- **Identify alternative means of meeting continuing education requirements.**

- **Understand the implications of noncompliance with continuing education requirements.**

- **Identify continuing education opportunities recognized by the ARRT as well as alternatives.**

- **Recognize cost-effective means of obtaining continuing education credits.**

- **Select the most productive way of obtaining continuing education credits.**

Most graduate technologists soon realize that although they have ended their formal education, they are at the beginning of what will prove to be a lifetime of learning.

KEY TERMS

academic course
biennial
Category A
Category B
certification
continuing education
  credit (CE credit)
in-service education
license
probation
Recognized Continuing
  Education Evaluation
  Mechanism (RCEEM)
registered technologist

CHAPTER OUTLINE

*National certification
  examination and
  registration
  Requirements
  Meeting the
    requirements
  Alternative means of
    meeting the
    requirements*

Continued

Renewal of registration
CE documentation
Noncompliance with CE
    requirements
Nonrenewal of
    registration
What to look for when
    seeking CE credits
    (Q & A)
Licensure requirements
Conclusion

Education presents itself in many forms. Day-to-day living provides many learning experiences that cause growth. Even when functioning within the specifics of a job description we are exposed to new experiences and questions for which our education has not provided answers. An educational program cannot possibly answer all questions or incorporate all potential experiences.

The profession, understanding the ever-changing needs of technologists, established mandatory continuing education in order to:

- Bridge the gap between entry-level formal education and advanced practice needs.
- Prevent professional obsolescence.
- Assure the public, our primary customers, that all technologists maintain competence.
- Demonstrate accountability to peers, physicians, health care facilities, and the public.
- Advance the profession through continuous growth of all technologists working in the field.
- Provide advanced growth opportunities for technologists through advanced preparation.
- Reinforce the Code of Ethics for all practicing professionals.

NATIONAL CERTIFICATION EXAMINATION AND REGISTRATION

After completion of a formal educational program in one of the primary disciplines in the radiologic sciences, the graduate technologist will take a national **certification** examination given by one of the following certification agencies:

American Registry of Radiologic Technologists (ARRT)
 Radiography
 Nuclear Medicine Technology or (NMTCB)
 Radiation Therapy
American Registry in Diagnostic Medical Sonography (ARDMS)
 Diagnostic Medical Sonography
 Vascular Technology
 Diagnostic Cardiac Sonography
Medical Dosimetry Certification Board (MDCB)
 Dosimetry
Nuclear Medicine Technology Certification Board
 Nuclear Medicine Technology or (ARRT)

For purposes of this discussion the ARRT requirements will be used.

By passing the ARRT examination, graduates are considered certified and may use RT(R) for radiographer; RT(N) for nuclear medicine technologist; or RT(T) for radiation therapist, as professional credentials following their names. The technologist is also placed on the registry or listing of **registered technologists**. It is from this listing that potential and/or current employers may determine whether a technologist is current with the national certification agency and compliant with mandatory continuing education requirements.

Although registered technologists must renew their ARRT registration annually, mandatory continuing education requirements and documentation that the required credits have been obtained are required on a **biennial** (2-year) basis.

Requirements

Newly (ARRT) registered technologists will have to begin accumulating credits on the first day of their next birth month after becoming certified. For example, a technologist certified in March of 2005, with a birth date of September 20, will need to begin acquiring **continuing education credits (CE credits)** on September 1, 2005. This will be the start date of that technologist's biennium. He or she may continue to accumulate the 24 required credits from September 1 through August 31, 2007, when all required credits must be completed.

A CE credit is a unit of measurement for continuing education activities. Each credit is based on a 50- to 60-minute contact hour. Programs longer than one hour are based on a 60-minute credit, with ½ credit awarded for an additional 30 to 49 minutes. Any activity under 30 minutes is not eligible to receive credit.

Obtaining the required number of CE credits necessary for the radiologic technologist to renew registration is easy if the following factors are remembered:

1. It is solely the technologist's responsibility to attend, obtain, and maintain documentation of attendance for each continuing education activity. This responsibility may not be delegated to anyone or any institution or organization.
2. 24 credits are required during each 24-month biennium.
3. A minimum of 12 CE credits must be identified as **Category A**. These activities have received approval *prior* to the activity by a Recognized Continuing Education Evaluation Mechanism (RCEEM). All 24 credits may be Category A.
4. A maximum of 12 CE credits may be identified as **Category B**. These activities have not obtained approval prior to the activity by an RCEEM.
5. Both Category A and Category B credits must be educational activities relevant to the radiologic sciences and/or patient care.
6. The same CE activity may not be used more than once in a biennium.

Meeting the Requirements

As previously noted, registered technologists must acquire 24 CE credits within their 24-month bienniums. Each CE activity must meet the ARRT's definition. They must be planned, organized, and administered to enhance the knowledge and skills underlying the professional performance that a technologist uses to provide services to patients, the public, or the medical profession. The most typical are:

- Professional society-offered activities
- In-service educational activities
- Directed readings
- Home-study
- Internet activities
- Basic Life Support (CPR) certification by the Red Cross, the Heart Association, or the American Safety and Health Institute equals 3 CE credits. NOTE: Can only be used once during biennium, in spite of the number of times the technologists may be required to participate).
- Advanced Life Support (ACLS), instructor or instructor trainer CPR certification is given 6 CE credits. NOTE: Can only be used once during biennium.
- Others may apply. Make certain to verify acceptance prior to participation.

ALTERNATIVE MEANS OF MEETING THE REQUIREMENTS

The 24-credit requirement may also be fulfilled in two other ways as long as these alternative methods are *completed within the individual's* biennium. These do not require prior approval of a RCEEM:

I. Radiologic technologists may decide to continue their formal education following graduation, certification, and registration in a primary discipline. They may choose to enroll in an additional accredited primary or postprimary discipline. This education will be considered to have met the CE requirements for the biennium. *It is important to note that the additional education must be completed and the certification examination must have been taken and passed prior to the end of the individual's biennium.*

A. Examples of additional primary education and examination are:
Radiographer (ARRT)
Nuclear Medicine Technology (ARRT or NMTCB)
Radiation Therapy (ARRT)
Dosimetry (MDCB)
Diagnostic Medical Sonography, Vascular Technology, or Diagnostic Cardiac Sonography (ARDMS)
Radiology Administration (AHRA)

B. Examples of approved postprimary examinations are:
Cardiovascular-Interventional Technology (ARRT)
Mammography (ARRT)
Computer Tomography (ARRT)
Magnetic Resonance Imaging (ARRT)
Quality Management (ARRT)
Sonography (ARRT)
Vascular Sonography (ARRT)
Bone Densitometry (ARRT)
Vascular-Interventional Technology (ARRT)

Cardiac-Interventional Technology (ARRT)
Breast Sonography (ARRT)
Nuclear Cardiology (NMTCB)
II. Academic Courses taken from an accredited postsecondary educational institution (college or university). The course must be relevant to the radiologic sciences and/or patient care. Relevant courses may be in:
Biologic sciences
Physical sciences
Radiologic sciences
Health and medical sciences
Social sciences
Communication (verbal and written)
Mathematics
Computers
Management
Education methodology
Courses that may NOT be applicable include:
Astronomy
Fine arts
Geography
Geology
History
Music
Philosophy
Religion

Renewal of Registration

When completing the ARRT renewal form, the technologist is asked to list the educational/learning activities attended during the biennium. Actual documentation should not accompany the renewal form. ARRT verification is performed by random sample. This means that the ARRT will request documentation from only a percentage of renewing technologists. A technologist may never, may periodically, or may biennially be requested to provide documentation of continuing education attendance. In any event, technologists are responsible for maintaining the necessary documentation for one year after the completion of their biennium.

Individuals certified in multiple modalities (e.g., radiography and radiation therapy) are not required to meet separate continuing education requirements for each modality. Twenty-four CE credits, with a minimum of 12 in Category A, and a maximum of 12 credits in Category B, obtained during the technologist's biennium, will meet the requirements of all disciplines of certification. It is important for technologists employed in licensing states to check the requirements outlined by their state law. Also, technologists who function in specific modalities, such as mammography, may have additional federal regulations.

CE Documentation

Proof of CE participation must be maintained by the registered technologist. Some ARRT-approved organizations will track CE credits for their members. Nonetheless, the technologist remains responsible for participating in, tracking, and maintaining documentation. Should the approved tracking organization make an error, the ARRT will not accept this as an excuse for the lack of documentation on the part of the technologist.

The sponsor of each program that technologists attend during their bienniums should provide documentation of attendance. This documentation MUST have the following:

1. Date(s) of attendance.
2. The topic/subject title.
3. Content of the educational opportunity.
4. Number of (50-60 minute) contact hours.
5. Name of speaker/presenter.
6. Name/signature of sponsor or authorized representative.
7. The RCEEM-approved reference number, when applicable.

This documentation must be maintained for 1 year beyond the end of each biennium.

NONCOMPLIANCE WITH CE REQUIREMENTS

Any technologist applying for renewal who has not obtained the necessary continuing education credits is considered on CE **probation**. These individuals receive a registration card with the probational status shown.

Probational status is granted only for the first year of the next biennium. If compliance does not occur during that 12 months, the individual is considered no longer registered by the ARRT.

Nonrenewal of Registration

As previously mentioned, potential and/or current employers, as well as state licensing agencies, may ask the ARRT about the current status of a technologist. If the technologist has not renewed her/his registration, the ARRT responds to any inquiry by stating that the individual in question is not registered by the ARRT.

Registration reinstatement may be requested by a delinquent technologist who is subject to compliance with CE requirements and submission with the appropriate fee. All other ARRT rules and regulations in effect at the time must be followed.

It is strongly suggested that technologists maintain current registration with the ARRT even if they are not currently functioning within the profession. If registration is allowed to lapse beyond the individual's biennium, no reinstatement is allowed without re-examination in one of the primary disciplines. The standard related examination fees must be paid.

WHAT TO LOOK FOR WHEN SEEKING CE CREDITS (Q & A)

Q. Is the program approved by a Recognized Continuing Education Evaluation Mechanism (RCEEM)?

A. Nonapproved continuing education may be costly in terms of time and money and may not meet the ARRT requirements, so exercise caution. The goal of each technologist should be to obtain 24 CE Category A credits, if some ultimately turn out to be in Category B, that will be acceptable.

The ASRT has been reviewing and approving CE programs since it established its ECE program in 1978. This program remains focused on enhancing the approval process to better identify high-quality learning opportunities for technologists attending their approved programs.

Q. What organizations are RCEEMs?

A. The following organizations are **Recognized Continuing Education Evaluation Mechanisms (RCEEMs)** approved by the ARRT:

American Society of Radiologic Technologists (ASRT)

Society of Nuclear Medicine Technologists Section's VOICE program

Society of Diagnostic Medical Sonography (SDMS)

American Healthcare Radiology Administrators (AHRA)

American College of Radiology (ACR)

Society of Vascular Technology (SVT)

Canadian Association of Medical Radiation Technologists (CAMRT)

Accredited Postsecondary Educational Institutions (e.g., colleges and universities—approved academic courses)

Q. What are the most cost-effective means of obtaining CE credits?

A. Typically the most cost-effective and beneficial methods are provided by the professional societies, such as the American Society of Radiologic Technology and your state affiliate society. The primary purpose of these organizations is to provide for the continuing educational needs of the professionals they represent.

Q. Why is this the most cost-effective method?

A. Any money spent on the endeavor of obtaining CE credits goes directly back into the profession itself. Like a "not-for-profit" hospital, all proceeds must be used directly by the organization to help keep it viable. Therefore, any money spent by a technologist to obtain continuing education from a professional society serves two purposes. Obviously, the first is the knowledge gained by the attendee. Secondly, monies spent are used by the society to help move the profession forward.

Q. What are in-service programs?

A. **In-service education** can be an effective low-cost method of obtaining CE credits. These are programs developed within the institution where the technologist is employed.

This type of continuing education may be used to address problems that affect the specific group's daily operation. For example, if repeat examinations are high within the department, an analysis may provide information with which to develop an in-service program.

It is not always necessary to look within the radiology realm. Patient care issues, phlebotomy, vital signs, and other basic services performed are appropriate expansions of technologists' scope of practice and benefit the patients for whom they are responsible.

The radiologist staff is an excellent resource for in-service programming. However, technologists themselves are the experts in the radiologic sciences and should be considered first whenever developing programs. Technologists in each of our disciplines are, in many ways, much better suited to address the continuing education needs of other technologists. In addition, technologists who prepare and present programs, if submitted and approved for Category A, will not only receive CE credits for the presentation (one credit for every 50 minutes contact hour) but also receive three (3) credits for preparation. This too is highly cost-effective.

Q. What is the method of obtaining the most CE credits?

A. Seminars where multiple credits may be obtained are obviously faster than any single-credit mechanism. However, the most productive method of obtaining many credits is **academic courses**. Credits are accumulated at the successful completion of the course based on the following credit calculations:

Twelve (12) credits per 1 quarter hour

Sixteen (16) credits per 1 semester hour

Continuing education should provide the technologist with new opportunities and knowledge. What better way to accomplish this than focusing these continuing education efforts toward obtaining a college or university degree? Technologists are strongly encouraged to consider using the academic means of CE credit compliance.

Q. I took a three-semester class on computer sciences. Using the calculation, I should have 48 CE credits. May I use 24 for my current biennium and the other 24 for my next biennium?

A. No. CE credits must be acquired and completed within the biennium. The technologist will need to begin acquiring new CE credits at the beginning of his or her next biennium.

Q. What are other sources to be considered?

A. Videotapes, audiotapes, and *directed readings,* provided in professional journals, are all methods of obtaining credits and can be obtained at home. You may contact the ASRT and state society for additional CE education opportunities.

LICENSURE REQUIREMENTS

At the printing of this text, more than half of the United States requires technologists to be licensed. The term **license** means that legal permission has been granted by a state allowing an individual to function as a technologist and administer ionizing radiation to human beings. Technologists must take the time necessary to familiarize themselves with all national and state requirements. By not doing so, they may seriously jeopardize their ability to work in their chosen professions.

The technologist must also learn whether separate mandatory continuing education requirements for license renewal exist within the state in which the technologist is employed. Typically, the same continuing education (CE) credits may be used for both the ARRT and the state; however this should never be assumed. It is the responsibility of the technologist to know when CE credits must be obtained, the number required, the acceptable types of continuing education, and any difference in renewal periods.

CONCLUSION

Although continuing education became mandatory for all ARRT-registered technologists in 1995, the technologists of today can consider themselves fortunate that many of their predecessors understood the value of continuing their education without mandate. These technologists, who helped themselves grow in turn helped the field grow.

Make certain to read the ARRT's Annual Report each year. Check for changes in the requirements that may affect your CE plan.

As with all fields of endeavor, it is only through the continued expansion of knowledge and questioning of "what could be" that a profession moves forward. Now, more than 100 years since the discovery of the x-ray, only the surface of our continually growing field has been scratched. With the need for mandatory continuing education, more technologists are participating in the profession's movement into the next century. By all technologists committing to personal growth, we guarantee that future generations of radiologic technologists will have new and even more exciting horizons to explore.

Review Questions

1. Continuing education for radiologic technologists is:
   a. Voluntary for entry level only
   b. Mandatory for advanced level only
   c. Mandatory for all registered technologists
   d. Voluntary for all registered technologists
2. The following educational activities are acceptable for CE credit except:
   a. Academic courses in an approved college or university
   b. In-service educational programs
   c. Local Radiologic Technology programs
   d. Registry review seminars
3. The organization requiring continuing education for renewal of certification is the:
   a. ASRT
   b. ARRT
   c. AERS
   d. RCEEM

4. The organization responsible for approving educational activities for CE credit is the:
   a. ARRT
   b. AERS
   c. RCEEM
   d. AHRA
5. The number of CE credits required for renewal of certification is:
   a. 12 units per year
   b. 24 units in a 2-year period
   c. 36 units in a 2-year period
   d. None are required; it is voluntary
6. CE credits may be obtained from an accredited postsecondary educational institution in:
   a. Courses of the learner's choice
   b. Courses carrying a minimum of 3 semester hours
   c. Courses in disciplines specified by the ARRT
   d. Radiologic technology courses only
7. For an academic course to be acceptable for CE credit, the course must be relevant to:
   a. The radiologic sciences
   b. Patient care
   c. The learner's culture
   d. A and B only
8. The ASRT established the ECE program in:
   a. 1968
   b. 1978
   c. 1985
   d. 1995
9. Continuing education programs meet the criteria for approved CE credit if:
   a. A fee or tuition is charged
   b. The program is at least 50 minutes
   c. The program is conducted by a physician
   d. None of the above
10. The main objective for continuing education is to:
    a. Enhance the public image of technologists
    b. Increase the technologist's self-esteem
    c. Provide efficient care for patients
    d. Foster creativity

BIBLIOGRAPHY

American Registry of Radiologic Technologists: *Annual report,* 1993, 1994, 1995, 2000, The Registry.

Gurley LT: Educational void, *Appl Radiol* 17:11, Nov 1988.

Nesbitt J: *Megatrends: 10 directions transforming our lives,* New York, 1982, Warner.

Status of Health Care Delivery

William J. Callaway

OBJECTIVES

On completion of this chapter, you should be able to:

- List key social forces that affect the health care system.
- Discuss the dominant ethical issues in medicine today.
- Explain the impact of an aging population on health care delivery.
- Describe the nation's health care expenditures.
- Explain prospective payment.
- Correlate defensive medicine, medical malpractice, and health care costs.
- Give the top five causes of death, and list the associated risk factors.
- Describe a typical wellness program.
- Describe the advantages of giving up smoking.
- Link poor diet to major causes of death.
- Outline dietary guidelines for good health.
- Discuss the role of the radiologic technologist in patient education.
- List alternate health care practices.
- Describe the overall goals of Healthy People 2010.

KEY TERMS

defensive medicine
diet
health maintenance
    organizations (HMOs)
Healthy People 2010
prospective payment
    system (PPS)
smoking

CHAPTER OUTLINE

*Social forces that affect
    health care
Ethical issues
Economic forces that
    affect health care
Need for health care
    management
Preventive medicine
    Healthy People 2010
The health care system
The beginning of your
    challenge
Conclusion*

As a radiologic technologist, you are part of a larger health care system that, in some way, touches the lives of everyone. As seen in Chapter 5, medicine has advanced from the occult to the scientific. The technologic advances alone have been dramatic. These improvements—coupled with a deeper understanding of the human being at the focus of our care—provide the basis for the continual evolution of health care delivery.

Economic and social forces not in existence in centuries past deeply affect the health care system today. As a key member of the health care team, you, too, are influenced. The quality of the care you provide is profoundly determined by the environment in which you practice and by your professional self-image. Chapter 1 discussed in detail the values you can add to the service you provide. Such values enhance not only the patient's experience but also your self-image. This final chapter presents the framework in which your professional career is being formed. The challenges are many; consequently, the opportunities for professional growth are plentiful. However, the radiologic technologist practicing at the turn of the millennium must have an understanding of the continually changing health care climate.

Social forces that affect health care

The aging of the population, increasing health care costs, and an upturn in the birth rate are key forces that are greatly changing health care delivery. Although diagnostic imaging will continue to play a prominent role in health care, its exact shape will continue to evolve. You have chosen a field of study that has a bright future but that will certainly have its peaks and valleys over time. The venues in which radiologic technologists practice continue to change, and the job market fluctuates constantly. However, radiologic technology will continue to be one of the fastest-growing occupations in the coming decades. Within the profession, individual fields will grow even faster than others, such as education and all forms of scanning and digital imaging.

Your patients and employers will expect and require the best of your talents and skills. They require a strong command of both the technical aspects of radiologic technology and the high-touch aspects of patient care and service. More work must be done with fewer caregivers when dealing with the realities of health care financing. You will also need a working knowledge of health care delivery issues.

Ethical issues

The advances in research and technology in medicine have prompted disagreement about ethical issues as never before. With all of its hope and ability to enhance the quality of life, health care has also raised questions that society must answer. Professionals and private citizens alike debate issues such as the patient's right to privacy and confidentiality of information. This topic has become particularly sensitive since the outbreak of acquired immunodeficiency syndrome (AIDS). Animal rights advocates decry the use of laboratory animals in medical experiments; other groups question whether new drugs are made available to humans too soon or not soon enough.

Health-care-related issues dominate the medical, religious, and political arenas. The elusive question of when life begins has yet to be answered by either science or the courts. At the other end of the life cycle is the debate over when life ends. Accompanying these controversies are the issues of abortion, active euthanasia (assisted suicide), passive euthanasia, and the right to die.

In vitro fertilization is a reality, and so is surrogate motherhood. Genetic engineering carries with it the hope for the elimination of inherited diseases as well as the specter of selecting which offspring to carry to term. Human cloning is near reality. Ultimately, the most sensitive ethical issue may be the rationing of health care.

Concern about long-term care for an aging population becomes greater with each passing year. At the beginning of the 21st century, more than 10 million older adults need care, and over 3 million are in institutions with the number growing. By the year 2025, half of all older Americans will be age 75 and older. Even now, more than two-thirds of those in nursing homes suffer from some form of cognitive disorder such as Alzheimer's disease. Most of the cost of long-term care is paid for by the nursing home residents and/or their families; it is not unusual for life savings to be depleted in a very short period of time. Some underwriters offer a form of long-term care insurance coverage, and the government is examining its role in funding such care.

Because of the sheer increase in the number of citizens in this age group, home care is on a steady increase. Home health care products cover simple hygiene as well as complex medical technology. In some areas, physicians and dentists make house calls. Mobile radiography services provide diagnostic testing in the community. Visiting nurses make their daily rounds in nearly every locale.

Serious ethical issues will likely be resolved by the judicial system long before science provides solutions. Indeed, science may not be able to answer the moral questions that have been raised. Discussion of these and other ethical controversies of the health care delivery system has an important place in your education.

The radiologic technologist must remember that these are times that require immense flexibility in dealing with all types of patients of all ages and in various clinical situations. It is a time of constant change and almost unlimited opportunity for professional challenge and personal growth.

ECONOMIC FORCES THAT AFFECT HEALTH CARE

Cost is a major issue in the status of health care delivery. Approximately 15% of the gross domestic product (GDP) of the United States is spent on health care; this figure amounts to well over $1 trillion annually. We spend more of our GDP on health care than any other nation in the world. The cost of health care in America has generally increased faster than the prevailing rate of inflation for more than three decades. Those who pay most of the nation's medical bills are the federal and state governments and private insurance companies. Historically, rates were set by the providers of health care (hospitals and physicians), and then third-party payers (e.g., insurance companies, the government) reimbursed the providers for that amount. With rising costs, this system could not continue.

A **prospective payment system (PPS)** is now in place. Under this structure, the government pays medical bills for older adults (Medicare) and the needy (Medicaid) based on diagnostic-related groups (DRGs). The cost for providing services, which is determined ahead of time by the government, is based on admitting diagnosis. Hospitals are pressed to provide the service at or below the level of payment. If costs exceed the predetermined amount, the hospital must absorb those costs. If care is provided at a lower cost, the hospital may keep the extra payment.

Most third-party payers now incorporate some form of prospective payment or negotiated fees as part of their contract for payment. Many patients are members of **health maintenance organizations (HMOs)** that offer, for a monthly fee, all necessary medical care at no additional charge. Some HMOs own their own hospitals or contract with others for the care of their members. Others are members of preferred provider organizations (PPOs) who negotiate lower fees with the patient's insurer. This entire system has forced hospitals to reduce overhead, examine cost schedules, and limit unnecessary medical care and services. The result has been a decline in the use of expensive inpatient services and greater use of cost-effective outpatient facilities. This change has greatly affected hospitals that historically relied on inpatient revenues, and some hospitals have not survived. Almost 500 hospitals have closed since the 1980s. The outlook at the start of the century indicates the closing or restructuring of at least 3,000 of the nation's 6,800 hospitals.

The political arena is congested with debate about the role of Medicare in health care financing. The 4.8 million citizens who will turn 65 years old in the year 2020 will, based on current dollars, spend $210 billion of the Medicare fund. The effect on the patients you serve can be profound. The older patient may be concerned that Medicare will not pay the entire bill. Early discharge from the hospital may be indicated because of limits on coverage for a given medical condition. Other patients have experienced medical insurance premiums rising 10% to 20% each year. Increased deductibles on insurance policies, whether they are individual or group plans, transfer more of the actual cost of care directly onto the patient. Such costs affect each patient as never before.

Trying to hold the line on health care costs is not easy. Just as some price controls are put into place, other factors cause fees to rise. Salaries, the highest single cost in health care, must be kept at competitive levels to attract and retain excellent clinicians. In fact, labor costs account for more than 70% of the average hospital's budget. Labor shortages in all areas of health care have put upward pressure on salaries. New technologies carry with them very high price tags; some estimate that the latest technology adds 50% to the patient's bill for each day in the hospital. Supplies for hospitals are costly, and new services must be offered to attract and serve patients. Finally, as the population ages and the majority of patients are over 75 years old, the medical care required increases because of a higher incidence of disability and chronic disease. Chronic disease consumes more than 80% of health care resources. Approximately 33% of the average American's lifetime health spending occurs during the final year of life, with almost half that amount spent in the last 2 months of life; along with this goes the total nation's health bill. In addition to fewer people in the work force to pay into government programs and group insurance, these factors are wreaking havoc with the delivery of health care.

There is no single answer to the problem of health care cost reimbursement. Hospitals and health care workers must do all they can to control costs. The question of who pays the bill must be answered. Many people carry no insurance at all or are not covered at their place of employment. The cost of medical care for them is absorbed by the hospital system or Medicaid. Furthermore, such individuals many times do not seek care at all, thus worsening their existing medical conditions, which ultimately results in higher costs for more serious problems. However, if employers are forced to cover all employees under group insurance, this can place a serious financial strain on their ability to compete with larger companies with greater resources or with foreign companies who carry no such burden. If all citizens were covered under a form of national health insurance, as is proposed by some, tax rates would skyrocket.

Another factor that affects the cost of health care is the practice of defensive medicine. **Defensive medicine** can be defined as any waste of resources (net excess of costs over benefits) that results from physicians changing their patterns of practice in response to the threat of malpractice liability (McLennan and Meyer, 1989). In a society that goes to court over almost anything, alleged medical malpractice is a high-visibility target. Defensive medicine, coupled with the dramatically increased cost of malpractice insurance premiums for physicians and hospitals alike, adds to the cost of providing services. Quality assurance has become a constant partner in the practice of medicine. Nevertheless, the overall cost is something that must be addressed sooner or later.

It seems that there is no easy answer. Suffice it to say that you as a health care worker will be affected by the system in which you work, both as an employee and as a patient. Your understanding of and involvement in the professional and political issues that affect your chosen career are vital. Keep abreast of these issues by maintaining membership and actively participating in your professional organizations.

NEED FOR HEALTH CARE MANAGEMENT

One of the best ways of holding down health care costs and improving the quality of life is the practice of preventive medicine. The impetus comes from business, which has seen rising medical care expenses reduce profits and inhibit the ability to compete in a global economy. Whether by directly paying expenses, suffering high absenteeism, or experiencing lower productivity, the business world has come to realize that managing the health of employees also allows it to maximize profits and benefits.

Companies report that most health care expenditures are directly connected to the lifestyle of their employees. According to the U.S. Centers for Disease Control and Prevention, more than half of early deaths are attributable to lifestyle. Box 26-1 correlates the risk factors with the top five causes of death (see Chapter 5). Sedentary lifestyle, not using seat belts, smoking, alcohol, and diet play a key role in more than 70% of the cases for each cause of death listed in Chapter 5.

BOX 26-1—RISK FACTORS AND PRIMARY CAUSES OF DEATH

Heart Disease

Sedentary lifestyle
Cigarette smoking
Hypertension
Obesity
Diabetes
High cholesterol

Cancer

Cigarette smoking
Positive stool occult blood
Failure to perform breast self-examination
Failure to have Pap smears

Cerebrovascular Disease

Cigarette smoking
Hypertension
High cholesterol

Accidents

Failure to use seat belts
High alcohol use

Chronic Lower Respiratory Disease

Cigarette smoking

PREVENTIVE MEDICINE

If most causes of disease, disability, and even death are directly related to lifestyle, then it is clear that wellness and health care costs can be managed. More and more employers now offer some form of wellness program to employees. This may take the form of in-house education and activities or memberships at local health and fitness facilities. Screening employees for high blood pressure, elevated cholesterol, abnormal glucose levels, and threatening lifestyle habits is commonplace. Counseling is provided in such areas as smoking cessation, proper nutrition, fitness, weight control, and stress management. Emphasis on prevention rather than medical intervention is the key to a healthy lifestyle as well as a healthy medical delivery system. An indication of the potential savings is reflected in the fact that smoking-related illnesses alone cost the health care system (that is, taxpayers and insurance premium payers) more than $65 billion annually. If tobacco use in the United States stopped entirely, an estimated 390,000 fewer Americans would die before their time each year. If alcohol were never carelessly used, about 100,000 fewer people would die from unnecessary illness and injury. AIDS—another almost entirely preventable disease—costs in excess of $13 billion annually to treat.

Two main lifestyle factors that are related to good health are **smoking** and **diet**. Many states have passed clean indoor air laws that prohibit or severely limit smoking in public places. In addition to the increased risk to the smoker, the effect on nonsmokers is serious. Secondhand smoke greatly increases the occurrence of cancer, heart disease, and lung illnesses, and it also aggravates preexisting conditions. Thirty-eight million American smokers who quit before they reach the age of 50 can reduce their risk of dying in the next 15 years by half; the risk of heart disease and lung cancer returns to the level of a nonsmoker in 5 to 10 years. Furthermore, data indicate that those who smoke spend nearly $1,000 more per year for medical care. In view of its link to virtually every major illness, it is surprising that 50 million people still smoke. However, a rapidly changing health care delivery system that is based on preventive care may change that figure as the century draws to a close.

According to the U.S. Senate Select Committee on Nutrition and Human Needs, which investigated American health: "Changes have occurred in the diet of Americans that could cause a wave of malnutrition (from both overconsumption and underconsumption) as damaging to health in the United States as the widespread, contagious diseases of the early part of the century. Overconsumption of fats, sugar, salt, and alcohol has been related to six of the ten leading causes of death. These six causes [of death] are heart disease and arteriosclerosis, stroke, cancer, diabetes, and cirrhosis of the liver. In addition, diet is thought to contribute to the development of conditions, such as hypertension, that [adversely] affect health."

Box 26-2 summarizes dietary guidelines from the U.S. Senate Select Committee, the American Heart Association, the National Cancer Institute, and the American Cancer Society.

BOX 26-2—UNITED STATES DIETARY GUIDELINES

- Eat a variety of foods.
- Maintain ideal weight.
- Limit daily total fat intake.
- Limit cholesterol intake.
- Increase protein intake.
- Limit sodium intake.
- Consume 25 to 35 grams of fiber each day from a variety of sources.
- Increase consumption of fruits, vegetables, and whole grains.
- Keep salt-cured, smoked, and nitrate-cured foods to a minimum.
- Decrease consumption of refined and other processed sugars and foods high in such sugars.
- Decrease consumption of animal fat; choose meats, poultry, and fish that reduce saturated fat intake.
- Except for young children, substitute low-fat and nonfat milk for whole milk and low-fat dairy products for high-fat dairy products.
- Decrease consumption of butterfat, eggs, and other high-cholesterol sources.

Chemicals, food additives, salt, sugar, and alcohol by themselves perhaps should not cause alarm. However, when you consider the combined effect of these factors, it is easy to understand how diet mismanagement leads to major health problems.

Healthy People 2010

The nation's health care goals are stated in a document entitled **Healthy People 2010**. It was compiled with the input of health care professionals, consumers, researchers, academic professionals, clergy, and policy makers. It targets the following 28 areas:

1. Access to quality health services
2. Arthritis, osteoporosis, and chronic back conditions
3. Cancer
4. Chronic kidney disease
5. Diabetes
6. Disability and secondary conditions
7. Educational and community-based programs
8. Environmental health
9. Family planning and sexual health
10. Food safety
11. Health communication
12. Heart disease and stroke
13. HIV
14. Immunization and infectious diseases
15. Injury and violence protection

16. Maternal, infant, and child health
17. Medical product safety
18. Mental health and mental disorders
19. Nutrition
20. Occupational safety and health
21. Oral health
22. Physical activity and fitness
23. Public health infrastructure
24. Respiratory diseases
25. Sexually transmitted diseases
26. Substance abuse
27. Tobacco use
28. Vision and hearing

Healthy People 2010 is a comprehensive, nationwide health promotion and disease prevention agenda. It contains 467 objectives for the 28 focus areas listed above. The primary goals are to increase quality and years of healthy life and to eliminate health disparities (Box 26-3).

Preventable conditions could save the nation billions at a time when there will be fewer workers to pay the bills for expensive diagnoses and treatment. Injuries cost more than $100 billion annually, cancer costs more than $70 billion, and cardiovascular disease costs more than $135 billion.

Good health comes from reducing unnecessary suffering, illness, and disability; it stresses improved quality of life and a sense of well-being. Renewed efforts on all fronts will help the nation achieve its goals. Ultimately, individual lifestyle choices will be the determining factor. For the student who is contemplating a career in health care, a healthy lifestyle will not only result in a happier, more productive education and working life, but it will also set an example for patients and coworkers.

THE HEALTH CARE SYSTEM

Our health care system is laden with the values of our society. In the United States our health care system has many components. According to Torrens (1978), 10 basic elements are necessary for any complete health care system:
1. Public health/preventive medicine
2. Emergency medical care
3. Simple, nonemergency, ambulatory patient care
4. Complex, ambulatory patient care
5. Simple, inpatient hospital care
6. Complex, inpatient hospital care
7. Long-term, continuing care and rehabilitation
8. Care for social, emotional, and developmental problems
9. Transportation
10. Financial compensations for disability

BOX 26-3—*HEALTHY PEOPLE 2010 GOALS*

1. Increase moderate daily physical activity to at least 30% of people
2. Reduce sedentary lifestyles to no more than 15% of people
3. Reduce overweight to a prevalence of no more than 20% of people
4. Reduce dietary fat intake to an average of 30% of calories
5. Reduce cigarette smoking to no more than 15% of adults
6. Reduce initiation of smoking to no more than 15% by age 20
7. Reduce alcohol-related crash deaths to no more than 8.5 per 100,000 people
8. Reduce alcohol use by school children age 12-17 to less than 13%; reduce marijuana use by youth age 18-25 to less than 8%; reduce cocaine use by youth age 18-25 to less than 3%
9. Reduce teen pregnancies to no more than 50 per 1000 girls age 17 and younger
10. Reduce suicides to no more than 10.5 per 100,000 people
11. Reduce adverse effects of stress to less than 35% of people
12. Reduce homicides to no more than 7.2 per 100,000 people
13. Provide quality health education in grades K-12 in at least 75% of schools
14. Provide employee health promotion activities in at least 86% of work-places with 50 or more employees
15. Reduce unintentional injury deaths to no more than 29.3 per 100,000 people
16. Increase automobile safety restraint use to at least 85% of occupants
17. Reduce work-related injury deaths to no more than 4 per 100,000 workers
18. Reduce work-related injuries to no more than 6 per 100 workers
19. Increase protection from air pollutants so that at least 85% of people live in counties that meet EPA standards
20. Increase protection from radon so that at least 40% of people live in homes found to be safe
21. Reduce the prevalence of dental caries to no more than 35% of children by age 8
22. Reduce infant mortality to no more than 7 deaths per 1,000 live births
23. Reduce coronary heart disease deaths to no more than 100 per 100,000 people
24. Reduce stroke deaths to no more than 20 per 100,000 people
25. Increase control of high blood pressure to at least 50% of people with the condition
26. Reduce blood cholesterol to an average of no more than 200 mg/100 ml
27. Reduce the rise in cancer deaths to no more than 130 per 100,000 people
28. Increase frequency of clinical breast examinations and mammography to every 2 years to at least 60% of women age 50 and older
29. Increase frequency of Pap tests to every 1-3 years to at least 85% of women age 18 and older
30. Increase frequency of fecal occult blood testing to every 1-2 years to at least 50% of people age 50 and older
31. Reduce disability from chronic conditions to no more than 8% of people
32. Reduce diabetes-related deaths to no more than 34 per 100,000 people
33. Confine HIV infection to no more than 800 per 100,000 people
34. Reduce gonorrhea infections to no more than 225 per 100,000 people

Continued

35. Reduce syphilis infections to no more than 10 per 100,000 people
36. Eliminate measles
37. Reduce epidemic-related pneumonia and influenza deaths to no more than 7.3 per 100,000 people age 65 and older
38. Increase childhood immunization levels to at least 90% of 2 year olds
39. Eliminate financial barriers to clinical preventive services
40. Develop and implement common health status indicators

Even with the necessary elements, such a system is useless unless the patient has the desire and confidence to use it. The patient's attitude is often determined by the demeanor and attitude of the health care provider. As a radiologic technologist, you have the opportunity to educate your patients about a particular radiologic examination and to inform them of other health care services, how they can be reached, and the value of the services. You can help educate people about their own health care and show them how to become more directly responsible for their lives and health; this is an example of total patient care and value-added service.

Traditionally, health care has been practiced in hospitals that offer a full range of services, from diagnostic testing to surgery and drug therapy. The emphasis has been on medical intervention. However, hospitals, along with businesses, are now heavily involved in wellness programs. They have also modified their traditional services to reflect a changing market. Outpatient clinics account for more diagnostic testing and simple treatment and cost far less than being admitted to a hospital emergency department. Many forms of surgery are performed on an outpatient basis. The graduate radiologic technologist of the near future will likely practice in an urgent care clinic, a group physicians imaging center, or an ambulatory care institution in addition to a conventional acute care hospital.

Hospitals respect the rights of their primary customer—the patient. It is recognized that patients are not just creatures to whom we are "doing things"; they are dignified individuals with emotions and feelings, likes and dislikes. In support of this attitude, the American Hospital Association adopted the *Patient's Bill of Rights*.

Alternate health care practices include acupuncture, touch therapy, and biofeedback. Many hospitals perform diagnostic radiologic examinations for chiropractic physicians.

The health care system in the United States is in a constant state of change as the new century dawns. Most of the issues presented in this chapter are being debated daily. Some will be resolved, and others will not. Many will be decided by the U.S. Congress and ruled on by the judiciary. Diagnostic procedures and methods of patient care are evolving as quickly as researchers can verify results. Health care delivery is changing faster than textbooks can be revised. Many of today's common treatments and procedures were at one time subject to ridicule, skepticism, and evaluation. Furthermore, approximately 85% of the technology in a hospital today had not been invented 10 years ago.

Radiologic technologists must draw on their years of education and experience to keep an open mind to the social and technologic changes as new methods of patient care and treatment enter the health care arena. It is hoped that all forms of medicine—preventive, interventional, and alternative—will come together for the benefit of all patients. You have chosen a career that can help fulfill this hope.

THE BEGINNING OF YOUR CHALLENGE

The status of health care delivery in no small part depends on you. Your work ethic, dedication to excellence, and unwillingness to provide anything but the best patient care and quality service are of paramount importance.

As you begin clinical education, establish your reputation immediately. Work hard, do more than is expected, and your patients and potential employers will take notice. Your patients will reward you with their gratitude, spoken or unspoken. Your potential employers, who are the clinical supervisors and department heads in radiology, begin making hiring decisions very early in the educational process; their reward may well be your first job in radiography. Most importantly, your dedication to excellence and hard work will build your self-esteem and confidence.

The challenge is there for those who want to meet it. As the web of health care delivery becomes more tangled, it will become more important for each health care worker to realize the important roles that all members of the team play. Professionalism should not be your goal; rather, professionalism is the path to follow toward your other goals. It is something to be practiced each and every day. True professionals rise to meet the challenges. They treat patients as guests and send them on their way feeling as if each one was the most important person cared for that day.

You are beginning a vitally important educational process. You are not "in training" for anything. Training tells you how to do something, but education tells you why you are doing it. Learning the technology that comprises radiography is essential to your practice. Dealing with patients and their families—and even your coworkers—with human warmth, understanding, and genuine caring will be vital to your satisfaction and the success of your career. Establishing good study habits and clinical behavior right from the start will help you greatly when the time comes to enter that job market.

CONCLUSION

The authors of this book hope to have gotten you off to a good start with this text, whether you are studying to make a career choice or are already beginning your radiography education. Thousands before you have used this book to begin their journey. Return to it again for reference or review; use it to explain to friends and family what it is you are studying to become; recruit new student radiologic technologists—the future of our profession—by sharing this book with them.

This is indeed the beginning of your challenge. You have many months of exciting work ahead of you. Hopefully, throughout your educational program or at least during the second year of your radiography education, you and I will interact again in *Mosby's Comprehensive Review of Radiography*. Until then, do more than is required during your educational process, and you will meet with a degree of success that you can only imagine today.

Review Questions

1. At the start of 2000, how many older adults required care in the United States?
   a. 1 million
   b. 5 million
   c. 7.2 million
   d. 10 million
2. What is a payment system that determines costs and payments before delivery of service called?
   a. Retrospective payment
   b. PPO
   c. Prospective payment
   d. Pay as you go
3. The single largest cost in providing medical care is:
   a. High-technology equipment.
   b. Computers.
   c. Disposable supplies.
   d. Labor.
4. When do most individuals incur the majority of their health care expenditures?
   a. Between the ages of 1 and 30
   b. During the final year of life
   c. Between the ages of 50 and 60
   d. If they are born premature
5. The number of workers available to pay into government or private health insurance plans is:
   a. Rising.
   b. At its highest point in history.
   c. Leveling.
   d. Falling.
6. Radiographic examinations performed for the sole purpose of avoiding litigation is an example of:
   a. Quality assurance.
   b. Defensive medicine.

c. Uncertain physicians.

    d. Total quality management (TQM).

7. Lifestyle choices account for what percentage of early deaths in the United States?

    a. 10%

    b. 25%

    c. More than 50%

    d. 75%

8. The lifestyle factor(s) that has/have the largest role in relation to the management of good health are:

    a. Diet and smoking.

    b. Exercise.

    c. Alcohol.

    d. Seat belts.

9. Annually, smoking-related illnesses cost Americans:

    a. More than $65 billion.

    b. Up to $25 billion.

    c. $1 billion.

    d. $13 billion.

10. Increasingly, entry-level radiologic technologists are working in:

    a. Imaging centers.

    b. Physician offices.

    c. Urgent care clinics.

    d. All of the above.

BIBLIOGRAPHY

Healthy People 2010: Data 2010, the *Healthy People 2010* database, National Center for Health Statistics, Centers for Disease Control and Prevention, United States Department of Health and Human Services, 2001, Atlanta, GA.

McLennan K, Meyer J: *Care and cost: current issues in health policy*, Boulder, CO, 1989, Westview Press.

Torrens PR: *The American health system issues and problems*, St. Louis, 1978, Mosby.

U.S. Select Committee on Nutrition and Human Needs, 1978.

Appendix

Answers to review questions

Chapter 1

1. d
2. c
3. b
4. c
5. d
6. a
7. c
8. b
9. b
10. a

Chapter 2

1. b
2. c
3. a
4. c
5. d
6. c
7. d
8. a
9. b
10. b
11. c
12. c
13. d

Chapter 3

1. b
2. c
3. c
4. c
5. a
6. d
7. c
8. a
9. d
10. d

Chapter 4

1. b
2. d
3. c
4. d
5. b
6. a
7. c
8. b
9. c
10. c

Chapter 5

1. a
2. e
3. d
4. c
5. b
6. c
7. a
8. c
9. b
10. b

Chapter 6

1. c
2. d
3. a
4. c
5. d
6. b
7. d
8. b
9. b
10. c

Chapter 7

1. b
2. h
3. d
4. a
5. c
6. b
7. a, b
8. a
9. c
10. b
11. d
12. c

Chapter 8

1. b
2. c
3. c
4. b
5. c
6. d
7. a
8. c
9. b
10. c

Chapter 9

1. c
2. e
3. c
4. d
5. b
6. c
7. b
8. d
9. e
10. a

Chapter 10

1. b
2. d
3. d
4. b
5. d
6. c
7. a
8. a
9. d
10. d

Chapter 11

1. d
2. a
3. a
4. d
5. d
6. b
7. c
8. c
9. d
10. c
11. d
12. b
13. d
14. b
15. b

Chapter 12

1. c
2. d
3. d
4. c
5. d
6. d
7. d
8. a
9. c
10. d

Chapter 13

1. c
2. c
3. b
4. b
5. d
6. a
7. d
8. c
9. c
10. a

Chapter 14

1. c
2. d

3. b
4. d
5. b
6. d
7. c
8. d
9. c
10. b
11. d

Chapter 15

1. d
2. c
3. c
4. d
5. c
6. a
7. d
8. b
9. b
10. c

Chapter 16

1. d
2. d
3. c
4. c
5. d
6. a
7. c
8. d
9. b
10. b

Chapter 17

1. d
2. d
3. b
4. b
5. c
6. c
7. a

8. d
9. b
10. c

Chapter 18

1. d
2. c
3. c
4. b
5. b
6. d
7. c
8. d
9. a
10. d
11. c
12. c
13. a
14. c
15. b

Chapter 19

1. d
2. c
3. b
4. d
5. a
6. b
7. b
8. d
9. c
10. a

Chapter 20

1. b
2. d
3. d
4. d
5. d
6. a
7. c
8. b

9. b
10. d

Chapter 21

1. d
2. d
3. d
4. d
5. d
6. d
7. b
8. a
9. c
10. a
11. d
12. d
13. a
14. a
15. d
16. d
17. d
18. a

Chapter 22

1. d
2. a
3. b
4. a
5. e
6. b
7. e
8. c
9. e
10. d

Chapter 23

1. d
2. b
3. c
4. b
5. c
6. d

7. d
8. c
9. c
10. d

Chapter 24

1. b
2. d
3. d
4. b
5. b
6. c
7. c
8. c
9. d
10. c
11. d
12. c

Chapter 25

1. c
2. d
3. b
4. c
5. b
6. c
7. d
8. b
9. d
10. c

Chapter 26

1. e
2. c
3. d
4. b
5. d
6. b
7. c
8. e
9. a
10. e

Glossary

academic course A course of study offered by an accredited postsecondary educational institution, such as a college

accreditation The process that a health care institution, provider, or program undergoes to demonstrate compliance with standards developed by an official agency

acquired immunodeficiency syndrome (AIDS) A contagious disease contracted through bodily fluids, sexual intercourse, and blood contamination

affective learning Relating to a person's feelings and emotions such as joy, sadness, evenness, or natural impulses

allied health A group of specialized and highly technical health care workers; professions resulting from specialization because of advancements in science and technology

American College of Radiology (ACR) A professional organization of physicians specializing in radiology

American Healthcare Radiology Administrators (AHRA) An organization that helps promote the common goal of safe radiology

American Registry of Radiologic Technologists (ARRT) The organization that certifies and registers qualified radiologic technologists

American Society of Radiologic Technologists (ASRT) The professional organization for radiologic technologists

angiographer A physician engaged in radiography of the blood vessels of the body

annihilation reaction The reaction that occurs when a positron collides with a negative electron; both particles give up their energy to form two high-energy photons that travel in opposite directions

anode An electrode toward which negatively charged ions migrate

antiseptics Substances that prevent or retard the growth of microorganisms

arteriogram A radiographic study of the arteries of a particular body region

arthrogram A radiographic study of the structures in and around a joint

as low as reasonably achievable (ALARA) The basis for the National Council on Radiation Protection and Measurements (NCRP) policies and regulations

Association of Collegiate Educators in Radiologic Technology (ACERT) A professional organization that exists to provide forums for educators to share ideas, strategies, and solutions in their quest for excellence in radiologic science education

Association of Educators in Radiological Sciences (AERS) A professional organization of educators representing all of the radiation sciences

attention Concentrating on one activity to the exclusion of others

attitudes A mental position with regard to a fact or state; a feeling or emotion

background radiation Refers to radiation from the sun and stars, radioactive elements in the earth, and radioactive substances found in food, water, and air

barium An element used to provide radiographic contrast of gastrointestinal structures

barium enema A radiographic examination of the colon involving the use of a contrast agent

biennial Every 2 years (24 months)

body mechanics The action of muscles in producing body motion or posture

bone densitometry Uses x-ray energy to measure bone mineral density

carcinogenic Cancer-causing

cardiac arrest A state of complete cessation of the heart's action

cardiopulmonary resuscitation (CPR) Restoration of function of the heart and lungs after apparent death

career mobility The progress of an individual from one career group to another

carte blanche credits Discretionary credits awarded by an institution of higher learning

case law The law that arises from interpretation of our constitutions, statutes, and administrative regulations by judges; these interpretations are set forth in court opinions that result from the litigation of disputes between two or more parties

Category A This learning activity designation is based solely on whether the activity meets the criteria established by a recognized continuing education evaluation mechanism (RCEEM) and receives that RCEEM's approval

Category B Those learning activities that have not received RCEEM approval

cathode A filament that gives off electrons when heated

certificate of need (CON) A certificate issued by a review committee to the purchaser or applicant after the need for the equipment or expansion has been established and well-documented

certification A guarantee of qualifications indicated by the issuance of a certificate

cholangiogram A radiographic study of the bile ducts

civil assault A tort resulting from intentional conduct; occurs when a person has a reasonable fear of physical touch or injury as a result of another person's use or threat of force (e.g., telling a patient in a threatening voice to hold still)

civil battery A tort resulting from intentional misconduct; occurs when a person intentionally and inappropriately touches another person without consent (e.g., health care professionals treating a patient without that patient's valid consent)

clinical competency evaluation The standard used for evaluation of a student's work performance within the clinical laboratory setting; based on clearly-defined levels of expected performance of various essential tasks

cognitive learning The intellectual process by which knowledge is gained through various methods such as books, classwork, judgment reasoning, lectures, memory, or perception

collimation The restriction of the primary radiation to a limited area

collimator A device attached to the x-ray tube to reduce the exposure field size to the size of the film, thus protecting the patient from unwanted radiation

compliance Agreement with published educational standards, validated by the evaluation process

compliance evaluations Inspection and testing of x-ray units to ensure that performance is within the mandated and recommended safety standards

Compton scatter An interaction in matter in which the incident photon ejects an electron from its orbit, giving up only part of its energy and resulting in the photon's change in direction with less energy

computed tomography (CT) A radiographic cross-sectional electronically created image using a very small beam of radiation

confidentiality Maintaining privacy and reliance with entrusted patient information

conflict Tension resulting from disagreements of incompatible inner needs or drives

conflict resolution The solving of provider-customer problems; the tools of conflict resolution include listening, emphasizing, building trust, and developing solutions; these tools can also be used to solve interdepartmental conflicts

contagious diseases Diseases that may be contracted by direct or indirect contact with the pathogen causing the disease

continuing education credit (CE credit) Unit of measurement for continuing education activities; these credits are based on 1 50-minute contact hour

contrast A difference in radiographic densities that makes differentiation of structures possible

contrast media Solutions or gases introduced into the body to provide radiographic contrast between an organ and its surrounding tissue

controlled environment An artificial environment to verify the results of an experiment

convulsions Violent, involuntary muscular contractions; spasms

creed A set of fundamental beliefs

critical thinking Making wise decisions based on a set of universally accepted values

curie (Ci) The amount of activity known as radioactive disintegration that a radionuclide gives off

customer service cycle The patient's entire care experience; the cycle includes any interaction the patient has with the radiology department

cystogram A radiographic study of the bladder

cytotechnologist One who stains, mounts, and evaluates human cells to determine cellular variations and abnormalities such as cancer and other physiologic changes

defendant The person being sued in a lawsuit

defensive medicine Any waste of resources that results from a change in physicians' patterns of practice due to the threat of malpractice

densitometer A device used to measure the density of a radiograph (i.e., the amount of light transmitted through the radiograph)

density The logarithm of opacity; the opacity is the ratio of the amount of light incident on the film to the amount of light transmitted by the film; a measure of the black metallic silver on the film after processing

deoxyribonucleic acid (DNA) A genetic material in the nucleus of all cellular organisms

detail The distinctness with which images of structures are recorded on the radiograph

developer solution A combination of chemicals in the film-processing unit to develop the latent image of a radiograph to a visible image

diagnosis-related groups (DRGs) Medicare's system of reimbursement; payment is limited to a set amount allocated to a specific diagnosis

diet A lifestyle factor relating to good health

dietitian One who applies the principles of nutrition and management in administering institutional food service programs, plans special diets at physicians' requests, and instructs individuals and groups about the application of nutrition principles in the selection of food

digital imaging Images generated by a computer where a numerical value is assigned to a color or shade of gray.

dignity The state of honor, esteem, or being worthy

disease Disorder of bodily functions; the pattern of response to an injury

disinfectants Substances used to destroy pathogens or render them inert

distortion Uneven magnification; a misrepresentation of the true shape of the object

diversity The condition of being different or having differences.

dosimetry A measure of radiation dose to an individual

educational standards The published standards providing the criteria with which educational programs must comply in achievement and maintenance of accreditation

effective dose equivalent (EDE) The absorbed dose multiplied by the appropriate quality factor and measured in rems or sieverts

effective listening An important tool in conflict resolution; effective listening includes establishing eye contact; using face, voice, and body to express concern; and avoiding interrupting

emancipation Freedom from restraint or influence

emancipatory learning Becoming aware of the forces that have created the circumstances in one's life and taking action to change them

emergency medical personnel Those who administer basic life-support skills and therapy in emergency situations through radio communication with a physician

emerging infectious diseases Diseases of infectious origin whose incidence in humans has either increased within the past two decades or threatens to increase in the near future

emotionality The quality or state of a sound emotional balance

empathy The understanding and acceptance of another person's feelings or experience

epidemic Affecting many persons at once. An outbreak or product of sudden rapid growth or development.

equated scores The taking into account of test-item difficulty and the ability level of each group taking the test

erythema dose An obsolete term describing the amount of radiation required to redden the skin

esophagram A radiographic study of the esophagus

events Those steps a patient takes to have a radiologic examination; these steps include making the appointment, arriving at the hospital, registering, having the examination performed, and being released

excretory urography Radiographic studies of the urinary system

exposure factors A term used to refer to the adjustment of voltage, amperage, distance, time, and other factors considered in the determination of producing a diagnostic radiographic study

external preparation Removing the patient's clothing and jewelry before radiography

fainting A sudden fall of blood pressure with a loss of consciousness

false imprisonment A tort resulting from intentional misconduct; occurs when a person is restrained or confined without proper authorization or consent

film badge A holder containing a strip of radiographic film worn by personnel to measure the occupational exposure by measuring the degree of blackening of the film

film processing equipment Equipment used for developing the latent image on a radiograph after exposure to radiation; usually refers to automatic film-developing units

filters Aluminum plates used in radiography to filter out soft radiation and allow the hard, more penetrating radiation to pass through; used to protect the patient from radiation that would not aid in the production of the image

fixer solution A combination of chemicals in the processing unit that removes unexposed silver bromide crystals from the film and hardens the film emulsion for preservation of the image

flowchart A chart used by administration to show pathways for routing or sequencing work unit activities; may be used to indicate personnel mobility or positions

fluoroscopic studies Radiographic studies obtained using a fluoroscope

fluoroscopy A procedure using x-rays to image inner parts of the body in movement and motion

focal spot The spot or source from which x-rays originate

formative evaluations In-depth individualized assessments of knowledge

gonad The general term describing both male and female reproductive organs

gravity line An imaginary vertical line that passes through the center of gravity; a term that refers to the center of gravity when a person is in the standing position

grid A device placed between the cassette and patient designed to absorb the multidirectional scatter radiation but allow the straight line radiation through to strike the film

health The state of complete physical, mental, and social well-being

health maintenance organizations (HMOs) Third-party payers that offer, for a monthly fee, all necessary medical care at no additional charge

Healthy People 2010 A document encompassing the nation's health care goals in 28 areas

herd instinct A natural cohesiveness within a social group

hierarchy of human needs An arrangement of needs into a graded or valued series, from the most basic to the highly complex

histologic technician One who sections, stains, mounts, and identifies human tissues for microscopic study

hospital safety committee A committee representative of a broad scope of activities for developing and monitoring safety in all areas of the hospital, such as electrical systems, sanitation and infection control, waste disposal, and fire and other disaster safety plans

human-made radiation Radiation emitted from human-made radioactive sources as developed at nuclear plants (e.g., ^{60}Co, ^{131}I)

hysterosalpingogram A radiographic study of the uterus and fallopian tubes

image intensifier A device that electronically improves and enhances radiographic images and transmits them to a television monitor

incidents Those steps the radiographer takes in performing an examination on a patient

independent clinical performance Work that is done by the individual without supervision; this may involve simple and/or complex levels of problem solving and decision making relative to completing the tasks

in-service education Education provided by the institution in knowledge, information, and skills related to specific tasks, policies, and procedures

inside customers Those patients who come to the radiology department from inside the hospital

intensifying screen A sheet of plastic embedded with phosphors

interaction To act on each other, often with reciprocal influence; may involve verbal and nonverbal communications systems with two or more individuals

internal preparation Using enemas to cleanse the abdomen so internal structures can be viewed radiographically

interventional radiography A growing subspecialty of special procedures that aids in patient treatment by taking the place of surgery or complementing the surgical process; certification by ARRT

iodine An element used to provide radiographic contrast between organs and blood vessels

ionizing radiation A term applied to radiation having sufficient energy to produce ions (i.e., displace electrons from atoms); x-rays are one form of ionizing radiation

isolation room A place to confine the diseased patient to protect the patient from microorganisms carried by people entering the room or to protect other patients or people working with the patient

kilovoltage An electrical factor that controls the energy of the x-ray beam; 1,000 volts

latent period The time between the initial irradiation and the occurrence of any biologic change

license Agency- or government-granted permission that is issued to an individual to engage in a given occupation on finding that the applicant has attained the degree of competency necessary to ensure that the public health, safety, and welfare are reasonably well-protected

life cycle cost The acquisition cost of the equipment plus the cost of maintaining it through its useful life

long-term memory The memory-storing process requiring organization and association of information

lymphocyte A mature white blood cell

magnetic resonance imaging (MRI) The cross-sectional/three-dimensional imaging modality that creates digital images by the use of a strong magnetic field and radio waves instead of radiation

mammogram A radiographic study of the breast

mammography Radiographic examination of the breast requiring the use of specialized equipment; certification by ARRT

maudlin Tearful, often weakly emotional; effusively or foolishly sentimental; lachrymose

Medicaid Government health insurance for the poor

medical records personnel Those who plan, design, develop, and manage patient-information systems, administrative and clinical statistical data, and patient medical records in all types of health care institutions

medical technologist One who is skilled in chemical laboratory analysis and complex and specialized tests for the diagnosis and treatment of disease

Medicare Government health insurance for older adults

memory retrieval Recalling, recovering, or obtaining events and experiences stored in memory

memory storage Recording of facts, images, sounds, pleasure, pain, other life experiences in the memory

milliamperage An electrical factor that controls the amount of x-ray produced; 1,000th of 1 ampere

milliampere-seconds (mAs) The term used to express the amount of radiation; milliamperage multiplied by time

mnemonics Assisting or intending to assist memory; a technique to improve memory

mobile unit An x-ray machine designed for easy movement for radiographing patients outside the radiology department (e.g., in surgery or on the wards)

modesty Propriety of dress, speech, or conduct

moments of truth Those times in which a patient forms an opinion concerning quality of service

morbidity The occurrence of disease; a diseased state

mortality The rate of death from various conditions

multiphase generator A generator operating on more than single-phase power; usually has three phases, which greatly increase the amount of x-ray produced per unit time

myelogram A radiographic study of the subarachnoid space of the spinal cord

negligence A breach or failure to fulfill a required standard of care; a medical standard of care is determined by the degree of care or skill a reasonable medical professional would have provided under the circumstances

nosocomial infection A hospital-related disease

nuclear medicine The diagnosis and/or treatment of a disease process by the administration of a radioactive material to a patient or patient's specimen

nuclear medicine technologist A health care professional whose duties include positioning and attending to patients undergoing nuclear medicine procedures, operating imaging devices, and other duties under the direction of a nuclear physician

nuclear radiology The branch of radiology that uses radioactive materials for diagnosis and treatment

nursing profession The oldest, largest, and most readily identified of the health professions, other than medicine

objectivity The quality or state of being able to interpret a situation from an unbiased point of view rather than from one's own subjective view

Occupational Safety and Health Administration (OSHA) A federal organization responsible for establishing safety standards for the workplace; an environmental watch to guard against pollution and waste-disposal hazards

occupational therapist One who evaluates the self-care, work-and-play/leisure tasks, and performance skills of disabled clients; plans and implements programs, social activities, and interpersonal activities designed to restore, develop, and maintain the client's ability to perform the daily-living tasks

organizational chart A chart depicting established lines of authority, responsibility, and accountability

outside customers Those patients that come to the radiology department from outside the hospital

pair production A photon of extremely high energy approaching the nucleus of an atom, which results in energy given up to form two particles—a positron and a negative electron

pandemic disease occuring over a wide geographic area and affecting an exceptionally high proportion of the population.

passive participation Present in a situation but not physically participating or contributing in any way other than as a listener or an observer

pathogen Any virus, microorganism, or other substance causing disease

peer review A characteristic of the program review process conducted by a qualified site visit team and accrediting agencies

perceptions Observations, mental images; a result of perceiving

personal obligation An obligation relating to an individual's character, conduct, motive, or private affairs as opposed to obligations expected of an institution or organization

personality The characteristics that define a person's identity as determined by heredity and environment, including personal attitudes, interests, values, and knowledge

personnel monitoring Measuring the radiation exposure received by personnel in the performance of their duties

photoelectric effect An interaction of a photon in which all its energy is absorbed by an electron, resulting in the ejection of the electron from its orbit

physical therapist One who uses physical agents, as well as biomechanical and neurophysiologic principle and assistive devices in relieving pain and restoring function following disease, injury, or loss of a body part

physician assistant A health professional who, under the supervision of a physician, performs tasks usually conducted by the physician

plaintiff The person who initiates the lawsuit in a civil case

position description A term synonymous with job description but that connotes a broader scope of activities; defines the place on the organizational chart based on tasks and duties

prefix An affix attached to the beginning of a word, base, or phrase to create a word or inflectional form

primal stresses Original, first, or fundamental fight-or-flight response

probation A status that denotes noncompliance with mandated requirements; in radiologic technology this status is extended for 1 year following the noncompliant biennium regarding CE credits

procedures manual An in-house procedure and policy manual designed to meet accreditation standards, state and federal standards, and hospital codes

processing A term in radiography that refers to the steps involved in converting the latent image to a visible image

prospective payment system (PPS) The government's response to the high cost of health care; reimburses hospitals for tests and treatments for Medicare and Medicaid patients

psychologic care Receiving care for developing and maintaining a healthy balance between rational thoughts and emotion

psychomotor learning The muscular action or practical execution of previously learned material that is believed to come from a conscious mental activity

quality assurance A term synonymous with quality control but usually used to refer to the monitoring and testing of imaging equipment, as well as the control of variables in the clinical setting

quality assurance technologist A person who oversees a system of activities whose purpose is to provide assurance that overall quality control is being done effectively

rad (radiation absorbed dose) A unit of absorbed dose of any type of radiation

radiation safety committee A committee responsible for monitoring and maintaining a radiation-safe environment

radiation therapy The treatment of disease, usually cancer, with ionizing radiation produced by a tube or a radioactive source; certification by ARRT

radiation therapy technologist A health care professional who delivers radiation therapy as prescribed by a radiation oncologist

radioactivity The property of certain elements to spontaneously emit rays or subatomic particles from matter

radiologic technologist A health care professional skilled in the theory and practice of the technical aspects of the use of x-rays and the diagnosis and treatment of diseases

Radiological Society of North America (RSNA) A professional organization for radiologists

radiologist A physician specializing in the medical science dealing with the use of x-rays, radioactive substances, and other forms of radiation energy in diagnosis and treatment of disease

radiologist assistant (RA) A supplement to radiologists assisting in fluoroscopy, special procedures, patient handling, and other tasks traditionally performed by radiologists

rare earth phosphors screens Screens made of phosphors such as lanthanum, gadolinium, lithium, and yttrium, which have to some extent replaced conventional screens made of calcium tungstate phosphors

Recognized Continuing Education Evaluation Mechanism (RCEEM) The control process for checking that educational activities meet certain standards; recognized RCEEM organizations have established programs for evaluating educational opportunities and activities

registered technologist A graduate technologist documented and officially qualified to practice radiography

registration An official entry on a list of people certified as eligible by qualifications

reinforcement behavior Shaping or modifying behavior by rewarding the desired behavior

rem (roentgen-equivalent-man) A unit measuring the biologic effect of x-, alpha, beta, and gamma radiation on humans

res ipsa loquitur "The thing speaks for itself"; this doctrine applies to a situation that suggests that an injury could not have occurred if there had been no negligence (e.g., leaving a pair of forceps in the patient's abdomen after surgery)

respiratory therapist A health care professional who administers respiratory therapy, testing, emergencies, and medication

respondeat superior "Let the master answer"; this doctrine requires that an employer pay victims for the torts committed by the employees

retakes A common term indicating a repeat of an examination because of inadequate technical quality

roentgen (R) A quantity of x-rays or gamma radiation that would produce ions in 1 cubic centimeter of air; one electrostatic unit of either sign

root The basis from which a word is derived

rote memorization To learn word by word; to learn by heart or repeat by heart or rote

scaled scores A process by which examination takers of comparable ability taking different versions of the examination can be given the same reported score

scope of practice A term used to describe, delineate, and define the boundaries of duties and responsibilities of the practicing professional

seizure An attack such as a convulsion

self-discipline Control over emotions and actions

self-study The period of time in which the program reviews all aspects of its operation and its outcomes to determine both its assessment of its degree of compliance with the standards as well as measuring its outcomes against its unique mission and goals

sensitometer A device used to expose films precisely so that each film will have the same density, provided the processor chemicals, temperature, and other variables remain constant

shock The profound depression of vital functions, with reduced blood volume and pressure

short-term memory Transient, fleeting memory that fades rapidly

sialogram A radiographic study of the salivary glands

silver reclamation The act of recovering silver from discarded radiographic film or from solutions (fixer) during the processing of the latent image

site visit The visit in which a JRCERT team is charged with verifying that the self-study report is an accurate portrayal of the program's operation and with evaluating the program's compliance with the established educational standards

smoking A lifestyle factor relating to good health

solicitous Full of fears, concerned, anxiously willing; manifesting or expressing solicitude or concern; may seem somewhat exaggerated in expression

sonography The diagnosis and/or treatment of a disease process, or the imaging of a certain condition such as pregnancy by the administration of high-frequency sound waves; certification by ARDMS

special procedures radiography The radiographic evaluation of the circulatory and nervous system by administering a contrast medium to demonstrate the anatomic structures not visualized on normal radiographs; certification by ARRT

sphygmomanometer An instrument used to measure blood pressure

Standards for an Accredited Program in Radiologic Sciences (STANDARDS) The standards that a program must meet to qualify for accreditation

standards of conduct Behavior established by custom or law; recognized and approved behavior

sterilization The destruction of all microorganisms in or about an object

stethoscope An instrument to aid in the respiratory and cardiac sounds in the chest or other body areas

stress A physical, chemical, or emotional factor that causes bodily or mental tension

subject contrast The contrast inherent in the anatomic part being radiographed; a factor of atomic number and the density or weight per unit mass

suffix An affix attached to the end of a word, base, or phrase

summative evaluations In-depth appraisals of knowledge resulting in final grades or certifying examination

Summit on Radiologic Sciences and Sonography A coalition of organizations that represents over 350,000 health care professionals

tomography A radiographic procedure in which the x-ray tube and film is set in motion during exposure to blur structures above and below the body part of interest

tort A civil wrong, as opposed to a criminal wrong, involving a breach of duty or standard of care that results in injury; can be intentional or unintentional

troubleshooting Solving problems by thinking of all possible causes and ruling them out individually

ultrasonography Radiologic technique in which deep structures of the body are visualized by recording the reflections (echoes) of ultrasonic waves directed into the tissues

upper gastrointestinal (GI) series Radiographic studies of the upper GI tract

U.S. Department of Health and Human Services A government department with the responsibility for providing health care and other human-needs services to citizens; also manages Medicare and Medicaid programs

venogram A radiographic study of the veins in a particular area of the body

vital signs Blood pressure, temperature, pulse, and respiration

x-ray film A sheet of polyester plastic, coated with a thin layer of gelatin and silver compounds

x-ray tube An evacuated glass bulb with positive (anode) and negative (cathode) electrodes

Index

A

Abbreviations, medical, 111-113
Abdomen, radiographic studies, 131
Academic courses, CE credits of, 378
Acceptance limits
  broad, 241f
  high, 241f
  on radiographs, 239-240
  of radiologic technologist, 240-241
  of radiologist, 230-240, 240f
Accreditation, 298, 363-364
  history of, 299-300
  by Joint Review Committee on
    Education in Radiologic
    Technology, 302-305
ACERT. *See* Association of Collegiate
    Educators in Radiologic
    Technology.
Acquired immunodeficiency syndrome
    (AIDS), 185
ACR. *See* American College of
    Radiology.
Acute radiation syndrome, 255
ADC (analog-to-digital converter), 115
Administrative radiology, in
    professional development, 319,
    359-360
Administrative responsibilities,
    radiology department, 206-207
Advanced life support certification, 374
AERS. *See* Association of Educators in
    Radiological Sciences.
Affective learning, 97
Agreement of Candidates, for ARRT
    certification, 289, 290b-291b
AHRA. *See* American Healthcare
    Radiology Administrators
    (AHRA).
AHRA Link, 319
AIDS (acquired immunodeficiency
    syndrome), 185, 382

Air
  as contrast agent, 129, 153-154
  radiographic density of, 146f
Air-contrast barium enema, 132
ALARA (as low as reasonably
    achievable), 249
Alcohol, risks associated with, 387
Allied health profession(s), 269-281
  bibliography on, 281
  cytotechnologist as, 273-274
  dental hygienist as, 278-279
  emergency medical
    technician/paramedic as, 277-278
  histotechnologist as, 273
  medical records administrator as,
    274-275
  medical technologist as, 271-273
  and nursing, 270-271
  nutritionist and dietetian as, 275-276
  occupational therapist, 276-277
  physical therapist as, 276
  physician assistant as, 277
  respiratory therapist as, 277
  review questions on, 280-281
  and team approach to health care,
    279-280
Alpha particles, 331
American Board of Health Physicists, 365
American Board of Radiology, 365
American College of Radiology (ACR),
    285, 299, 316, 318
  radiologist assistant program
    developed by, 385-359
American Healthcare Radiology
    Administrators (AHRA), 318, 319
American Medical Association, Council
    on Medical Education and
    Hospitals, 299
American Registry of Diagnostic
    Medical Sonographers
    (ARDMS), 337, 372
American Registry of Radiologic
    Technologists (ARRT), 100,
    285-296
  agreement signing with, 289

American Registry of Radiologic
    Technologists (ARRT)—cont'd
  application forms from, 289
  bibliography on, 296
  certification examination of, 100,
    285-296, 372-374
  certification examination procedures
    of, 287
  certification examination scheduling
    with, 289
  certification handbook of, 287
  continuing education requirements of,
    371-376. *See also* Continuing
    education.
    noncompliance with, 376
  history of, 286-287, 361
  organization of, 287
  registry examination creation by, 289,
    292
  renewal of registration with, 373-376
  review questions on, 295-296
  score report from, 292-294
  specialty certification with, 294,
    328-329
American Society for Therapeutic
    Radiology and Oncology, 318
American Society of Radiologic
    Technologists (ASRT), 285, 299,
    314-316, 361
  affiliates of, state and local,
    317-318
  annual conference of, 315
  Clinical Competency Evaluation of,
    97-104
  curriculum guide published by, 93-96
  Job Description and Scope of
    Practice of
    for Diagnostic Medical
      Sonographer, 338b-339b
    for Nuclear Medicine Technologist,
      334b-335b
    for Radiation Therapist, 330b-331b
    for Radiologic Technologist, 326b-
      327b
  licensing legislation promoted by, 317

American Society of Radiologic
    Technologists—cont'd
organization of, 314-316
position descriptions of, 206-207
practice standards of, 316-317
publications of, 315
radiologist assistant program
    developed by, 358-359
representation of, in other
    professional organizations,
    315-316
staffing and compensation of, 317
Amperage, 143-144
Analog-to-digital converter (ADC), 115
Analytical thinking, 51
Angiocardiography, 341
Angiographic suite, 219f
Angiography, 133, 340, 340f
Annihilation reaction, 252
Anode, 115, 119
Antiseptics, 185
Aortography, 341
Application form, for certification
    examination, 289
Application status report, ARRT
    certification, 289
Apprehension, patient, 231-232
Archimedes, 76
ARDMS. See American Registry of
    Diagnostic Medical
    Sonographers.
ARRT. See American Registry of
    Radiologic Technologists.
ARRT Certification Handbook, 287, 288
rules and regulations in, 289
Arteriography, 133, 340-341
Arthrogram, 133
Aseptic technique(s), 186-187
ASRT. See American Society of
    Radiologic Technologists.
Association of Collegiate Educators in
    Radiologic Technology
    (ACERT), 318-319
Association of Educators in
    Radiological Sciences (AERS),
    318
Atomic Energy Commission (AEC),
    248
Attention, 37-39
Attitudes, and reactions, patient,
    171-173
Automatic collimation, 115
Automatic exposure devices, 236-238,
    237f

B

Background radiation, 246
Barium, as contrast agent, 129, 153
Barium enema, 132
Barium platinocyanide coating, 77, 78,
    83

Barnard, Christiaan, 64
Basic life support certification, 182, 374
Beam alignment, x-ray, in radiographic
    quality, 156-157
Beam angle, x-ray, and film contrast,
    155-156, 156f
Beam-limiting devices, 149
    and image contrast, 155
Beaumont, William, 63
Becquerel, Henri, 83, 329
Becquerel (Bq) (unit), 247
Beliefs, personal, 52-54
Bergonie and Tribondeau
    findings of, in tissue response to
        radiation, 328
    law of, 254
Bernard, Claude, 63
Beta particles, 331
Bibliography for the Radiology
    Administrator, 319
Biologic effects, of ionizing radiation,
    252-257
Biotechnology, 66
Bloyd, Michael, 187
Blur, 115
Body mechanics, in patient transfer,
    183-184
Bone, radiographic density of, 145, 146f
Bone densitometry, 348
Boyle, Robert, 76
Breast tissue, lack of contrast in, 153f
Bucky, 115
Bucky slot, as source of scatter
    radiation, 263
Bureau of Radiological Health (FDA),
    248
Burger, Hans, 64

C

Calcium tungstate coating, 83
Cannon, Walter Bradford, 337
Carcinogenic effects, of ionizing
    radiation, 255-256
Cardiac arrest, 184
Cardiopulmonary resuscitation (CPR),
    182, 374
Cardiovascular interventional
    radiography, 133, 135,
    339-342
Cardiovascular interventional
    technology (CIT), practice
    standards in, 316-317
Career advancement. See Professional
    development opportunities.
Career mobility, 356
Carte blanche credits, 357
Case law, 192
Cassette, 115, 120, 120f, 121
Cassette holders, safe use of, 263
Category A, continuing education
    credits, 373

Category B, continuing education
    credits, 373
Cathode, 115, 119
Cathode ray development, 76-77
Cathode ray tube (CRT), 115
CE credits, 373-375. See also
    Continuing education.
    documentation of, 376
Cellular reaction, to ionizing radiation,
    252, 254
Centers for Disease Control and
    Prevention (CDC), 67
    emerging infectious disease control
        by, 72-73
    guidelines for isolation precautions
        of, 185-187
    as source of health statistics, 67-68
Cerebral angiographic study, 340f
Cerebral angiography, 341
Certificate of need, 218
Certification examination, ARRT,
    287-294, 372-374
    organizations creating, 289, 292
    qualifications and application for,
        287-289
    requirements of, 373-374
        meeting, 373-375
    scheduling, 289
    score report for, 292-294
    specialty, 293t, 294
Chemical solutions, maintaining, 233-234
China, medicine in ancient, 60
Christianity, beginnings of, and
    medicine, 61
Civil assault, 193
Civil battery, 193
Clinical Competency Evaluation
    (ASRT), 97-104
    criteria of, 100-104
    definition of, 97-98
    flow chart of process of, 101f
    grade sheet of, 102f
    sample checklist for, 99b-100f
Clinical participation, 98
Cobalt-60, 258
Code of ethics, 5
Cognitive learning, 97
Collimation, reducing radiation
    exposure with, 260-261
Collimator(s), 115, 119
    and radiographic density, 149
Communication
    and interaction, in patient care, 9b,
        12-16, 173
    in quality assurance, 242
Competency evaluation, American
    Society of Radiologic
    Technologists, 97-104
Competency requirements, for radiologic
    technologists, 238, 288
Complaint systems, 7

Compliance evaluations, radiologic, 211
Compromise, 29
Compton scatter, 251-252, 253f
Computed radiography (CR), 115
Computed tomography (CT), 84
  equipment used in, 121-122, 122f, 344-345
  history of, 343
  image production in, 85f
  practice standards in, 316-317
Computed tomography (CT) scan, 345f
Computed tomography (CT) scanner, 121-122, 122f, 344-345
  cost of, 219
Computed tomography (CT) technologist, 343
  education of, 345
  employment opportunities for, 346
  responsibilities of, 343-344
Computer science
  introduction to, course description, 96
  professional development in, 363
Concentration, mental, improving, 38-39
Cones, and radiographic density, 149
Confidentiality, patient, 173-174
  form for, 175f
Conflict, 29
  internal, 30
  management and resolution of, 16-18, 30-31
  reactions to, 30
Consent, patient, 198-200, 200-201
Consent form, 199f
Constantine (Emperor), 61
Consumer, patient as, 6-7, 10
Consumer trends, survey in health care, 10-12, 11b
Contagious disease(s), 185-186
Continuing education in radiology, 84-85, 104, 238, 313-323, 353-355, 371-372
  American Registry of Radiologic Technologist requirements for, 371-376
    approved programs, 377-378
    noncompliance, 376
  American Society of Radiologic Technologists in, 318
  areas of
    administrative radiology, 359-360
    commercial representative, 366
    computer science, 363
    equipment specialist, 365-366
    quality assurance, 363-364
    radiation safety, 364-365
    radiologic technologist educator, 360-363
    radiologist assistant, 358-359

Continuing education in radiology—cont'd
  associations supporting, 318-319
  bibliography on, 369
  and licensure requirements, 378-379
  noncompliance with, 376
  postgraduate
    certification and, 374-375
    long term, 357-358
    short term, 355-357
  review questions on, 367-368
Contrast, radiographic, 115, 151-156
  enhancement of, with contrast media, 153-155
  other factors in, 155-156
  and perceptibility of detail, 159
  radiation penetration and, 152
  short scale and long scale, 155
  in specialized radiographic procedures, 341
  tissue density and, 151-152
Contrast media, 128-129
  purpose of, 153-155
Control features, of radiographic machine, 141-144, 142f
Controlled environment, 28
Convulsion, 184
Cost, of health care. *See* Economics.
Cost-effectiveness, 223
coulomb/kg (C/kg), 247
CPR (cardiopulmonary resuscitation) certification, 182, 374
CR. *See* Computed radiography.
Creed, 172
Critical thinker
  description of, 51b
  qualities of, 50-52
Critical thinking, 49-50
  bibliography on, 56
  developing skills of, 49, 54-55
  influencing factors in, 52-54
  review questions on, 55-56
Crookes, William, 76-77
CRT (cathode ray tube), 115
CT. *See* Computed tomography.
CT technologist. *See* Computed tomography (CT) technologist.
Cultural diversity, 8
Curie, Marie, 63-64, 329
  research and medical advances of, 83, 360
Curie, Pierre, 63-64, 329
  research of, 83
curie (Ci), 247
Customer
  outside and inside, 10-12
  patient as, 6-7, 10-12. *See also* Customer service.

Customer service, patient care and, 6-9
  bibliography on, 19-20
  communication and interaction in, 9b, 12-16
  conflict resolution in, 16-18
  customer satisfaction in, 6-7, 10-12
  diversity in, human and cultural, 8-9
  empathy and effective listening in, 17-18
  events in, 13-15
  moments of truth in, 12
  quality of, 10
  review questions on, 19-20
  telephone communication in, 15-16
Customer service cycles, 12-15, 13b
Cyclotron, 84
Cystogram, 133
Cytotechnologist, 274
Cytotechnology, 273-274

D

da Vinci, Leonardo, 62
Davy, Humphry, 63
Defamation, 193
Defendant, 200
Defensive medicine, 385
Democritus, 76
Densitometer, 233, 233f
Density(ies), radiographic, 115, 144-145
  beam limiting devices and, 149, 150f
  definition of, 144
  detail and, 159
  distance from radiation source and, 147
  film characteristics and, 148, 148f
  filters and, 150-151
  fog and, 149
  grid use and, 150
  of human body, 145-146
  intensifying screens and, 148-149
  kilovoltage effect on, 146
  of metals, 145-146
  milliamperage effect on, 146-147
  processing method and, 149
  subject thickness and, 145-151
  time-of-exposure effect on, 147
Dental hygiene, 278-279
Dental hygienist, 278-279
Deoxyribonucleic acid (DNA), 252, 254
Detail, radiographic
  definition of, 158
  and quality of radiograph, 158-159
  factors in, 159-163
Detail visibility, 158
Developer, 140
Developer solution, 234
Diagnosis, radiologist responsibility for, 239

Diagnosis-related groups (DRGs), 222, 384
and efficiency of radiology department, 223
Diagnostic imaging, principles of, course description, 94
Diagnostic medical sonographer (RDMS)(ARDMS)
education and certification of, 337
Job Description and Scope of Practice of, ASRT, 338b-339b
responsibilities of, 336
Dietary guidelines, U. S., 388b
Dietitian, 275-276
Digital fluoroscopy, 121
Digital imaging, 84
Digital imaging and communications (DICOM), 115, 125
Digital imaging equipment, 119
Direct digital radiography (DR), 115
Direct-hit theory, 252
Directory of Registered Radiologic Technologists, 287
Disease, definition of, 67
Disinfectants, 185
Distance, from radiation source, and radiographic density, 147
Distortion, 115
and radiographic quality, 156-158
Divergent x-rays, and distance from radiation source, 147, 147f
Diversity, human and cultural, 8-9
DNA (deoxyribonucleic acid), 252, 254
Doppler sonography, 124
Dosimetry, 264
Dosimetry device, personal, 264, 264f
DR (direct digital radiography), 115
DRGs. *See* Diagnosis-related groups (DRGs).
DuFay, Charles, 76

E

Eastman, George, 77
Economics
of health care delivery, 382, 383-385
managing, 385-386
preventive medicine in, 387-389
of radiology department, 217-225
bibliography on, 225
certificate of need in, 218
equipment costs in, 219-220
Medicare prospective payment in, 222-223
radiographic quality in, 220-221
review questions on, 223-224
silver recovery in, 221-222
staffing in, 218-219
Edison, Thomas A., 80, 81, 83
Education, in-service, 377-378

Educational preparation, 93-96, 288.
See also American Registry of Radiologic Technologists; American Society of Radiologic Technologists; Continuing education.
bibliography on, 107
clinical, and training, 97-104
history of, 299-300
review questions on, 105-107
Educator, radiologic technology, 318-319, 360-363
Educator standards, of Joint Review Committee on Education in Radiologic Technology, 362-363
Effective dose equivalent (EDE), 248-249
maximum, for occupational exposure, 249t
Effective dose equivalent limits, 248-249
Effective listening, 17, 17b
patient response to, 18
Egypt, medicine in ancient, 59
Ehrlich, Paul, 64
Eighteenth century medicine, 62-63
Einstein, Albert, 83
Einthoven, Willem, 64
Electrical safety, 212
Electricity, experimentation with, 76
Electromagnetic induction, discovery of, 76
Electron microscope, 64, 65f
Electroscope, 76
Emancipatory learning, 50
Embalming practices, of Egyptians, 59
Emergency medical personnel, 277-278
Emergency medical technician, 277-278
Emerging infectious diseases, 71-73
outside United States, 72b
in United States, 72b
Emotional balance, 25
Emotional response, 53-54
Empathy, 17-18, 17b
Emulsion, film, 148, 148f
Endoscopic retrograde cholangiopancreatography (ERCP), 133
Entrepreneurs, professional, 177
Epidemic, definition of, 71
Equated scores, 292-293
Equipment, 84, 85f, 119
bibliography on, 126
for computed tomography, 121-122, 344-345
cost and economics of, 219-220
course description, 84, 85f, 94
digital imaging, 119
for film processing, 233-234

Equipment—cont'd
film-screen, 119-120
fluoroscopic, 121
imaging, 119-126, 340-341
for magnetic resonance imaging, 122
maintenance of, 213-214, 234
in nuclear medicine, 123, 332
orientation to, and handling of, 103, 235-236
pathogens on, 185
picture archiving and communication system with, 124-125
portable, 123-124
for positron emission tomography, 122-123
quality assurance assessment of, 232-235
radiographic, 234-235
review questions on, 125-126
for sonography, 124, 335-336
for specialized imaging, 121-125, 340-341
tomographic, 124
Equipment maintenance contracts, types of, 220
Erythema dose, 247
Esophagram, 132
Ethical aspects. *See also* Patient care.
of health care delivery, 66, 382-383
Evaluation, of radiologic technologists, 232, 238
Event(s), in patient care, 13-15, 13b
Examination for certification, ARRT, 287-294
creation of, 289, 292
qualifications and application for, 287-289
scheduling, 289
score report for, 292-294
specialty, 293t, 294
Examinations, radiographic, 127-137
Excretory urography, 131
Exercise, for optimal health, 25
Exposure
film (radiographic)
automatic devices for, 236-238, 237f
control of factors affecting, 236-238, 259
factors affecting, 141-144, 142f
and image evaluation, 104
and milliamperage, 146-147
principles of, course description, 95
and radiographic density, 148
speed of film and intensifying screens in, 148-149
to radiation, human. *See* Radiation exposure.
Exposure devices, film, automatic, 236-238, 237f

Exposure indicator, 115
External preparation, 128
Extremities, radiographic studies, 130-131

F

Fahrenheit, Gabriel Daniel, 62
Fainting, 184
False imprisonment, 193
  case example of, 198
Faraday, Michael, 76
Fat, radiographic density of, 145, 146f
Fermi, Enrico, 84
Fernel, Jean, 62
Fetus, exposure to radiation, 250, 250f
Fiber optics, 84
Film(s), radiographic, 84, 115, 120. *See also* Film exposure; Film processing.
  double emulsion, cross section of, 148
  evaluation of, course description, 95-96
  and screen combinations, 119-120
    reducing radiation exposure in, 260-261
  type of
    and contrast, 155
    and radiographic detail, 161
Film badge, 264, 264f
Film exposure
  automatic devices for, 236-238, 237f
  factors affecting, 141-144, 142f
    control of, 236-238
  and milliamperage, 146-147
  and radiographic density, 148
  speed of film and intensifying screens in, 148-149
Film processing, 140-141
  course description, 94
  detail in film, 159
  equipment for, 233-234
  and image contrast, 155
  method of, and radiographic density, 149
Film processor, 116, 140-141
Film-screen combinations, reducing radiation exposure in, 260-261
Film-screen system, 119-120
Film speed, 148
Filters (filtration), use of
  and image contrast, 155
  and radiographic density, 150-151
  reducing radiation exposure with, 259-261
Five rights, of giving medication, 187
Fixer, 141
Fixer solution, 234
Flanders, Ned, 39
Flow charts, radiology department, 207-208, 208f

Fluoroscopic studies, 131-133
  barium enema, 132
  endoscopic retrograde cholangiopancreatography, 133
  esophagogram, 132
  upper gastrointestinal series, 132
  urinary system studies, 133
Fluoroscopic x-ray tube, 257-258
Fluoroscopy, 121
  development of, 83
  portable, 123-124
Focal film distance. *See* Source-to-image distance.
Focal object distance. *See* Source-to-object distance.
Focal spot (focal track), 115, 159
  and radiographic detail, 159-160
Focus unsharpness, 160
Fog
  and detail, 159
  and image contrast, 155
  and radiographic density, 149, 150f
Forgetting, 43-44
Formative evaluations, 362
Franklin, Benjamin, 76
Frozen mindset, 53

G

Gadolinium, 149
Galileo, 62
Gamma rays, 331
Gas, radiographic density of, 145
Geiger-Muller counter, for radiation dosimetry, 264
Genetic effects, of ionizing radiation, 256-257
Genetic material, 252, 254
Genetics, current research in, 66
GI (upper gastrointestinal) series, 132
Gilbert, William, 76
Glucagon, 132
Gonad, 261
Gonad shielding devices, 261-262
Goodspeed, William, 77
Gravity line, and base support, 183
gray (Gy), 247
Greek medicine, ancient, 59, 60-61
Grid(s), 115
  and absorption of scattered radiation, 260
  image contrast, use of, 155
  and radiographic density, 150
Group loyalty, 53
Grubbe, Emil H., 327

H

Hales, Stephen, 62
Hand, radiograph of, 145f
Harvey, William, 62
Health, definition of, 67

Health and Human Services, U. S. Department of, 270
Health care and health care delivery, 6, 7, 381-382
  advances in, 5
  allied health professions in, 279-280
  bibliography on, 394
  economic aspects of, 222, 383-385
    managing, 385-386
    preventive medicine in managing, 387-389
  ethical aspects of, 66, 382-383
  population dynamics affecting, 382
  review questions on, 393-394
  system providing, 389, 391-392
  team approach to, 279-280
Health care service, 6-7, 10
  marketing of, 10-12
  National Consumer Trends Survey of, 10, 11b
  quality of, 12
Health care system, U. S., 389, 391-392
Health maintenance organizations (HMOs), 384-385
Health physicist, 364-365
Health statistics, 67-71
  sources of, 67-68
Healthy People 2010, 388-389
  goals of, 390b-391b
Heart, electrical conduction system of, 67
Hebrew medicine, 59
Hepatoscopy, 58
Heraclitus, 60
Herd instinct, 53
Hippocrates, 61
Histogram, 115
Histologic technician, 273
Histotechnology, 273
Hittorf, Johann Wilhelm, 76
HMOs (health maintenance organizations), 384-385
Hospice development, 66
Hospital safety committee, 211
Hospitals, in Christian Rome, 61
Hounsfield, G. N., 343
How to Get Control of Your Time and Your Life (Lakein), 31
Human needs, hierarchy of, 22-24, 23f
Human structure, and function, course description, 94
Humane values, 51
Humility, in learning, 54
Humors, of body, 59
Hunter, John, 62
Hunter, William, 62
Huygens, Christian, 62
Hysterosalpingogram, 133-134

I

Image, professional, 174-176
Image intensifier, 121. *See also*
    Intensifying screen(s).
Image receptor, 115
Imaging equipment, 119-126
    bibliography on, 126
    course description, 84, 85f, 94
    digital, 119
    film-screen, 119-120
    fluoroscopic, 121
    pathogens on, 185
    picture archiving and communication
        system with, 124-125
    quality assurance evaluation of,
        234-235
    review questions on, 125-126
    sonographic, 124, 335-336
    specialized, 121-125, 340-341
        for computed tomography,
            121-122, 344-345
        for magnetic resonance imaging,
            122
        in nuclear medicine, 123, 332
        portable, 123-124
        for positron emission tomography,
            122-123
    tomographic, 124
    x-ray, 119
Imaging plate (IP), 115
Implied consent, 198
In-service education, 377-378
Incidents, in patient care, 13-15
Independent clinical performance,
    98
Independent service organization (ISO)
    contract, 220
India, medicine in ancient, 59-60
Indirect hit theory, 252
Infection control, sanitation and, 212
Infectious diseases, 71
Injury
    to patient, case examples of, 196-197
    from radiation exposure. *See*
        Radiation exposure; Radiation-
        induced injury.
    to radiologic technologists, case
        example of, 197-198
Inquisitiveness, 52
Institutional accreditation, 298
Intensifying screen(s), 115, 119-120, 121
    contact with film, and radiographic
        detail quality, 162-163
    and cost of radiographic unit
        generator replacement, 115
    and image contrast, 155
    and radiographic density, 148-149
    and radiographic detail, 161, 162
Intentional memorization, 36-37
Intentional misconduct, 193

Internal preparation, 128
International System of Units (SI), 247
Interpersonal relationships, in
    radiologic technology
    with patient, 167-168, 171-173
    professional, 169-171
Interventional radiography, 133-135,
    339
    cardiovascular, 133, 135, 339-342
    career mobility in, 356-357
Intravenous pyelogram (IVP), 131
Intravenous urography, 131
Invasion of privacy, 193
Inverse square law, 259, 260f
Iodine, as contrast agent, 129
Ion pair, 251
Ionizing chamber, for radiation
    dosimetry, 264
Ionizing radiation, 246. *See also*
    Radiation.
IP (imaging plate), 115
ISO (independent service organization)
    contract, 220
Isolation precautions, 185-187
Isolation room, 185

J

Jenner, Edward, 62
Jerman, Eddy Clarence, 360-361
Jesus, as healer, 61
Job Description and Scope of Practice,
    ASRT
    for Diagnostic Medical Sonographer,
        338b-339b
    for Nuclear Medicine Technologist,
        334b-335b
    for Radiation Therapist, 330b-331b
    for Radiologic Technologist, 326b-327b
John Gaston Hospital, 83
Joint Commission on Accreditation of
    Healthcare Organization
    (JCAHO), 7, 211-212, 364
Joint Review Committee on Education
    in Radiologic Technology
    (JRCERT), 297-298
    accreditation by
        categories of, 305-306
        maintenance of, 306
        noncompliance and investigation
            of, 307
        process of, 302-305
        value of, 307-308
    bibliography on, 311
    contact information for, 308-309
    educator standards of, 362-363
    history of, 299-300
    mission statement of, 300
    organization of, 301-302
    programs accredited by, 301
    review questions on, 309-311

Joint Review Committee on Education
    in Radiologic Technology
    —cont'd
    standards of, 302
Joint Review Committee on Education
    Programs in Nuclear Medicine
    Technology, education program
    of, 332-333

K

Kilovoltage, 142-143, 257
    and contrast in radiographic density,
        146, 152, 154f
Koch, Robert, 63
kVp (peak kilovoltage), 115

L

Lainnec, Rene-Theophile Hyacinthe,
    63
Laird, Donald and Elanor, 42
Lanthanum, 149
Latent period, 254
Law, 191-192
    bibliography on, 203-204
    case, 192
    and medicine, 191-192
    review questions on, 202-203
    tort, 192-193
        case examples of, 196-198
        and intentional misconduct, 193
        and medical malpractice, 192
        and patient consent, 198-200
        and payment of settlements, 200
        and unintentional misconduct,
            193-198
Lawrence, Ernest, 84
Lawson, Sonya, 185
Lead apron, 116
Lead shielding devices, 262
Legal aspects, of practicing as
    radiologic technologist, 201. *See
    also* Law.
Lenard, Philipp, 77
Licensure requirements, 317, 378-379
Life cycle cost, 220
Life expectancy, in United States, 70-71
Lifestyle
    and medical costs, 385-386
    preventive medicine, 387-389
Lifting patients, body mechanics in,
    183-184
Listening skills, improving, 39
Lister, Joseph, 63
Lithotripsy, 134
Long, Crawford W., 63
Long scale contrast, 155
Long term effects, of ionizing radiation,
    255
Long term memory, 41-42
Loritsch, Mary, 185

Lymphocytes, sensitivity to ionizing radiation, 254
Lymphography, 341

M

Maddox, R. L., 77
Magnetic resonance imaging (MRI), 84, 346-347
  equipment used in, 122, 123f, 346-347
  history of, 346
  image production in, 85f
  practice standards in, 316-317
Magnetic resonance imaging (MRI) scan, 347f
Magnetic resonance imaging (MRI) scanner, 122, 123f, 346-347f
  cost of, 219
Magnetic resonance imaging (MRI) technologist
  education of, and employment opportunities, 347
  responsibilities of, 346
Magnification, and radiographic quality, 156-158
Malphigi, Marcello, 62
Malpractice, medical, 192
Malpractice insurance, medical, 201-202, 385
Mammogram, 134, 342f
Mammography
  practice standards in, 316-317
  special procedures radiography in, 342-343
Managers, in radiologic technology, 206-207, 319, 359-360
mAs. *See* Milliampere-seconds.
Maslow, Abraham H., 22
Matrix, 116
McDowell, Ephraim, 63
MDCB. *See* Medical Dosimetrist Certification Board.
Meaning, search for, 42
Medicaid program, 222, 384, 385
Medical Dosimetrist Certification Board (MDCB), 329, 372
Medical ethics and law, course description, 94
Medical knowledge, of radiologic technologist, 182-184
Medical malpractice, 192
Medical records administration, 274-275
Medical technologist, 271, 272f
Medical technology, 271-273
Medical terminology, 109-118
  abbreviations in, 111-113
  bibliography on, 118
  course description, 95
  prefixes in, 110b
  radiographic nomenclature in, 114-116
  review questions on, 117-118

Medical terminology—cont'd
  roots in, 110b-111b
  suffixes in, 111b
  word parts in, 110-111
Medical titles, and organizations, 113-114
Medicare program, in health care delivery, 384-385
Medicare prospective reimbursement, 222-223
Medicine
  ancient practice of, 58-61
    in China, 60
    in Egypt, 59
    in Greece, 60-61
    in India, 59-60
  bibliography on, 74
  early Christian practice of, 61
  eighteenth century practice of, 62-63
  health statistics in, 67-71
  Hippocratic practice of, 60
  infectious disease control in, 71-73
  nineteenth century practice of, 63-64
  pre-Hippocratic practice of, 60
  prehistoric practice of, 58-59
  Renaissance contributions to, 62
  review questions on, 73-74
  statistics in, health and disease, 67-71
  twentieth century practice of, 64-65
  twenty-first century practice of, 65-67
Memorization, 35-37
  attention and, 37-39
  bibliography on, 47
  and forgetting, 43-44
  and listening skills, 39
  of nonsensical material, 44
  perception and, 36-37
  and reading skills, 40-41
  and retrieving from memory, 41-42
  review questions on, 46-47
Memory
  distortion of, 44-45
  long term and short term, 41-42
Memory retrieval, 41-42
Memory storage, 41-42
Mendel, Gregor, 63
Mental set, 42
Metals, radiographic densities of, 145-146, 146f, 153-155
Microminiaturization, development of, 64
Military radiologic technologists, 83, 288
Milliamperage, 142, 257
  and effect on radiographic density, 146-147
Milliampere-seconds (mAs), 116, 143-144
Minnesota, University of, 39

Misconduct
  intentional, 193
  unintentional, 193-198
Mnemonics, 44
Mobile fluoroscopy (C-arm), 123-124
Mobile unit, high output, cost of, 219
Modesty, patient, 172-173
Moments of truth, 12
Moral obligation, 176
Morbidity, 67
  in United States, leading causes of, 70
Morgagni, Giovanni Battista, 62
Morgan, William, 76
Mortality, 67
  risk factors and primary causes of, 386b
  in United States
    in Black population, 69
    due to specific causes, 69-70
    in general population, 68-69
    in Hispanic population, 69
    leading causes of, 68
Mortality statistics, 67-70
Motion, patient, and radiographic detail, 159, 160f
Motion picture radiography, 341
Moving patients, body mechanics in, 183-184
Moxibustion, 60
MRI. *See* Magnetic resonance imaging.
MRI (magnetic resonance imaging) scanner, cost of, 219
Muscle, radiographic density of, 145, 146f
Mutations, genetic, 256-257
Myelogram, 134-135

N

National Center for Health Statistics, 67
National certification examination, 372-374. *See also* Certification examination, ARRT.
National Consumer Trends Survey (in health care), results of, 10, 11b
National Council on Radiation Protection and Measurements (NCRP), 247-248
  guidelines on radiation exposure, 249-250
National Society of Radiology Practitioner Assistants (NSRPA), 358
Negligence, 193-194
  case examples of, 196-198
  definition of, 194-195
  payment of court settlements, 200
  proof of innocence of, 200-201
Nei Ching, 60
Neurovascular radiology, 84
Newton, Isaac, 62, 76

Nichols, Ralph, 39
Nineteenth century medicine, 63-64
No-threshold concept, 248-249, 258
Nollet, Jean Antoine, 76
Nomenclature, radiographic, 114-116
Noncompliance
  with continuing education
    requirements, 376
  with JRCERT accreditation
    requirements, 376
Nosocomial infections, preventing,
  184-187
Notes, written, 39
NSRPA. *See* National Society of
  Radiology Practitioner
  Assistants.
Nuclear magnetic resonance scanner,
  346
Nuclear medicine, 84, 299, 329,
  331-333
  employment opportunities in, 333
  equipment and procedures used in,
    123, 332
  image production in, 85f, 123
  practice standards in, 316-317
Nuclear medicine technologist
  RT(N)(ARRT)
  education and certification of,
    332-333, 356
  Job Description and Scope of
    Practice of, ASRT, 334b-335b
  responsibilities of, 332
Nuclear Medicine Technology
  Certification Board, 333,
  372
Nuclear radiology, 84
Numbers, remembering, 44
Nursing profession, 270-271
Nutrition
  and dietetics, 275-276
  for optimal health, 24
Nutritionist, 275-276

O

Object-to-image distance (OID), 116
  in detail quality, 161, 161f
  in radiographic quality, 157, 158f
Objectivity, 25-26
Occupational therapist, 276-277
Occupational therapy, 276-277
Open mind
  listening with, 39
  thinking with, 51
Organization, importance of, 31
Organizational charts, radiology
  department, 207-208, 209f
Organizations, medical, 113-114
Organized thinking, 51
Original equipment manufacturer
  (OEM) contract, 220

P

PACS (picture archiving and
  communications system), 116,
  124-125
Pair production, 252, 253f
Pandemic, definition of, 71
Paracelsus, 62
Pare, Ambroise, 62
Particles, high speed, 84
Passive participation, 98
Pasteur, Louis, 63
Pathogens, 185
Pathology, course description, 96
Patience, in thinking, 51
Patient
  assessment of, 231-232
  attitudes and reactions of, 171-173
Patient care, 92, 181-182
  administrative evaluation of, 232
  bibliography on, 189
  communication in, 173, 242
  and customer service, 6-9
    bibliography on, 19-20
    communication and interaction in,
      9b, 12-16
    conflict resolution in, 16-18
    customer satisfaction in, 6-7, 10-12
    diversity in, human and cultural,
      8-9
    empathy and effective listening in,
      17-18
    events in, 13-15
    moments of truth in, 12
    quality of, 10
    review questions on, 19-20
    telephone communication in, 15-16
  medical monitoring and resuscitation
    procedures in, 182-184
  methods of, course description, 96
  and prevention of nosocomial
    infections, 184-187
  professional relationship in, 167-168,
    171-173
  and quality assurance of radiologic
    care, 231-232
  reducing radiation exposure in,
    258-262
  review questions on, 188-189
  transfer of patient in, 182-184
  verification of patient identification
    in, 182
  verification of procedures requested
    in, 182
Patient consent, 198-200
Patient identification, verification of,
  182
Patient information disclosure, liability
  for, 200-201
Patient preparation, for diagnostic
  radiography, 128-129, 172-173

Patient-technologist relationship,
  evaluation of, 102
Patient transfer, body mechanics in,
  183-184
Patient's Bill of Rights, 391
Pavlov, 64
Peak kilovoltage (kVp), 115
Perception, 36-37
Personal dosimetry device, 264, 264f
Personal obligations, 176-177
Personality, components of, 22
Personnel, radiology department,
  economics of, 218-219
Personnel monitoring, for radiation
  exposure, 211, 249, 249t, 264
Personnel procedures, radiologic
  department, 210-213
Personnel records, 210
PET (positron emission tomography),
  122-123, 332
Pharmacology, and drug
  administration, course
  description, 96
Phosphors, rare earth, 119-120, 220. *See
  also* Intensifying screen(s).
  effects of, on intensifying screens, 148,
    149f
  in intensifying screens, 148-149
Photoelectric effect, 251, 253f
Photographic copy, first, 77
Photon(s), 250-251
Photon interactions, 251-252
Physical facilities readiness, evaluation
  of, 101
Physical therapist, 276
Physical therapy, 276
Physician assistant, 277
Physiologic needs, for optimal health,
  24-25
Picture archiving and communications
  system (PACS), 116, 124-125
Pinel, Phillipe, 63
Pixel, 116
Plaintiff, 200
Planning, importance of, 31
Pocket ionization chamber, for radiation
  dosimetry, 264
Policies and procedures, of radiology
  department, 207-210
Portable imaging technology, 123-124
Position, radiographic, definition of, 116
Position description(s), of American
  Society of Radiologic
  Technologists, 206-207. *See also*
  Job Description and Scope of
  Practice, ASRT.
Positioning, patient, importance of, 142f
Positioning skills
  developing, 236
  evaluation of, 103

Positron emission tomography (PET), imaging equipment for, 122-123, 332
Postgraduate education, 355-358, 374-375
Postprocessing image enhancement, 116
Practice standards, of American Society of Radiologic Technologists, 316-317
Prefixes, in medical terminology, 110b
Pregnant women, exposure to radiation, limits for, 250, 250f
Preparation, patient, for diagnostic radiography, 128-129
Pressure injector, 341
Preventive medicine, 387-389
Priestly, Joseph, 63
Primal stresses, 26-28
Privacy
    invasion of, 193
    of medical information, liability for disclosure, 200-201
Probational status, 376
Procedures, radiographic, course description, 95
Procedures manual(s), radiologic department, 208, 210
Procedures requested, verification of, 182
Processing. See Film processing.
Processor. See Film processor.
Professional associations, and organizations, 313-314
    American Society of Radiologic Technologists in, 314-320
    bibliography on, 323
    for radiologists and physicists, 320-321
    review questions on, 322-323
    Summit on Radiologic Sciences and Sonography as coalition of, 321-322
    for technologists, 320
Professional development opportunities, 353-355
    in administrative radiology, 359-360
    bibliography on, 369
    as commercial representative, 366
    in computer science, 363
    as equipment specialist, 365-366
    in postgraduate education. See also Specialized radiology.
        long term, 357-358
        short term, 355-357
    in quality assurance, 343, 363-364
    in radiation safety, 364-365
    as radiologic technologist educator, 318-319, 360-363
    as radiologist assistant, 347-349, 358-359
    review questions on, 367-368

Professionalism, aspect(s) of, 167-179, 316-317
    bibliography on, 179
    confidentiality as, 173-174
    entrepreneurship as, 177
    goals as, 168-169
    image as, 174-176
    patient relationship as, 171-173
    personal obligations as, 176-177
    professional relationships as, 169-171
    review questions on, 178-179
Projection, radiographic, 116
Prospective payment system (PPS), 383-385
Prospective reimbursement, Medicare, 222-223
Prostheses, development of, 65
Protection, from radiation. See Radiation exposure, protection from.
Psychologic care, 25
Psychologic needs, for optimal health, 25-26
Psychomotor learning, 97
Public exposure, to radiation, limits for, 249, 249t
Pupin, Michael Idvorsky, 83
Pyramid
    administrative, 228, 229f
    of radiograph production, 228-229, 230f, 231

Q

Quality, 230f
    definition of, 228
    radiographic, 141-144
        bibliography on, 165
        checking, 143f
        contrast in, 151-156
        cost of, in radiology department, 220-221
        density in, 144-151
        detail in, 158-163
        distortion and magnification in, 156-158
        radiation control in, 141-144
        review questions on, 163-164
        subject thickness in, 145-151
Quality assurance, 213, 227-228
    bibliography on, 244
    and communication, 242
    course description, 96
    equipment assessment in, 232-235
    patient considerations in, 231
    patient's assessments in, 232
    professional development in, 343, 363-364
    pyramidal structure of, 228-231
    radiologic technologist in, assessment of, 235-238

Quality assurance—cont'd
    radiologic technologist's role in, 235-238
    radiologist in, assessment of, 239-242
    review of, 242
    review questions on, 243-244
Quality assurance technologist, 364

R

rad (unit), 247
Radiation, ionizing
    background, 246
    bibliography on, 267
    biologic effects of, 252-257
        on germ cells, 256-257
        on somatic cells, 255-256
    carcinogenic effects of, 255-256
    effective dose equivalents of, 248-249
    external medical sources of, 257-258
    human-made sources of, 246
    interaction of, with matter, 250-252, 253f
    internal medical sources of, 258
    long-term biologic effects of, 255-257
    medical sources of, 257-258
    regulation of exposure to, 236-238, 247-250, 259. See also Radiation exposure.
    remnant, 144-145
    review questions on, 265-267
    scatter, 149, 150f, 151f
    sources of, 246
    units of measurement of, 246-247, 248t
Radiation Control for Health and Safety Act (1968), 248
Radiation exposure
    adverse effects of, 81-83, 258-267. See also Radiation, ionizing.
    control of, 236-238, 247-250, 259
    guidelines on, National Council on Radiation Protection and Measurements, 249-250
    medical sources of, 257-258
    occupational limits of, 249, 249t
    patient, and use of filters, 150-151
    personnel monitoring for, 211, 249, 249t, 264
    principles of, and patient safety, 259
    protection from, 246-250
        evaluation of, 103
        for patient, 258-262
        principles of, course description, 95
        for radiologic technologists, 263-265
    regulation of, 247-248
Radiation exposure limits
    for fetus, 250, 250f
    for pregnant women, 250, 250f
    for radiologic technologists, 249, 249t
Radiation-induced injury, 246

Radiation physics, course description, 96
Radiation safety committee, 211-212
Radiation safety officer, 364-365
Radiation therapist RT(T)(ARRT)
  education and certification of, 328-
    329, 355-356
  Job Description and Scope of
    Practice of, ASRT, 330b-331b
  responsibilities of, 328
Radiation therapy, 84, 299, 327
  employment opportunities in, 329
  history of, 327-328
  practice standards in, 316-317
Radioactive elements, 331
Radioactivity, 83
  scientists prominent in discovery of,
    83
Radiobiology, course description, 96
Radiograph(s)
  acceptance limits of, 239-240
  definition of, 116
  first, 77, 78-79, 79f
    in United States, 83
  interpretation of, 143f, 239
  life cycle of, 139-141
  and privacy of information, legal
    aspects of, 200-201
  quality of, factors affecting, 141-144.
    See also Quality, radiographic.
  useful life of, 141
Radiograph demonstration/image
    evaluation, evaluation of, 103-104
Radiographer, 4
Radiographic rooms, cost of
    maintaining, 219
Radiography, diagnostic, 4, 84, 127-137
  bibliography on, 137
  early development of, 79-83
  equipment for. See Equipment.
  fluoroscopic studies in, 131-133
  introduction to, course description,
    94
  motion picture, 341
  patient preparation for, 128-129
  portable, 123-124
  practice standards in, 316-317
  radiographic studies in, 130-131
  review questions on, 136-137
  scientific discoveries in development
    of, 76-79
  special procedure(s) in, 133-135, 337,
    339-349
    bone densitometry as, 347
    computed tomography as, 135,
      343-346
    history of, 337
    interventional cardiovascular, 133,
      135, 339-342
    interventional radiologic, 133-135,
      339

Radiography, diagnostic—cont'd
    mammography as, 134, 342-343
Radioisotopes, medical use of, 84
Radiologic sciences education, history
    of, 298
Radiologic technologist(s) RT(ARRT),
    4, 140. See also Radiology, and
    radiologic technology.
  acceptance limits of, 240-241
  certification of, 100, 285-296. See also
    American Registry of Radiologic
    Technologists; Certification
    examination.
  clinical education and training of,
    97-104
  competency evaluation of, 97-104
  competency requirements of, 238, 288
  continuing education of, 84-85, 104,
    238, 371-381. See also
    Continuing education.
  educational preparation as, 93-96, 288
    bibliography on, 107
    review questions on, 105-107
  evaluation of, 232, 238
  injury to, case example of, 197-198
  Job Description and Scope of
    Practice of, ASRT, 326b-327b
  legal aspects of practicing as, 201. See
    also Law.
  medical knowledge of, 182-184
  military, 83, 288
  professional associations for, 320. See
    also Professional associations.
  professional development
    opportunities for, 353-369
  professional status of, 316
  protection of, from radiation
    exposure, 263-265
  quality assurance role of, 235-238
  radiation exposure limits for, 249,
    249t
  registered, 294, 372-374. See also
    American Registry of Radiologic
    Technologists; Certification
    examination.
    bibliography on, 380
    continuing education programs
      approved for, 377-378
    and licensure requirements,
      378-379
    requirements for, and renewal,
      373-376
      noncompliance with, 376
    review questions on, 379-380
  responsibilities of, 92-93
  specialization areas for, 325-351. See
    also Specialized radiology.
Radiologic Technology, 315
Radiological Society of North America
    (RSNA), 286, 318

Radiologist(s), 360
  assistants to, 348-349, 358-359
  professional associations for,
    320-321
  quality assurance role of, 239-242
    acceptance limits in, 239-240
Radiologist assistant (RA), 347-349
  education programs for, 358-359
Radiology, and radiologic technology, 4,
    91-92
  basic curriculum of, 94-96
  career advancement in, 6, 353-369
  certification and registration in,
    285-296. See also American
    Registry of Radiologic
    Technologists.
  certifying and accrediting
    organizations in
    American Registry of Radiologic
      Technologists, 285-296
    Joint Review Committee on
      Education in Radiologic
      Technology, 297-311
  continuing education in, 84-85, 104,
    238. See also Continuing
    education.
  development of, historical, 77-85
  educational preparation in, 4-6,
    93-96. See also Certification
    examination; Educational
    preparation.
  history of, 299-300
  educators in, 318-319, 360-363
  equipment used in, 84, 85f. See also
    Equipment.
  ethics in, 167-179
  historical development of, 75-87
    bibliography on, 87
    review questions on, 85-87
  interventional, 133-135, 339
  managers and supervisors in, 319
  modern medical application of,
    84-85
  nuclear, 84
  patient care and customer satisfaction
    in, 3-20. See also Patient care.
  people prominent in, 76-84
  personal preparation for vocation in,
    21-34
  practice standards for, 316-317
  professional associations in, 313-323.
    See also Professional
    associations.
  professional goals in, 168-169
  professionalism in, 5, 167-179. See
    also Professionalism.
  scope of, 4
  specialized areas in, 325-351. See also
    Specialized radiology.
  technical advances in, 79-84

Radiology, and radiologic technology—cont'd
tort law applicable to practice of, 192-201. *See also* Law.
vocational choice of, 21-22
Radiology department, 205-206
administrative responsibilities in, 206-207
administrator's role in, 359-360
bibliography on, 215-216
economics of, 217-225
equipment maintenance in, 213-214
policies and procedures of, 207-210
quality assurance maintenance in, 213, 227-244
review questions on, 214-215
safety procedures of, 211-213
safety training within, 213
staff activities within, 207
and working relationship with other hospital departments, 207
Radiology information system (RIS), 116
Radiology Management, 319
Radionuclides, 258, 331
Radiopharmaceuticals, 331
Radium, 258
Rare earth minerals, 149
Rational thinking, 51
RCEEM. *See* Recognized Continuing Education Evaluation Mechanism.
React actively, 42
Reading efficiency, 40-41
Reading skills, improving, 40-41
Reasoning, faulty, 52
Recognized Continuing Education Evaluation Mechanism (RCEEM), 373-374
approved programs for, 377-378
Recorded detail, 116
Reed, Walter, 64
Refresh memory, 42
Registered radiologic technologist RT(ARRT), 294, 372-374. *See also* Certification examination, ARRT.
bibliography on, 380
continuing education programs approved for, 377-378
and licensure requirements, 378-379
registration and renewal requirements for, 373-374
noncompliance with, 376
review questions on, 379-380
Regulation of radiation exposure, for public health, 247-248
Reinforcement behavior, 28
rem (unit), 247

Remembering information, 41-42, 43-44
inaccuracy in, 44-45
methods of, 44
optimizing practices for, 45
Remnant beam (exit radiation), 116
Remnant radiation, 144-145
Renaissance medicine, 62
Renewal. *See* Registered radiologic technologist RT(ARRT).
Repeat exposure, avoiding, 261
Requesting radiologic service, 208
Requisition, evaluation of, 100-101
res ipsa loquitur, 197, 200-201
Respect, for other opinions, 54
Respiratory therapist, 277
Respiratory therapy, 277
respondeat superior, 200
Responsibilities, of radiologic technologists, 92-93
Restraining devices, for patients, 263
Retakes, cost of, 221
Rhyming, in memorization, 44
RIS (radiology information system), 116
Risks-versus-benefits relationship, 248
Robotic surgery, 66-67
Roentgen, Wilhelm Conrad, 63, 77, 78f
early life of, 77
x-ray discovery by, 77-79
roentgen (R), 247
Roentgen rays. *See* X-rays.
Rokitansky, Carl, 63
Roots, word, in medical terminology, 110b-111b
Rote memorization, 35-36
RSNA. *See* Radiological Society of North America.
Ruhmkorff, H. D., 76
Rush, Benjamin, 63

S

Safety standards, and procedures, of radiology department, 211-213, 254-265
Safety training, within radiology department, 213, 264-265
Salk, Jonas, 64
Sanitation, and infection control, 212
Scaled scores, 293
Scanner, 317
Scatter radiation, 149, 150f, 151f
and radiographic density, 149, 150f, 151f
Scattering, electron, 251-252
Scholtz, J. H., 77
Scintillation counter, for radiation dosimetry, 264
Score report, for ARRT certification examination, 292-294

Screen. *See* Intensifying screen(s).
Seizure, 184
Self-awareness, 54-55
Self-discipline, 25, 31
Self-study, 303
Sensitivity of cells, to ionizing radiation, 254
Sensitometer, 233
Sensitometric monitoring, 233
Service, patient expectations of, 6-7, 10
Shielded booth, for radiographic machine operator, 263
Shielding devices, reducing radiation exposure with, 261-262
Shielding evaluation, 211
Shock, 184
Short scale contrast, 155
Short term memory, 41-42
SI (International System of) units, 247
Sialogram, 135
SID (source-to-image distance), 116
in radiographic detail quality, 158, 161, 162f
sievert (Sv), 247
Silver bromide, in film emulsion, 148
Silver reclamation, 221-222
methods available for, 222
Sims, J. Marion, 63
Single phase generator, image quality, using intensifying screens, 220
Skinner, B. F., 28
Skull and headwork, radiographic studies, 130
Sleep, for optimal health, 24-25
Smoking, risks associated with, 387
Social and economic aspects, of health care delivery, 382-385
Sonographer, diagnostic medical education and certification of, 337, 356
Job Description and Scope of Practice of, ASRT, 338b-339b
responsibilities of, 336
Sonographic scan, 357f
Sonography, 124, 333
employment opportunities in, 337
equipment used in, 124, 335-336
history of, 333
practice standards in, 316-317
Source-to-image distance (SID), 116
in radiographic detail quality, 158, 161, 162f
Source-to-object distance (SOD), 116
and radiographic detail quality, 161
Space, physiologic and pharmacologic research in, 67
Spallanzani, Lazzaro, 62

Special procedures radiography, 133-135, 337, 339
bone densitometry in, 348
cardiovascular interventional radiography in, 133, 135, 339-342
computed tomography in, 135, 343-346
magnetic resonance imaging in, 346-348
mammography in, 134, 342-343
Special procedures technologist(s)
in bone densitometry, 348
in cardiovascular intervention technology, RT (R)(CV) (ARRT), 341
education and certification of, 341
employment opportunities as, 341-342
responsibilities of, 339-340
in computed tomography, 343-346
education of, 345
employment as, 346
responsibilities of, 343-344
in magnetic resonance imaging, 346-347
in mammography, RT (R)(M)(ARRT), 342-343
in quality management, RT (R)(QM)(ARRT), 343
Specialized imaging equipment, 121-125
for computed tomography, 121-122, 344-345
for magnetic resonance imaging, 122, 346-347
in nuclear medicine, 123, 332
portable, 123-124
for positron emission tomography, 122-123, 332
Specialized radiology, 325-327
accreditation in, 294, 298
bibliography on, 350-351
certification in, 293t, 294
educator in radiologic technology in, 318-319
nuclear medicine as, 329, 331-333
practice standards for, 316-317
radiation therapy as, 327-329
radiologist's assistant in, 347-349
review questions on, 349-350
sonography as, 333, 335-337
special procedures radiography in, 337, 339-349. See also Special procedures technologist(s).
Sphygmomanometer, use of, 184
Spine, radiographic studies, 131
Sprengel, Herman, 76
Staff activities, within radiology department, 207
Staffing, radiology department, economics of, 218-219

Standard of care, 194
breach of, 194, 195
Standard Six, 362
Standards, practice, of American Society of Radiologic Technologists, 316-317
STANDARDS-MD, 302
STANDARDS-MR, 302
Standards of conduct, 167
STANDARDS-RS, 302
Statistics, health, 67-71
sources of, 67-68
Sterile package, 186f
Sterile technique(s), 186-187
Sterilization, of equipment, 186
Stethoscope, use of, 184
Stratton v Swanlond, 193
Stress(es), 28-29
and conflict, 28-31
coping with, 28
organization and reduction of, 31
primal, 26-28
Student exposure, to radiation, limits for, 249
Studies, radiographic, 130-131
Subject contrast, and radiographic density, 151-152
Subject thickness, and radiographic density, 145-151
Suffixes, in medical terminology, 111b
Summative evaluations, 362
Summit on Radiologic Sciences and Sonography, 321-322
Supervisors, in radiologic technology, 319

T

Tao, 60
Tax Equity and Fiscal Responsibility Act (TEFRA), 222
Techniques for Efficient Remembering (Laird), 42
Telephone interaction, with patient, 15-16
Thales, 60, 76
Thermoluminescent dosimetry (TLD), 264
Tholos, 60
Thoracic cavity, radiographic studies, 130
Time, of exposure, 147
Time and materials (T&M) contract, 220
Timer, 142
Tissue damage, by ionizing radiation, mechanisms of, 252-257
Tissue density(ies), 145-146
contrast of, 151-152, 152f, 153f, 154f
Titles, and organizations, medical, 113-114

TLD (thermoluminescent dosimetry), 264
Tomography, 124, 135
Torricelli, Evangelista, 76
Torts, and tort law, 192-193
applicable to practice of radiologic technology, 193-201
proof of innocence in, 197, 200-201
Transfer of patient, 182-184
Transplant surgery, development of, 64-65
Troubleshooting techniques, for equipment problems, 232
Twentieth century medicine, 64-65
Twenty-first century medicine, 65-67

U

U. S. Air Force, programs in radiography, 288
U. S. Army School of Roentgenology, 83
U. S. Navy, programs in radiography and nuclear medicine technology, 288
Ultrasound, 84, 333. *See also* Sonography.
Unintentional misconduct, 193-198. *See also* Negligence.
Units of measurement, for radiation, 246-247, 248t
University of Tennessee, 83
Upper gastrointestinal (GI) series, 132
Urinary system, radiographic studies, 131, 133

V

Vacuum tubes, first creators of, 76
van Guericke, Otto, 76
van Helmont, Jan Baptisa, 62
van Leeuwenhoek, Antonie, 62
Venogram, 135
Venography, 341
Versallus, Andreas, 62
Victor X-ray Corporation, 361
View, radiographic, definition of, 116
Virchow, Rudolf, 63
Visibility of detail, 158
Vital signs, monitoring, 184
Voiding cystourethrogram, 133
Voltage, 142-143
von Haller, Albrecht, 62
Voxel, 116

W

Watson, William, 76
Weber State University (Utah), 358
Window level, 116
Window width, 116
Word parts, in medical terminology, 110-111

Working relationships, with other hospital departments, 207

X

X-ray film, 120. *See also* Film(s).
X-ray tube, 119
   fluoroscopic, 257-258
X-rays. *See also* Beam angle.
   adverse effects of exposure to, 81-82, 83. *See also* Radiation, ionizing.

X-rays—cont'd
   discovery of, 75
      by Roentgen, 77-79
      scientific discoveries enabling, 76
   early development of technology with, 82-84
   early uses of, 79-82
   first application of, 78-79, 79f
   interaction of, with matter, 250-252, 253f

X-rays—cont'd
   medical sources of, 257-258

Y

Yttrium, 149